A·H·T· ROBB-SMITH

& C·R· TAYLOR

LYMPH NODE BIOPSY

A DIAGNOSTIC ATLAS

Lymph Node Biopsy

BY A·H·T· ROBB-SMITH

EMERITUS NUFFIELD READER IN PATHOLOGY,
UNIVERSITY OF OXFORD · HONORARY CONSULTING PATHOLOGIST
UNITED OXFORD HOSPITALS

AND C·R· TAYLOR

PROFESSOR OF PATHOLOGY, UNIVERSITY OF SOUTHERN CALIFORNIA
HEAD, SECTION OF IMMUNOPATHOLOGY,
LOS ANGELES COUNTY MEDICAL CENTER

A DIAGNOSTIC ATLAS
WITH 300 PHOTO-MICROGRAPHS
IN FULL COLOR

OXFORD UNIVERSITY PRESS ~ NEW YORK

PUBLISHED IN THE UNITED STATES AND CANADA BY
OXFORD UNIVERSITY PRESS · 200 MADISON AVENUE · NEW YORK, NY 10016 · USA

Library of Congress Cataloging in Publication Data

Robb-Smith, Alastair Hamish Tearloch.
  Lymph node biopsy.

  Bibliography: p.
  Includes index
  1. Lymph nodes—Biopsy. 2. Lymph nodes—Diseases—
Diagnosis. 3. Histology, Pathological. I. Taylor, Clive Roy,
joint author. II. Title. [DNLM: 1. Lymph nodes—
Pathology—Atlases. 2. Lymphatic diseases—Diagnosis—
Atlases. 3. Biopsy—Atlases. WH 17 R631L]

RC646.R58   616.4′20758   80-26505

ISBN 0–19–520247–3

MADE IN SWITZERLAND
PRINTED AND BOUND BY ARTS GRAPHIQUES COOP SUISSE · BASLE
ILLUSTRATIONS ORIGINATED BY SCHWITTER AG · BASLE
TEXT SET BY INPUT TYPESETTING · LONDON SW19 8DR · ENGLAND

CONTENTS

(Chapter II continued)

CHAPTER III · PSEUDO-FOLLICLES   97

CHAPTER IV · SINUS PROLIFERATION   127

(Chapter V continued)

PREFACE

IT IS GENERALLY AGREED that the interpretation of a lymph node biopsy is one of the more difficult aspects of histopathology and yet a precise diagnosis is of paramount importance both to clinician and patient. The powerful therapeutic armamentarium available for the treatment of Hodgkin's Disease and kindred conditions can have serious effects if administered to a patient with a simple reactive lymphadenopathy, while prompt treatment is essential if complete remission is to be achieved in cases of lymphoreticular malignancies.

This monograph is an attempt to assist pathologists in lymph node diagnosis and is grounded on experience gained from the follow-up studies of the Oxford Lymph Node Registry, the section of Hematopathology and Immunopathology of the School of Medicine of the University of Southern California and other collaborative enquiries in this country and abroad.

In recent years there has been considerable interest in decision theory and the principles of the diagnostic process, with discussion of the relative merits of flow charts, decision trees and clustering techniques in simulated models. It is clear that the histopathologist utilizes, knowingly or not, some form of decision tree or dendrogram in the initial assessment of biopsy diagnosis. Some years ago a pilot scheme using this approach in the diagnosis of lymph node abnormalities was presented in outline and proved popular. It has been greatly expanded in this book with two significant advances:– the provision of coloured photomicrographs of the more important conditions and the introduction of specific methods for cell identification. In conformity with the concept that histological diagnosis is largely a matter of pattern recognition, the photomicrographs are either low power survey views (usually ×40) or high power details (of the order of ×750) of selected fields in which the characters of individual cells can be recognized; it is here that the histochemical and immunohistological techniques are of value in the precise identification of functional cell types which might otherwise be confused.

As this monograph has been written primarily for the hospital pathologist concerned with lymph node diagnosis, rather than for research workers investigating lymphoproliferative disorders, greater emphasis has been placed on classical histology than on electron micrographs or the use of membrane markers in cell identification as these are complex and time-consuming techniques while their interpretation is often far from simple. Nevertheless, a few electron micrographs and illustrations of 'rosetting' have been included where they are really of significance in interpretation.

Presented with a diagnostic biopsy, the first essential is a familiarity with the ordinary appearance of the tissue and the range of variability that can be accepted as 'normal', and the next is the differentiation of physiological reactive processes from pathological changes. In the case of lymphoreticular tissue, this demands a basic knowledge of 'normal' lymph node architecture and a clear definition of the individual cell types present within the lymph node. Our understanding of lymph node architecture and the response to antigenic stimulation has been much influenced by advances in the theoretical and practical aspects of immunology. In addition there is also an increasing awareness of the radical changes in lymphocyte morphology which may occur as part of the 'normal' response of the lymphocyte to antigenic stimuli. These aspects of lymph node pathology are considered in the first chapter which is primarily concerned with the functional anatomy of the lymph node and the definition of the principal component cells.

Following this there is a discussion of those lymph node structures – cortex and paracortical tissue, follicles, medulla, sinuses etc., – which can be regarded as histological landmarks in the process of diagnosis. These must be looked for and their presence or absence determined: if they are present, whether they are normal or abnormal structurally and in cell content; and if they are absent, how this has occurred. These are the principles adopted here for the recognition of the various pattern of lymph node disease. In addition there may be specific features which enable the pathologist to assign a particular process to a defined disease group or diagnostic entity. Thus certain of the lymphadenopathies possess histological or cytological features which are sufficiently characteristic to allow the distinction of a particular pathological process from other forms of reactive hyperplasia. Similarly some neoplasms possess distinctive histological features which enable the pathologist to make the diagnosis with some certainty.

However, the lymph node has only a limited repertoire of responses to a wide variety of stimuli, and in some cases a reactive condition may simulate a lymphoreticular neoplasm, or vice versa, and so a critical appraisal of all the relevant histological and cytological evidence is of great importance in arriving at a diagnosis.

The application of this approach to a lymph node biopsy forms the major part of this book, in which the different pathological processes encountered are described and illustrated in relation to the diagnostic schema, rather than ordered according to any arbitrary classification. To facilitate orientation, there is, at the beginning of each chapter, an analytical summary with which are linked the running headings together with marginal headings and figure references. As this is primarily a manual of diagnostic histology, it seemed inadvisable to attempt a comprehensive review of the clinical features, natural history and therapeutic response of the various identifiable lymphoreticular disorders, but reference is made to authoritative studies where they exist. On the other hand, it was impossible to evade some discussion of the various nomenclatures and classifications that have come to the fore in recent years. Unhappily, the diverse terminology results in great conceptual difficulties, and forms an impediment to communication amongst clinicians and pathologists. No attempt is made in this book to propound any new classification or even to champion an existing one, but to avoid confusion the common alternative terms are given wherever this is possible. We have avoided acronyms or abbreviations but have used 'lymphoma' qualified by a suitable morphological epithet for the low grade conditions, restricting the use of 'malignant lymphoma' to those with sarcomatous characters. This approach should assist pathologists and clinicians in integrating published reports, based on one terminology, with their own experience, which may be founded on a distinct system of classification. In this way it is hoped that not only will this monograph assist the diagnostic pathologist, but will also reveal to oncologists, whatever their particular expertise, the problems facing the histopathologist.

THIS BOOK could not have been written without the help and support of many people to whom we should wish to express our thanks.

First to the patients, whose biopsies we studied and then learnt from our clinical colleagues the degree of accuracy and value of our histological interpretations, interpretations that were often influenced by discussion with other pathologists. There are many colleagues who, knowingly or not, have contributed to the observations and concepts set out here, sometimes as joint authors of papers from which quotations appear, and to all of these we are very grateful.

In addition we would wish to express our appreciation of the permission given to us by Professor Saul Rosenberg and Dr. Costan Berard, to include in the Appendix the classification scheme or 'working formulation for clinical usage' which is being put forward by the international panel of the U.S. National Cancer Institute's Non-Hodgkin Lymphoma Study, in the hope that it may reduce the babel of confusion that is hampering lymphoma discussions.

We have been fortunate over the years to have had working with us histological technicians who recognized the importance to our patients of providing preparations of the highest quality, if a reliable diagnosis was to be achieved; it is impossible to clepe all these, but it would be churlish if we failed to acknowledge the help we received from the late Mr. Reginald Duffett, Mrs. Ruby Hughes, Mr. Anthony Chaplin, Miss Maria Hambridge and Mrs. Ysanne Smart. The immunological advances were the result of Mr. J. Burns' initiative and collaboration, while the masterly electron microscopy of Mr. D. Jerome was always available to us.

Our imperturbable secretaries, Mrs. Joan Braidwood and Mrs. Vera MacIntosh typed and re-typed our original manuscripts, each in its own way almost indecipherable, and subsequently a host of secretary cryptographers have unravelled scarcely legible amendments and alterations. We are grateful to Dr. Anita Borges for reading the book in manuscript and also deeply indebted to Dr. Parry, Messrs. Cousin and Reed, who prepared with infinite care the photomicrographs which were translated into admirable coloured illustrations by the skill of Cliché Schwitter of Basle.

However, this book would never have been completed but for the enthusiasm, knowledge and tolerance of Mr. Harvey Miller, whose sensibility was able to translate all our ill-defined ideas into the reality of print, while accepting with tranquility our over-enthusiastic estimates of the time involved in consummation.

In the later stages, when galley proofs and photographs were changing into pages of type and plates, it was the artistic precision of Mrs. Elly Miller, who could turn with equanimity from miniatures in illuminated manuscripts to colour requirements of immunoperoxidase preparations, that ensured that the book was both typographically and orthographically correct; indeed, we often felt that her name should appear on the title page as editor, if not co-author.

The research work which generated this book was originally supported by the British Empire Cancer Campaign and the Lady Tata Memorial Fund, and more recently by the Leukaemia Research Fund, the research funds of the United Oxford Hospitals, the Medical Research Council of the United Kingdom as well as groups from the National Institute of Health in the United States of America. We can only hope that it may play some part in the achievement of the objectives for which these charitable and governmental funds were established.

We dedicate this book to our families
who have given us support and encouragement
during the years that this incubus was nurtured

CHAPTER I

THE HUMAN LYMPH NODE

Component cells and functional anatomy; Principles of lymph node diagnosis

ANALYTICAL
SUMMARY

1. **Technique of Lymph Node Biopsy**

   Aspiration and Drill Biopsy – handling of lymph node biopsies in the laboratory – preparation of bone marrow – preparation of spleen – staining techniques

2. **General Structure of the Lymph Node**

   Component cells – general anatomy of the node

3. **Patterns of Lymph Node response**

   Humoral immune response – cellular immune responses – histiocytic responses

4. **General Principles in the Examination of a Lymph Node Biopsy**

THE ASSESSMENT AND DIAGNOSIS of lymph node disorders must be based upon a sound knowledge of the basic nodal architecture and a recognition of the morphological changes occurring during the normal functioning of the lymph node. Traditionally, the 'range' of reactive responses has been determined by experience and one of us has maintained an active interest in lymph node pathology for more than forty years. However, advances in experimental immunology during the past decade have profoundly influenced our concepts of lymph node function and anatomy. Generally, histopathology has been slow to assimilate this new information and, until recently, little account has been taken of the radical changes in morphology occurring during 'transformation' of the small lymphocyte in response to contact with specific antigen.

In this chapter the component cells and architectural features of the resting lymph node will be related to current immunological concepts, and the basic patterns of the immune responses will be examined.

1. Technique of Lymph Node Biopsy

Recognition of the more subtle elements which are of value in the diagnosis of lymph node disorders, is vitally dependent on adequate biopsy and on proper fixation and processing.

The *Selection of the Biopsy Site* is to a large extent determined by the location of the enlarged nodes, or by an abnormal lymphangiogram. However, in the absence of definite clinical indication, the nodes of election for histological diagnosis are from the low cervical region or axilla. Inguinal nodes are commonly scarred, while upper cervical nodes frequently show some degree of reactive hyperplasia which may obscure a more significant change. These difficulties were clearly illustrated in a study reported by Saltzstein (1965). In biopsies of sixty-eight patients a diagnosis was reached in 64% of supra-clavicular nodes, and in nodes from other sites as follows: cervical 46%, scalene 36%, axillary 27% and inguinal 22%. Of thirty-five patients in whom the biopsy was not diagnostic, six were subsequently shown to have a serious lymph node disorder, emphasizing the importance of selecting the biopsy site, even if lymphadenopathy is widespread.

The ultimate decision is of course the prerogative of the surgeon, but certain principles apply. One or more nodes should be removed intact with a minimum of trauma. If possible the surgeon should be dissuaded from a close dissection of the nodes, as this can result in the capsule remaining within the wound while the pathologist only receives fragments of lymphoid tissue. It is much to be preferred if a reasonable amount of the periadenoid tissue is included in the biopsy. This procedure requires an adequate incision with good exposure, and small biopsies taken under local anaesthesia are seldom satisfactory.

When a group of nodes is involved, it is advisable to remove both superficial and deep nodes, for the former may show only reactive features, while the deeper and less accessible nodes are involved by some process of serious clinical import; Slaughter et al (1958) displayed this in their studies of cervical block dissection in Hodgkin's disease.

Aspiration and Drill Biopsy have their advocates, but have proved unrewarding in our hands. It is true that, by these methods, samples of tissue can be obtained under local anaesthesia with little inconvenience to the patient, and there is no doubt that lymph node aspirates, if handled properly, can provide excellent cytological detail. However, this can equally well be achieved by making imprints from excised nodes as will be described later. The major disadvantages of these techniques are the risk of cellular trauma and distortion, and the possibility that the fragments obtained could be too small to reveal the relationship of the various cellular and structural elements, on which accurate diagnosis largely depends. It may be possible to state that the sample includes malignant cells, and that these are from a carcinomatous metastasis or malignant lymphoma, and on occasion it is possible to diagnose a particular granulomatous process. However, in our experience this type of biopsy is quite unsuitable for recognition of the subtle features of many lymph node disorders, and all too frequently microscopical examination fails to achieve a definite diagnosis. Thus, the patient, having suffered the discomfort of aspiration, must then be subjected to a full surgical procedure.

The Handling of Lymph Node Biopsies in the Laboratory

Ideally the intact unfixed lymph node should be presented immediately to the pathologist, who then has the opportunity of selecting suitable portions for

Diagram 1

TRANSFORMATION CYCLE
Detail of postulated relation of lymphocyte cell types

Transformation

[2]DNA synthesis
– decreased chromatin clumping
– increased prominence of nucleolus
– incorporation of tritium labelled thymidine (Henry et al 1972).

Maturation

[2] DNA and RNA synthesis
– increased chromatin clumping
– decreased prominence of nucleolus
– decreased cytoplasmic basophilia[2]

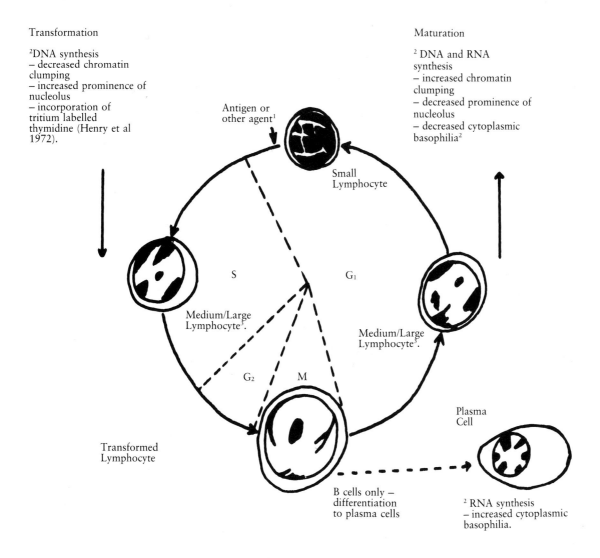

Antigen or other agent[1]

Small Lymphocyte

S

G_1

Medium/Large Lymphocyte[3].

Medium/Large Lymphocyte[3].

G_2

M

Transformed Lymphocyte

Plasma Cell

B cells only – differentiation to plasma cells

[2] RNA synthesis
– increased cytoplasmic basophilia.

The phases of the cell cycle are reprensented by the lettered segments: G_1 – Presynthetic Gap; S – Period of DNA synthesis; G_2 – Post-synthetic gap; M – Mitosis
[1] Other agents include PHA, pokeweed, streptolysin S, staphylococcal filtrate, trypsin, mixed lymphocyte culture, anti-lymphocyte sera (see Henry et al 1972).

[2] Basophilia persists in plasma cells. Also some lymphocytes of the B cell series produce significant amounts of immunoglobulin and show corresponding basophilia of the cytoplasm.

[3] Possibly including the cleaved cell or centrocyte: the uncertain position of the cleaved cell or centrocyte reflects the lack of precise knowledge of the sequence of changes in B lymphocyte transformation in reactive centres (Lukes, Collins, 1975: Lennert, et al 1975).

Diagram 2

The Two-Component Concept of Development
and Function of the Lymphoid System[1]

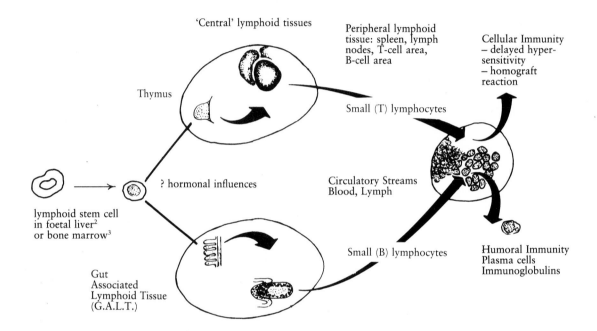

'Central' lymphoid tissues

Peripheral lymphoid
tissue: spleen, lymph
nodes, T-cell area,
B-cell area

Cellular Immunity
– delayed hyper-
sensitivity
– homograft
reaction

Thymus

Small (T) lymphocytes

lymphoid stem cell
in foetal liver[2]
or bone marrow[3]

? hormonal influences

Circulatory Streams
Blood, Lymph

Gut
Associated
Lymphoid Tissue
(G.A.L.T.)

Small (B) lymphocytes

Humoral Immunity
Plasma cells
Immunoglobulins

[1] For detailed discussion see Burnet, 1969; Nossal and Ada, 1971; Good, 1973.

[2] Taylor, 1965.

[3] Van Bekkum et al, 1971; Nossal and Ada, 1971.

Table 1

Methods for distinguishing T- and B-cells in man, and the corresponding reactions of monocytes in suspension

	T-Lymphocyte	B-Lymphocyte	Monocyte
Transformation studies using mitogens (e.g PHA, periodate)	+	−[1]	−
E rosette (sheep red cell rosette)	+	−	−
Fc Receptor			
Aggregated immunoglobulin adsorption	−[2]	+[3]	+
EA rosette (sheep[4] red cell − antibody rosette)	−[2]	+	+[3]
C₃ Receptor:			
EAC rosette (sheep[4] red cell − antibody − complement rosette)	−	+	−
Surface immunoglobulin (immunofluorescence or immunoperoxidase methods)	−	+	(+)[5] (−)
Cytoplasmic immunoglobulin (immunofluorescence or immunoperoxidase methods)	−	+[6]	(+)[7] (−)
Scanning electron microscopy	Usually smooth, lack microvilli	Usually 'hairy', possess microvilli	Undulating or rippled surface

[1] A variable proportion of B-cells also transform with different mitogens, but generally only T-cells show stimulated thymidine uptake.

[2] Occasionally positive on T-cells (probably activated or transforming cells); helper and suppresser T-cell subsets.

[3] Aggregated immunoglobulin procedure preferential for B-lymphocytes, EA rosette procedure for monocytes (Warner, 1974).

[4] Species of red cells, other than sheep, may be preferable in the EA and EAC rosette methods to avoid the possibility of spontaneous E-rosette formation by the sheep red cells.

[5] Monocytes and granulocytes possess Fc receptors and may adsorb surface immunoglobulin. T- and B-cells may be distinguished by their capacity to resynthesise surface immunoglobulin in culture following enzymatic stripping (Brouet et al, 1975, 1976). Some T-cell subsets express C₃ receptor activity.

[6] Only a small proportion of circulating B-cells contain demonstrable immunoglobulin.

[7] Monocytes and granulocytes may contain variable amounts of immunoglobulin from phagocytosis of immune complexes.

From the general literature − see Möller (ed.), 1973: 'T- and B-lymphocytes in Humans'; Polliack et al 1973, 1975; Polliack and De Harven, 1975; for electron microscopic study − Aiuti et al, 1974; reviews − Braylan et al, 1975; Preud'homme and Labaume, 1975; Taylor, 1977, 1978, 1979.

while others are positive by the E-rosette method and also bear surface immuno-globulin (mixed T- and B-cell features). In addition, using the usual immuno-fluorescence methods for surface immunoglobulin, it is often difficult or impossible to distinguish between B-lymphocytes bearing synthesised surface immuno-globulin and monocytes bearing immunoglobulin adsorbed by Fc receptors (Table 1, p. 17). The experiments of Haegert and Coombs (1979) and their concept of 'B-major' and 'B-minor' lymphocytes have resolved many of these difficulties. For the histopathologist these methods also leave much to be desired, in that it is difficult to relate findings to cell morphology. In this context peroxidase labelled antibody methods have some application, as exemplified by the demonstration of fine morphological detail, surface immunoglobulin, and E-rosettes in a single *Fig. 1.5* preparation. Finally, these methods are generally not applicable to lymphocytes in section, though some success has been claimed for the complement and Fc receptor rosette methods with frozen sections (Jaffe et al, 1974; Brubacker and Whiteside, 1977).

The proportion of T- and B-lymphocytes in cell suspensions of peripheral lymphoid organs of the mouse is shown in Table 2 (below), and similar figures

Table 2

Distribution of B- and T-lymphocytes in the peripheral lymphoid organs of the mouse

Cell suspension from	% T-(Thymus dependent) cells	% B-(Thymus independent) cells
Thymus	100	0
Lymph	85	17 – 28
Spleen	35	42 – 56
Peyer's Patches	30 – 90[1]	61
Bone Marrow	0	15 – 39
Thoracic Duct	85	5 – 14
Blood	70	19 – 33

Table compiled from: Raff (1970, 1971), Raff et al (1970, 1971), Basten et al (1972)

The range of figures given partly reflects the different techniques used:
cytotoxicity testing and surface immunofluorescence methods,
for Thy (θ) antigen, surface immunoglobulin determinants, and
MBLA (mouse bone marrow lymphocyte antigen).

[1] Chanana et al (1973) in newborn mice.

have been obtained for man. In addition T- and B-lymphocytes localize or 'home' to separate distinct areas of the lymph node (ecotaxis; de Sousa, 1971, 1978), and recognition of the significance of these areas in the human lymph node constitutes a notable advance.

Morphology of the Lymphocyte

Small Lymphocyte

Some of the morphological features are depicted in Diagram 1, in which the metamorphosis to large forms occurring during transformation is also illustrated.

The small lymphocyte in sections has a nuclear diameter of 6–8μm. The nucleus is round in shape and may show an indentation or deep cleft in cells sectioned in the appropriate plane, although it is not possible to be as definite as Maximow who, in 1928, stated that 'the nucleus always shows a deep irregular fold of the membrane'. Dense areas of blue-black chromatin are distributed randomly and usually no nucleolus is visible. The cytoplasm is limited to a small annulus of variable staining reaction from pale eosinophilia to distinct basophilia.

Normal T- and B-lymphocytes are not readily distinguishable morphologically. However, certain neoplastic T-cells possess a striking multiple folding of the nuclear membrane, more easily seen under the electron microscope (variously known as a cerebriform, Sézary or Lutzner cell – see p. 153). There have also been claims distinguishing a further variety of neoplastic T-lymphocyte by virtue of its scanty cytoplasm, finely dispersed chromatin and irregular or convoluted nuclear outline (convoluted lymphoma, p. 162). In certain conditions (T-cell chronic lymphocytic leukaemia, T-zone lymphoma), where marker studies have confirmed that the majority of the small lymphocytes were of T-cell type, it is possible to recognize that these lymphocytes show rather more size variation than B-lymphocytes, with an irregular, somewhat angular nuclear outline, often showing small projections and may rarely be convoluted, but the chromatin remains dense; sometimes there is a significant rim of very pale cytoplasm which may contain small vacuoles (Shimoyama and Watanabe, 1979). Lennert and colleagues and Lukes and Collins also distinguish the neoplastic B-lymphocytes of some follicular lymphomas according to the presence of a single deep nuclear cleft (centrocytes: Lennert; cleaved cells: Lukes and Collins).

The lymphocyte has no characteristic histochemical reactions demonstrable in paraffin sections, though reports of intra-nuclear aryl sulphatase (Lawrinson and Gross, 1964) and of focal cytoplasmic acid phosphatase (Catovsky et al, 1974, Stein et al, 1976) staining are of potential value in smears or frozen sections. The PAS reaction is used by haematologists to assist in identification of the 'malignant lymphocytes' of acute lymphoblastic leukaemia, but is of limited value in distinguishing lymphocytes in histological sections, though there is some evidence that PAS staining increases in the early stage of lymphocyte transformation (Douglas,

1971), and Lennert and colleagues have claimed that immunoglobulin secreting neoplasms are frequently PAS positive (Lennert et al, 1973). In addition, a characteristic necklace of beaded PAS positivity occurs frequently in Sézary cells (Claudy, 1974), and may be of value in identifying this cell type. Potentially useful cytochemical reactions are summarised in Table 3 (below), and are classified more fully in Appendix II (pp. 267–270).

Table 3

Cytochemical procedures of possible value in the distinction of T-cells, B-cells and monocytes (modified from Taylor, 1977)

	T-lymphocyte	B-lymphocyte	monocyte	other cells giving a positive reaction
chloroacetate esterase	–	–	+ –	mast cells, granulocytes
non-specific esterase	–[1]	–	+++	histiocytes[2]
acid phosphatase	– → ++ focal	–[3]	++	histiocytes 'hairy' cells[4]
methyl-green pyronine	– → ++	– → ++++	– → ++	any cell with active protein synthesis, including dividing cells
PAS	– → ++[5]	– → +++[6]	– → ++	many cell types

[1] Focal positivity has been reported in lymphocytes using modified procedures.
[2] Fluoride resistant in histiocytes, labile in monocytes.
[3] Positive in plasma cells, B-lymphocyte negative.
[4] Generally tartrate labile, partly resistant in histiocytes, resistant in hairy cells.
[5] Beaded positivity in Sézary cells.
[6] Among B-cells those secreting IgA and IgM often positive.

Transformed Lymphocyte (lymphoblast, immunoblast, centroblast, non-cleaved cell, basophilic stem cell, activated reticulum cell, large lymphoid cell)

It has recently been recognized that radical morphological changes occur during the process of lymphocyte transformation following stimulation by antigen, and there have been attempts to apply these observations to the interpretation of histological material. In the progression from the small 'dormant' lymphocyte to the large activated or transformed cell, there is a gradual change in morphological characters (Diagram 1), and most observers are agreed that particular cell types can be identified during the transformation process.

The *fully transformed lymphocyte* appears as a large cell, with a rounded, or oval, vesicular nucleus of 15–25 μm diameter, containing one or two distinct nucleoli and small chromatin masses arranged peripherally. The cytoplasm appears basophilic (and pyroninophilic), and the nuclear membrane is clearly defined. Outside reactive centre areas, transformed B-cells are only distinguishable with certainty from transformed T-cells by the presence of intracellular immunoglobulin in the B-cell types. These cells can be identified in formalin-paraffin section by the use of immunoperoxidase methods, specifically staining the intracellular immunoglobulin. The morphology of these cells is shown in Figs. I.1f-i and all gradations towards the mature plasma cell can be seen. Previously a number of different terms had been applied to this cell type, as its true nature was unrecognized, or only dimly seen; thus the transformed lymphocyte corresponds to the activated reticulum cell of Marshall (1956), the reticulum cell (stem cell) of Gall (1958), the immunoblast of Dameshek (1963), Lukes and colleagues (1973), and Lennert (1974), the large lymphoid cells of André-Schwartz (1964) and Cottier et al (1972), the reticular lymphoblasts of Hartsock (1968), the non-cleaved follicular centre cells of Lukes and Collins (1974, 1975), and the centroblasts of Lennert et al (1975).

Within the reactive centres certain morphological expressions of the intermediate phases of B-lymphocyte transformation have been identified by name.

The *centroblast* (formerly germinoblast of Lennert 1973, 1975) is equivalent to the *non-cleaved follicular centre cell* of Lukes and Collins (1973, 1974, Diagram 3, p. 22). It has a basophilic (and pyroninophilic) cytoplasm, with a round to oval vesicular nucleus containing small masses of chromatin and one or more small nucleoli, usually arranged peripherally at the distinct nuclear membrane.

The *centrocyte* (formerly germinocyte) of Lennert (1973, 1974) is equivalent to the *cleaved follicular centre cell* of Lukes and Collins (1973, 1974, Diagram 3), and varies in size with a nuclear diameter of 12 μm up to 25 or 30 μm. The nucleus is characteristically polymorphous or cleaved and possesses a delicate nuclear membrane with compact basichromatin; nucleoli, if present, are small and inconspicuous. The cytoplasm appears as an ill-defined rim and is usually faintly basophilic.

In their morphological descriptions Lukes and Collins and Lennert agree, but they differ in their interpretation of the temporal relationship of these cells one to another during the process of B-cell transformation in the reactive centre; a difference which, due to the cyclical nature of the transformation process (see Diagrams 1 and 3), is perhaps less significant than might at first be supposed.

The *B-immunoblast* is equivalent to the fully transformed B-lymphocyte and its partially differentiated progeny (*plasmablast*); it is usually found outside the germinal centre areas, though identical cells may be found within. The nuclear membrane is particularly distinct, the nucleolus conspicuous and usually central, and the cytoplasm strongly basophilic (pyroninophilic). A juxta-nuclear hof is often present, and the cell cytoplasm may have a clearly defined ovoid or polygonal outline.

The postulated sequence of morphological changes according to Lukes and Collins is illustrated in Diagram 3, in which the phase of immunoglobulin pro-

Diagram 3

Scheme of 'B'- and 'T'-Cell Transformation (from Taylor, 1976)

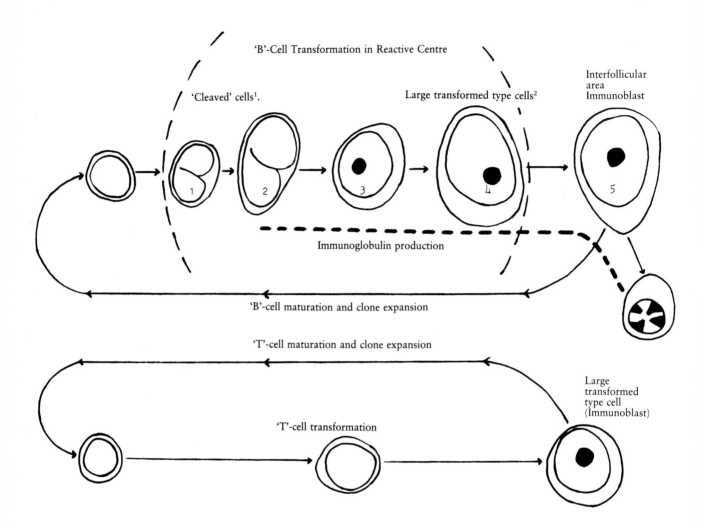

'B'-Cell Transformation in Reactive Centre

'Cleaved' cells[1].

Large transformed type cells[2]

Interfollicular area Immunoblast

Immunoglobulin production

'B'-cell maturation and clone expansion

'T'-cell maturation and clone expansion

Large transformed type cell (Immunoblast)

'T'-cell transformation

[1] Cleaved cell (Lukes, Collins), centrocyte (Lennert)

[2] Non-cleaved cell (Luke, Collins), centroblast (Lennert).

duction is also depicted. Concurrent with evidence of intracellular immunoglobulin production there is loss of the surface immunoglobulin normally carried by B-cells, and mature plasma cells have none. These cells are regarded by the present authors as different morphological phases of B-lymphocyte transformation in the reactive centre areas, and of maturation in the diffuse cortex, paracortex, and medulla.

The term *lymphoblast* has been widely used by haematologists and histologists and unfortunately no precise description can be given for this term, since its usage has been so variable, and the morphological features have not usually been defined. Generally, the term lymphoblast implies a large obviously lymphoid cell, with an overall diameter of 15–20 μm. The cytoplasm shows moderate basophilia and appears as a uniform rim around the centrally placed nucleus. The nucleus itself is round or oval, with a distinct but small nucleolus and scattered basichromatin. The term lymphoblast has been applied to reactive cells (transforming cells – 'blast cell' transformation), but especially to neoplastic cells, as in acute lymphoblastic leukaemia and 'lymphoblastic lymphoma'. Lennert has given some definition to his usage of the term: 'the so-called lymphoblasts of chronic lymphocytic leukaemia are quite different from basophilic germinal centre cells (germinoblasts or centroblasts)' (Lennert et al, 1975), and he assigns various malignant lymphomas to a 'lymphoblastic' group, including those forms related to acute lymphoblastic leukaemia, Burkitt's lymphoma, and convoluted cell lymphoma (see chapter V). The subtle characteristics described by Lennert and colleagues are of limited value to the ordinary histologist, and we prefer to regard those cells which may be termed lymphoblasts as nothing more than different stages in the transformation process, though quite how they relate to the cleaved cell (centrocyte), the non-cleaved cell (centroblast), the fully transformed lymphocyte (immunoblast) and the differentiating transformed lymphocyte (plasmablast), remains to be resolved. Consequently, there may still be a justification for using 'lymphoblastic' as an adjectival qualifier to characterise a malignant lymphoid neoplasm, provided the usage of the term is clearly defined. For example, both Lennert (Stein et al, 1976) and Rappaport (Nathwani et al, 1976) have used the term lymphoblastic lymphoma in this context (corresponding at least in part to convoluted cell lymphoma, p. 162).

Plasma Cells

The distinctive morphological features of mature plasma cells were recognized long before their function became apparent, and the descriptions of Marschalko have not been bettered:

> 'das der Kern nicht in der Mitte der Zelle, sondern excentrisch und bei den ovalen zellen in dem einen Pole derselben liegte. . . . In der Mitte des Zellleibes aber ensteht ein hellerhof. . . .'   *Thomas v Marschalko, 1895.*

Mature plasma cells have a spherical nuclear diameter of 8–12μm with characteristic peripheral clumped chromatin (clock-face). Within the basophilic (and pyroninophilic) cytoplasm there may be a 'heller hof' together with accumulated secretions constituting Russell bodies (Russell, 1890). Mott cells (Mott, 1905), thesaurocytes and the flame cells of Undritz (1952) are all thought to be variants of this 'storage cell' type (Maldonado et al, 1965).

Cells termed *plasmablasts* represent B-immunoblasts having morphological evidence of differentiation towards plasma cells. They contain demonstrable immunoglobulin. Cells having mixed features of the small lymphocyte and the plasma cell are termed *lympho-plasmacytoid cells*, and like plasma cells they are derived by differentiation and maturation of the B-immunoblast. Typically lympho-plasmacytoid cells contain IgM, and are an especial feature of Waldenström's disease (p. 196).

Plasma Cell Origin and Function

The origin of plasma cells from small lymphocytes by antigen induced transformation is generally accepted (Nossal and Ada, 1971). Much of the controversy in the literature as to the origin of plasma cells from reticulum cells may be resolved by the recognition that in many instances the term reticulum cell was applied to the large transformed B-lymphocyte, prior to the realisation of the relationship of this cell type with the small lymphocyte. This is of particular relevance to the diagnosis of plasmacytoma and multiple myeloma, and the observation of progression of these neoplasms to tumours resembling so-called reticulum cell sarcomas.

The only ascribed function of the plasma cell is the production of antibody, first convincingly demonstrated by Amano et al (1944) and Fagraeus (1948). Immunocytochemical methods show that the first traces of antibody are found in the nucleolus of immature cells (plasmablasts), prior to the appearance of significant amounts in the perinuclear space, then the ergastoplasm, and finally, the saccules of the Golgi apparatus, prior to its secretion from the cell (Straus, 1968; Sordat, 1970; Murphy et al, 1972). This sequence of events may be followed under light microscopy, by the demonstration, using immunoperoxidase methods, of immunoglobulin in a spectrum of cell types from the large transformed B-lymphocyte (plasmablast) to the mature plasma cell. The work of Takahashi et al (1969) suggested that immunoglobulin synthesis is maximal during the G_1 and early S phase of the lymphocyte cell cycle. This would agree with the observations of Hay et al (1972), who found that during secondary immune responses to horseradish peroxidase antigen, the predominant antibody forming cells were 'large blast cells' (as in Figs I.1f and 1g).

Histiocyte Series. Cells of the Reticulo-endothelial System

Due in part to morphological variability in relation to physiological activity, and confusion between transformed lymphocytes and certain cells of the histiocytic series, nomenclature and cell identification are far from simple. Furthermore, there is the problem of the relationship between tissue histiocytes and blood monocytes. Present evidence is that tissue histiocytes are derived partly by recruitment of monocytes and partly by mitotic division of histiocytes in response to various stimuli (Spector et al, 1966, 1968, 1970).

Histiocyte

Unhappily, the term 'histiocyte' has been applied to a wide range of cell types, and has also been used collectively for tissue cells which store vital dyes and may show active phagocytic powers.

The nucleus of the tissue histiocyte is oval or kidney shaped, measuring up to 12μm in the long axis. The nuclear membrane though fine is distinct and somewhat wrinkled. The chromatin appears dispersed with a tendency to peripheral clumping and, together with an inconspicuous nucleolus, gives the nucleus an overall vesicular appearance. The cellular outline may be variable, but is often spindle shaped with finely branched processes. The cytoplasm is variable in amount and, when the cells are unstimulated and free from particulate matter, is inconspicuous. On activation, the cytoplasm increases in volume and varies from a pale hue to intense eosinophilia. Often it assumes a granular appearance and may contain particulate matter or vacuoles.

These features contrast with the more rounded nucleus, prominent nucleolus and basophilic cytoplasm of the transformed lymphocyte. However, it is recognized that in some instances there may be local proliferation of histiocytes in the tissue (Spector et al, 1966, 1968, 1970) in which the cells may be rounded, developing cytoplasmic basophilia and prominent nucleoli, so that they resemble to some extent transformed lymphocytes.

Various histochemical reactions have been described as relatively specific for histiocytes (acid phosphatase, alkaline phosphatase, non-specific esterase – Yam et al, 1971; Li et al, 1972; Niemi and Korhonen, 1972), while by the Hortega microglia methods the cytoplasm is black to grey, with coarse granules, and the fine cytoplasmic processes are clearly demonstrated. Unfortunately these techniques cannot be applied effectively to formalin-paraffin sections and the muramidase technique (Appendix II, p. 281), which is applicable to paraffin sections, only marks a proportion of histiocytes. However, Isaacson et al (1979) have found that α^1-antitrypsin is present in the cytoplasm of normal and malignant histiocytes and can be displayed with the immunoperoxidase technique.

Histiocytes in special situations may show distinctive features and are specifically named.

Littoral Cells (Sinus Histiocytes)

These are specialised histiocytes which lie upon the margin and reticulin fibrils of the lymph sinuses of the lymph nodes. Similar cells line the venous sinuses of the spleen, bone marrow and liver (Kupffer cells). Cytologically they are identical with the histiocyte described above. In the resting phase they are markedly spindle-shaped and may be difficult to distinguish unless thick sections are examined. On stimulation they assume an arachnoid form with projecting cytoplasmic processes, and may evolve to rounded macrophages within the sinus lumen.

Dendritic and Interdigitating Reticular Cells – Dendritic Macrophages

Present knowledge of 'dendritic reticular cells' owes much to the independent studies of Hanna and Nossal (Nossal and Ada, 1971), following upon the observations by various authors of intercellular deposits of antigen in germinal centres (Sainte-Marie, 1962; Mellors and Korngold, 1963).

The dendritic reticular cell is present both in primary and secondary centres and is morphologically distinct from the tingible body macrophage. In some centres the dendritic reticular cells are extremely prominent and form a distinct 'peripheral cap' to the reactive centre.

Antigen trapping by the numerous fine cytoplasmic process of the dendritic reticular cells is believed to play a vital part in the immune response, and the possible mechanisms of antigen trapping, dependent upon surface receptors for the Fc component of immunoglobulin, have been discussed by Nossal and Ada (1971). Active phagocytosis of antigen by dendritic reticular cells does not occur though antigen may be retained at the cell surface for long periods, and serve to initiate lymphocyte transformation. These cells are difficult to identify with certainty in haematoxylin and eosin sections as the cytoplasm stains poorly. Silver impregnation methods may be used to demonstrate the dendritic cell processes, or alternatively they can be displayed by histochemical methods for acid phosphatase. While it seems possible that tingible body macrophages and dendritic reticular cells are related, there is no direct evidence for this. The interdigitating reticular cell of the paracortex is probably related to the dendritic cell though morphologically and functionally distinct (Rausch et al, 1977).

Monocyte

The circulating blood monocyte is thought to be derived from the bone marrow and certainly a large proportion of the macrophages in an inflammatory reaction are derived from blood monocytes (Spector et al, 1968, 1970). In the tissues they appear as rounded or oval cells having an eosinophilic cytoplasm and an indented, chromatin-rich, nucleus with an inconspicuous nucleolus.

Epithelioid Histiocytes

This is a descriptive term applied to a variety of histiocytes found in certain granulomatous reactions, probably developing in response to certain non-degradable materials. The cytoplasm is large in amount, the cell measuring 20–30 μm, and appears eosinophilic and granular. Large amounts of lysozyme are demonstrable within such cells (see Figs. II.4d; II.8 and II.25c) by the immunoperoxidase method using antisera to purified lysozyme (muramidase – Mason and Taylor, 1975). The nucleus resembles that of the histiocyte and is round or oval, vesicular in appearance, with a well marked nuclear membrane and distinct nucleolus.

Macrophage

The term macrophage has come to be applied to free rounded histiocytes found in zones of phagocytic activity, and in particular sites may have special designations (e.g. tingible body macrophage of germinal centre, compound granular corpuscle in the brain, Hofbauer cells of the placenta etc.).

The appearance in section is very variable and they range in size from 20μm to 40μm or more. The cell ouline is sharp though pseudopodia may be observed, and the cytoplasm is faintly eosinophil. Older forms may appear more granular, apart from containing particulate material, vacuoles and lipids. The nucleus is similar to that of the histiocyte, but may be somewhat larger.

In argyrophil preparations the cytoplasm varies in colour from grey black to brown, and cytoplasmic processes are easily seen. Generally cells showing evidence of phagocytosis do not contain demonstrable lysozyme (muramidase).

The Tingible Body Macrophage ('Der tingible Körper' of Flemming, 1885)

Tingible body macrophages are regarded as characteristic features of reactive germinal centres, but are probably nothing more than ordinary macrophages in a special site. They are first observed in developing secondary follicles (reactive or germinal centres) approximately four days after exposure to antigen, and appear to be phagocytic cells containing nuclear debris which is generally supposed to be derived from degenerating lymphocytes. There is some evidence that the proliferation of the monocyte-histiocyte series precedes and accompanies the lymphoid proliferation in the immune responses, but probably only as a reflection of the great proliferative activity and associated cell death of lymphocytes undergoing transformation and cell division (Fliedner, 1964; Hinrichson, 1967).

In regressing centres the tingible body macrophages may persist for a considerable time, and so appear relatively prominent as the lymphocyte complement decreases.

Giant Cells

Both Langhans' giant cells and ordinary foreign body type giant cells are derived from mononuclear cells of the histiocyte – monocyte series by a process of nuclear division in the absence of corresponding cytoplasmic cleavage.

Some giant cells show a granular eosinophilic cytoplasm resembling that of epithelioid cells, and many contain lysozyme in high concentrations.

'Reticulum Cells' – 'Reticular Cells'

Like democracy, the terms 'reticulum cell' and 'reticular cell' have many meanings and are often used in a loose or undefined way for any large cell having a vesicular nucleus with prominent nucleolus, occurring in lympho-reticular tissues. In the majority of instances, when the intentions of the users have been defined, these terms have been applied to cells believed to belong to the histiocyte series, though in a quiescent potentially phagocytic stage. However there is no doubt that cells designated by some observers as reticulum cells are in fact transformed lymphocytes. Less commonly the terms reticulum or reticular cell have been applied to cells believed to be involved in the formation of reticulin fibrils and possibly related to fibroblasts.

It is undeniable that throughout the cortex, paracortex, follicles and medulla of the node cells may occur which cannot be assigned with certainty to the various cell types already described, and such cells of uncertain nature are common in some lympho-proliferative conditions. These are the cells which have often been loosely termed reticular or reticulum cells, and may in reality be pluripotent stem cells, histiocytes, transformed lymphocytes or fibroblasts. We must await extension of histochemical and immunohistological methods for the demonstration of other cellular products, before a more definite identification of such cells can be achieved.

Accordingly the terms reticulum cell and reticular cell will not be used here, except in reference to the work of other authors, and in these circumstances the precise usage of the term will be qualified wherever possible. It will be necessary to return to these problems of nomenclature in the discussion of various types of malignant lymphomata and the varied usage of terms such as reticulosarcoma, reticulum cell sarcoma etc. (see Appendix I).

Fibroblasts, endothelial cells and other connective tissue elements

Endothelial cells in section may be confused with 'reticulum cells' (in the sense of transformed lymphocytes), and Söderström (1967) noted that in reactive hyperplasia, the swollen endothelial cell of the post-capillary venules may appear as solid cords of cells, having a remarkable resemblance to small reactive centres. Such resemblance is enhanced by the vesicular nucleus of the endothelial cell, and the frequent presence of a distinct nucleolus, producing a nuclear configuration not unlike that of follicle centre cells. The true nature of the endothelial cell is generally apparent from its position within the basement membrane of the blood vessel. However, tangential cutting of post-capillary venules may result in the appearance of endothelial cells scattered within the paracortical area without obvious relation to vessels; small clusters of such cells may be misinterpreted as transformed lymphocytes (immunoblasts) or even as Reed-Sternberg cells, causing confusion which can be serious.

Fibroblasts (fibrocytes) appear as small inconspicuous cells with a slender elongated nucleus and a small nucleolus. It is obvious that such cells cannot clearly be distinguished from other cell types ('reticular cell' group). Indeed in the literature there has been considerable discussion as to the possibility of transformation of cells of the reticular-histiocyte series and fibrogenic cells (Davis, 1967). Further examination of these possibilities with additional references may be found in the papers of Ross, 1968 and Spector, 1969.

Granulocytes – Polymorphonuclear leucocytes

The basic physiological reactions of these cells will be described briefly as the appearance of these cells in association with a lymphomatous process, exemplified by the eosinophils in Hodgkin's disease, is probably nothing more than the usual physiological response of these cells to a concurrent immunological reaction.

Neutrophils. Mature segmented polymorphonuclear neutrophil leucocytes are readily recognisable in sections, and in addition show a number of histochemical reactions. The primary azurophilic granules contain lysosomal enzymes (including peroxidase and lysozyme itself) and the secondary specific granules contain other enzymes including alkaline phosphatase. A positive PAS reaction (abolished by diastase digestion) results from the glycogen within the granules. More primitive cells of the neutrophil series show diminished or absent reactivity for some enzymes; the myeloblast is PAS negative and gives a variable chloro-acetate esterase and peroxidase staining reaction. These stains are of great value in facilitating the recognition of solid masses of cells in myelogenous leukaemias.

Eosinophil. The mature eosinophil is slightly larger than the corresponding neutrophil (diameter 12–15 μm) and has a characteristic bi-lobed 'spectacle' nucleus. The specific granules are fewer in number and larger, while eosinophil peroxidase can be distinguished from the verdoperoxidase of neutrophils as it is insensitive to cyanide blocking.

The roles of the neutrophil and eosinophil granulocytes in immune responses have been extensively investigated, but definitive conclusions have not resulted (Spiers, 1958; Archer, 1968). Both types of granulocyte respond to the chemotactic activity of the products of complement fixation and possibly also to chemotactic factors (lymphokines) isolated from lymphocytes (Cohen and Ward, 1971). These responses may be relevant to the occurrence of granulocytes in association with certain of the lymphomas.

Basophils and Mast Cells. Mast cells were first described by Ehrlich in 1877 and the basophil leucocyte of the blood was distinguished by him two years later. Subsequently mast cells and basophils have been established as separate cell lines which appear however to have some reciprocal relationship. Basophils are rarely observed in tissues. The physiological role of mast cells has been extensively investigated and they have been shown to contain many enzymes, together with biogenic amines, including histamine, and heparin (Selye, 1965, Bessis, 1973). In addition the numbers of mast cells are increased in the vicinity of some neoplasms and in the bone marrow in some lympho-proliferative disorders (Nixon, 1966). Mast cells give a positive reaction for chloro-acetate esterase, and stain metachromatically with toluidine blue and similar dyes.

In addition to the cell types described in this chapter, there may occasionally be found other cells which are more or less closely related to either the lymphocyte or the histiocyte, but are not a 'normal' component of the lymph node. These pathological cells are often of sufficiently distinctive form that their presence may justify the diagnosis of a specific lymphoproliferative or lymphomatous disorder, and are described in detail in the appropriate place; Reed-Sternberg cells, lacunar cells, Sézary cells or cerebriform lymphocytes, convoluted lymphocytes, Burkitt cells.

Lymphokines

In order to appreciate better the complex interaction of the various normal cell types, some reference should be made to the possible role of lymphokines in mediating the immune response. Lymphokines are biologically active substances normally released by lymphocytes in response to stimulation by specific antigen. Individual lymphokines are usually defined by their biological activity, which also serves as an assay for the presence of the lymphokine in question. The principal lymphokines recognized to date include chemotactic factors for neutrophils, basophils, eosinophils, monocytes and lymphocytes, as well as macrophage migration inhibitory factor (MIF), macrophage activating factor and specific macrophage arming factor (MAF and SMAF), mitogenic factor (MIT) and transfer factor (TF) (reviews – Granger, 1972; Cohen, 1976; Waksman and Namba, 1976).

2b. General Anatomy of the Lymph Node

Having considered the various cells which may be found in lymphoid tissue, it is proper to relate these to the nodal architecture and its reactive mutability. Much of the experimental work relating to lymph node function and morphology has been performed in animals, particularly inbred strains of mice. In many animals, including the mouse, the nodes are large and few in number; but in primates the nodes are relatively smaller and more numerous, occurring in chains or arcades. However, the general topography and architecture of the lymph node is really quite similar in all mammals, though fine structural details may vary with any of several factors, of which age, anatomical site, and any current or previous antigenic stimulation are the most important for the diagnostic pathologist.

Diagram 4

Anatomical Diagram of normal lymph node
modified from Heudorfer (1921)

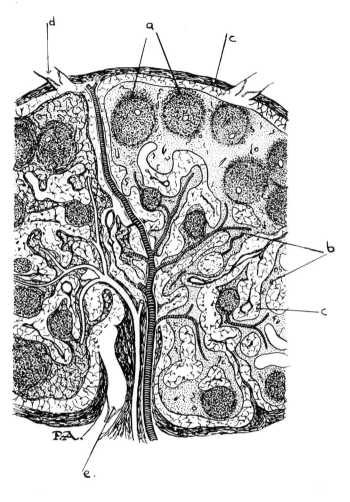

(a) Primary follicles

(b) Medullary pulp (c) Sinuses

(d) Afferent lymphatic (e) Efferent lymphatic.

The reticulin framework of the node is shown on the left side of the diagram.

Basic Structure

A number of authors have presented stylised diagrams of the minute structure of
the resting lymph node, as examplified by that of Heudorfer in 1921 (Diagram
4, above), and indeed the basic microscopical anatomy has been established in
principle since 1862 when His distinguished a peripheral cortex of dense lymphoid tissue and a medullary area traversed by sinusoids. The variability observed
in lymph node structure was discussed by von Recklinghausen (1862) and the
general structure, reticulum, and germinal centres reviewed by Job (1922).

Unfortunately, the nomenclature is less clear than this would suggest, and the

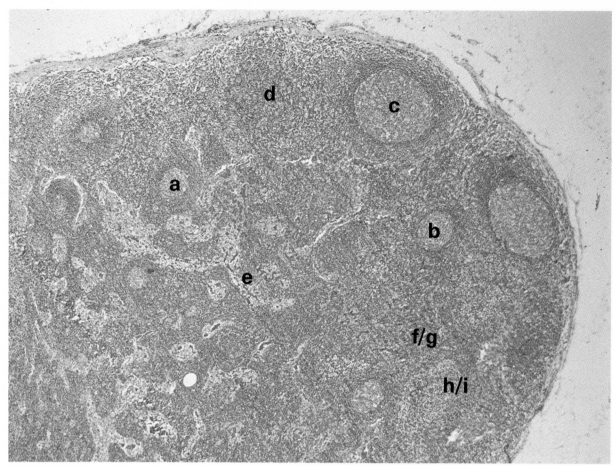

I.1 The Normal Lymph Node   (The letters indicate the location of the high power fields shown opposite.)

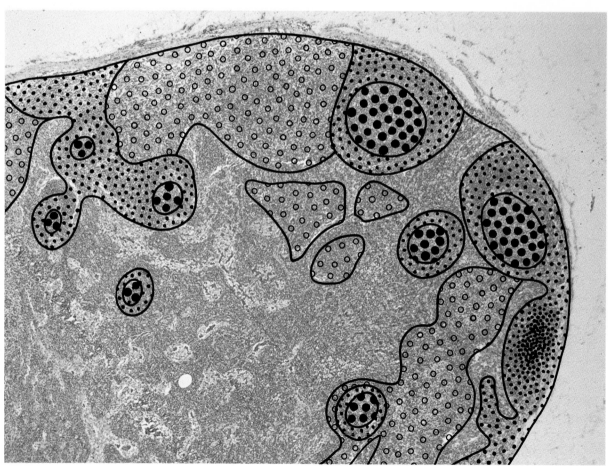

Key to Figure I.1 (above) The Normal Lymph Node,
to show the demarcation of the functional areas

Cortex (outer cortex). Follicles
Paracortex (cortico-medullary junction area). The
Medullary cords and sinuses.

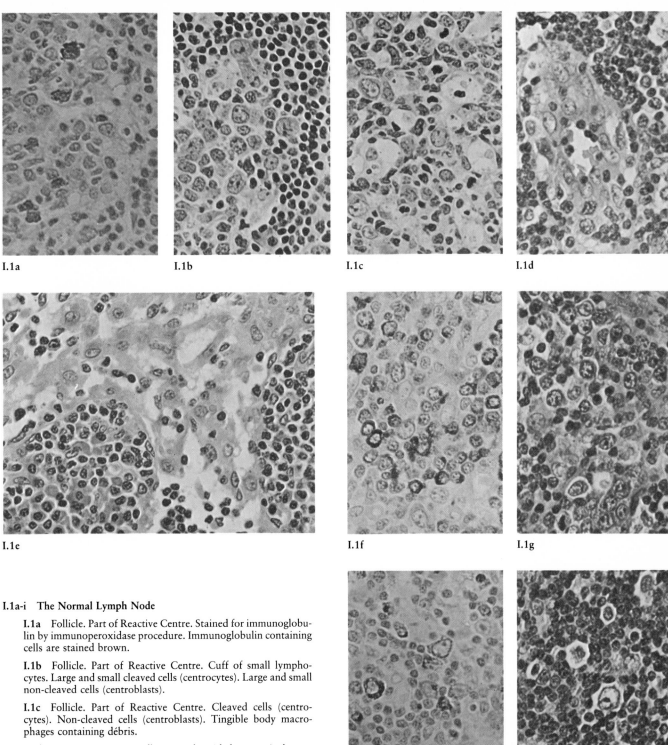

I.1a

I.1b

I.1c

I.1d

I.1e

I.1f

I.1g

I.1h

I.1i

I.1a–i   The Normal Lymph Node

I.1a   Follicle. Part of Reactive Centre. Stained for immunoglobulin by immunoperoxidase procedure. Immunoglobulin containing cells are stained brown.

I.1b   Follicle. Part of Reactive Centre. Cuff of small lymphocytes. Large and small cleaved cells (centrocytes). Large and small non-cleaved cells (centroblasts).

I.1c   Follicle. Part of Reactive Centre. Cleaved cells (centrocytes). Non-cleaved cells (centroblasts). Tingible body macrophages containing débris.

I.1d   Paracortex. Post-capillary venule with large vesicular endothelial cells surrounded by small and transformed lymphocytes.

I.1e   Medullary sinus and cord. The sinus shows the histiocytes and littoral cells while the medullary cord consists largely of plasma cells with the occasional small lymphocyte and immunoblast.

I.1f–g   Paracortex. Stained for immunoglobulin and haematoxylin and eosin. Transformed lymphocytes (immunoblasts), plasmablasts. Mature plasma cells. Immunoglobulin appears brown. Immunoglobulin containing cells are migrating through paracortex.

I.1h–i   Paracortex. Stained for immunoglobulin and haematoxylin and eosin. Transformed lymphocytes. Plasma Cells. Lymphocytes. Immunoglobulin appears brown.

inconsistency in identification and naming of the cells of the lympho-reticular system is also to be found in definitions proposed for the principal regions of the lymph node.

It is unnecessary to embark upon an examination of the prior usage of the terms cortex and medulla; suffice it to say that the term medulla has been variously applied to represent only the central region of the node, or alternatively to include all of the substance of the node excepting the follicles, and this has naturally led to confusion.

The terminology used in this book is based upon current concepts of distinct functional areas within the lymph node, which show correspondence to the areas of distribution of the T- and B-lymphocytes (Parrott, de Sousa and East, 1966; Parrott and de Sousa, 1971).

These areas have largely been defined through experimental work in animals, involving thymic ablation in the foetus or neonate (and bursectomy in birds), or reconstitution of thymectomised lethally irradiated animals with thymic cells or marrow lymphocytes, with concurrent observations of the resulting histological changes in the peripheral lymphoid organs. Alternatively H^3 thymidine labelled thymic (T) or bone marrow (B, bursal, or thymic independent) lymphocytes may be injected, and the sites of localisation examined by autoradiography of organs removed at autopsy. In addition fresh organs may be taken, cell suspensions prepared, and the percentage of B- or T-cells determined by surface markers (see Tables 1 and 2, pp. 17, 18). The distribution of T- and B-lymphocytes is similar in most mammalian species for which information is available.

As distinctive types of immune responses were assigned to either the T - or B-cell system (Diagram 2, p. 16), so these experimental observations were extended by correlating the areas of marked reactive change in the lymphoid organs with the type of immune response in progress (Turk, 1967). Thus the T-cell areas show marked hyperplasia in a response of a primarily cell mediated immune type; and the B-cell areas in humoral immune reactions.

Evidence that T- and B-cell areas are present in human lymph nodes has been provided by various authors in detailed studies of naturally occurring immune deficiency diseases of man, which have been considered analogous to some of the animal experiments previously described. The morphological features of immune deficiency diseases will be discussed in later chapters.

As a result of these experimental studies it is possible to map out areas of the human lymph node corresponding to those demonstrated in experimental animals. It must be emphasized that the demarcation between the medullary and paracortical areas is less distinct in man than in some of the animals in which much of the experimental work has been performed. The basic schemes suggested by Nossal and Ada (1972) and Cottier et al (1972) are entirely satisfactory, but for the purposes of this text it seemed more useful to pencil in the different functional areas of the lymph node upon a map of the 'normal' lymph node depicted in Figure I (p. 32). According to this scheme five principal regions may be distinguished:

The cortex (outer cortex)

The follicles (including germinal centres, part of the outer cortex)

The paracortex (cortico-medullary junction area)

The medullary cords

The sinus system

The Cortex (outer) is situated immediately internal to the subcapsular (marginal) sinus. It consists predominantly of densely crowded small lymphocytes in which are scattered a small number of histiocytes and larger lymphoid cells.

The distinction from the subjacent para-cortical area is neither abrupt nor absolute. In some sections collections of densely packed small lymphocytes may appear isolated in the deep parts of the node, and may contain germinal centres. This apparent discontinuity from the major part of the cortex is probably an artefact of the plane of section.

Situated within the outer cortex are the various forms of lymphoid follicles.

The Follicles. Flemming (1885) described focal collections of cells within the lymphoid tissues and believing them to be the chief (though not exclusive) places of multiplication of lymphocytes, he introduced the term 'germinal centre'. This theory was supported by the observation of frequent mitotic figures within the 'germinal centre', and the nascent lymphocytes were believed to move centrifugally into the surrounding diffuse lymphoid tissue. Maximow (1932) illustrated the concept in detail, though he noted the uncertainty which existed regarding the exact nature of the lymphocyte progenitor cells. Further, Maximow elaborated upon the phasic changes in germinal centres, previously noted by Flemming in his original description.

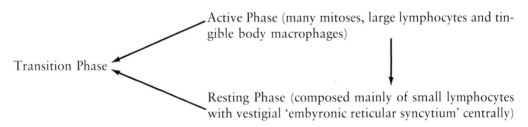

Transition Phase

Active Phase (many mitoses, large lymphocytes and tingible body macrophages)

Resting Phase (composed mainly of small lymphocytes with vestigial 'embyronic reticular syncytium' centrally)

An alternative view of the nature of the follicles had developed from the critical observations of Marchand (1913) and Hellman (1921, 1930), who proposed that the lymph follicles were in reality centres of reaction to noxious agents, and argued that the lack of intermediate forms was against the concept of a primary lymphopoietic role. Also, Flemming's centres were not observed in the foetus

35

when lymphocytes were actively forming (Cooper et al, 1967). Congdon and Hannan (1967) briefly discussed these theories of the function of the secondary follicles.

This latter concept of 'reactive centres' is now generally accepted, and such reactive centres may be seen to develop de novo following antigenic stimulation (Ringertz and Adamson, 1950; Turk and Stone, 1963; Cottier et al, 1964). Also in favour of the reactive nature of the follicles were the several observations of absence, or partial development, of follicles in 'germ-free' animals (Thorbecke, 1959; Gordon and Wostmann, 1960; Ernström, 1965; Pollard, 1967).

Yoffey (Yoffey and Courtice, 1970), in studies using H^3 labelled thymidine, noted the presence of small clusters of labelled cells deep within the lymph node, and explored the possibility that these might represent reactive centre formation by expanding lymphocyte clones, in accordance with the clonal selection theory advanced by Burnet (1969). Yoffey observed that as these new centres enlarged they appeared to occupy a more peripheral position in the lymph node. Against this concept of the reactive centre as a product of a single clone are the observations within a single centre of different immunoglobulin types and classes (Pernis, 1967), although other reports have supported the proposition that germinal centres are monospecific (Sordat, 1970; Hay et al, 1972).

The 'reactive' and 'germinal' theories are not incompatible. The present supposition is that considerable lymphopoiesis does occur in germinal centres, but that this occurs in response to antigenic stimulation, when the characteristic germinal (reactive) centres are seen. Such centres are the site of B-lymphocyte transformation and the large lymphoid germinal centre cells (variously termed centroblasts, centrocytes, large cleaved and non-cleaved cells, reticulum cells, etc.) represent phases in the transformation of the B-lymphocyte and its maturation to the plasma cell (Diagrams 1 and 3, pp. 15, 22).

Only two morphological forms of the follicle warrant separate description, being at either end of a continuous spectrum of appearances from the inactive follicle to the florid reactive centre.

(i) PRIMARY FOLLICLE. This appears as a dense condensation of small lymphocytes within the cortex (100–400μm in diameter in man), generally in a peripheral position. In the centre of the follicle there may be relatively more medium sized lymphocytes, dendritic reticular cells and macrophages. This represents the non-stimulated follicle and may become the site of a characteristic secondary follicle following exposure to an antigen. Alternatively some secondary follicles probably arise de novo.

(ii) SECONDARY FOLLICLES. (Flemming's centre, reactive centre, germinal centre, including developing and regressing forms.) In the classical florid form the secondary nodule measures 100–600 μm in diameter and is composed of a peripheral annulus of dense small lymphocytes (mantle), with a central paler area (the germinal/reactive centre), consisting of differing proportions of large

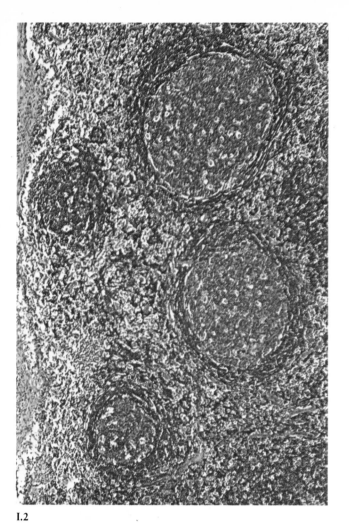

I.2

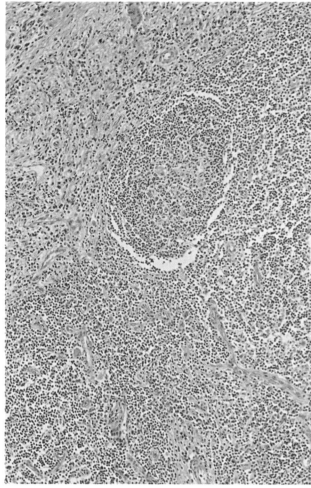

I.3

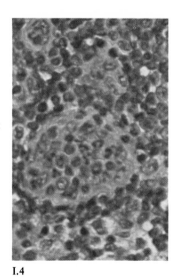

I.4

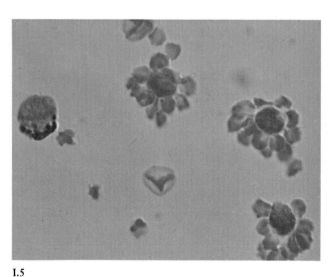

I.5

I.2 Various Stages in the Development of Secondary (reactive) Follicles in the Cortex

Note the ring of small lymphocytes and tingible body macrophages in the reactive centre.

I.3 Regressed Secondary Follicle

There is an absence of transformed lymphocytes and no lymphocytic cuff, but histiocytes are numerous and some hyalinization of the centre. The thickened capsule and prominent hyalinized vessels in the paracortex are quite characteristic.

I.4 Paracortex in Acute Reactive Hyperplasia

Swollen post-capillary venules containing eosinophils, neutrophils and lymphocytes.

I.5 Preparation of Lymphocytes combining Techniques for Surface Immunoglobulin by Immunoperoxidase and Spontaneous Sheep Red Cell Rosetting

The B cell shows intense brown surface staining for immunoglobulin with capping, while three T-cells show red cell rosetting.

37

lymphoid cells (transformed lymphocytes, previously known by many names including reticulum cell), medium lymphocytes, immature plasma cells, tingible body macrophages, and dendritic reticular cells. In some secondary nodules the transformed lymphocytes are particularly concentrated within the deep aspect of the nodule. 'Flash' labelling with tritiated thymidine reveals that many of the cells of an active secondary nodule are in DNA synthesis (Hinrichson, 1967), and the newly formed cells do not seem to remain in the mantle zone. The route of emigration of these numerous newly formed lymphocytes, including immature large lymphocytes and recognisable plasma cell precursors, is a matter of speculation, as is their ultimate fate. Nossal described a procession of 'blast cells' (again meaning transformed lymphocytes) between the reactive centres and the medullary cords (Nossal and Ada, 1971).

Fig. 1.2

(iii) R E G R E S S I V E   F O L L I C L E. Following cessation of antigenic stimulation there is a progressive decrease in lymphocyte transformation within the follicle, and consequently fewer of the large transformed type cells (large cleaved and non-cleaved follicle centre cells) are present. The histiocytes (tingible body macrophages) tend to persist for longer periods and may be relatively prominent, appearing as angular cells with pale cytoplasmic eosinophilia. Such follicles often show stromal hyaline change. These features are believed to signify 'regressed' secondary follicles.

Fig. 1.3

The Paracortex is that part of the cellular lymphoid tissue lying internal to the cortex, but excluding the medullary cords. It consists, like the cortex, predominantly of small lymphocytes, but these are less densely packed, and there are variable numbers of larger lymphocytes and histiocytes. Groups of plasma cells, of varying maturity, may also be found in relation to adjacent reactive centres and medullary cords. The paracortex may show very great variation in extent, and in cell population, during immune responses.

A distinctive feature of the paracortex is the presence of a number of specialized small blood vessels, the post-capillary venules. These are characterised by a tall endothelium and are thought to allow the passage across their walls of large numbers of small lymphocytes. Frequently lymphocytes may be seen in the vessel wall, or actually within the endothelial cells (Marchesi and Gowans, 1964). The majority favour the view that the direction of lymphocyte migration is from blood to lymph (Gowans and Knight, 1964), and see this as the major source of the small lymphocytes of the paracortex. Sainte-Marie et al (1967) proposed that lymphocyte passage occurs in the reverse direction.

Fig. 1.4

Söderström (1967) has presented a detailed study of the development of the post-capillary venules (or high endothelial venules to use his terminology), and believes that they play an important role in the organisation of the lymph node, appearing as central vessels within a substantial lymphocyte sheath. Generally, a lumen can be observed within the venule, but in some instances the endothelium is tall and the venule appears as a solid cord of pale cells with a surrounding cuff of small lymphocytes. This appearance may be difficult to distinguish morphologically from a developing germinal centre. Post-capillary venules are most prominent in the young and regress with old age.

The Medullary Cords. The true medulla may be considered to consist of many cords of lymphoid cells, together with variable numbers of plasma cells, extending centrally towards the hilum of the lymph node. The complex spaces between these cords constitute the medullary sinuses, and are of varying proportions in different species and different anatomical regions. In man the medullary cords are usually less clearly defined, unless abnormally expanded by accumulated plasma cells in a long standing hyperplasia. The histiocytic sinus lining cells partially separate the lymphocytes of the cords from the sinus contents.

Running in the core of many of the cords are small arteries, radiating from the hilum, together with their concomitant veins.

The cell population of the medullary cords and sinuses is dependent upon the phase of reaction of the lymph node. In the short term the cell population of the sinuses may change quite rapidly. This aspect is considered further in the discussion of functional responses of the lymph node.

The Sinuses. A variable number of afferent lymphatics drain into the marginal (cortical or subcapsular) sinus which almost totally surrounds the cellular part of the lymph node. The marginal sinus is continuous with the network of cortical sinuses and the confluence of medullary sinuses. In a median section, the medullary sinuses may be observed to merge into one or more efferent lymphatics.

Anatomically the sinus lining layer is defective, and the lymphoid cells of the cortex and medulla have direct contact with the contents of the sinuses. Thus the lymphocytes may be regarded as forming part of the sinus wall, throughout the lymph node.

A further feature of the sinuses is that they are traversed not only by numerous reticulin fibres, but also by fixed sinus histiocytes. These may detach to become free active histiocytes.

The sinus contents are fluid lymph draining from the tissues into the afferent lymphatics, in which are suspended varying numbers of lymphocytes, histiocytes and other cells. The cellular contents of the sinuses are greatly modified during passage through the node, and the efferent lymph has a remarkably different cell population. The sinus contents also vary greatly according to the reactivity of the node (Diagram 5, Table 4, p. 41) e.g. sinus histiocytosis, or many polymorphonuclear leucocytes during the hours immediately following antigen injection.

Capsule, Trabeculae and Reticulin Lattice

The capsule is composed of fibrous connective tissue, principally of mature collagen, and may be quite thin in small lymph nodes. However, the fibrous elements may be greatly increased by disease. Generally very few lymphoid cells are seen within the capsule.

The fibres of the capsule extend centripetally in some areas, forming varying numbers of fine trabeculae, which partially subdivide the cortex. The trabeculae may also carry fine vessels in from the capsule and in addition, small arteries extend from the hilum of the node to supply paracortex and cortex, and fine branches to reactive centre areas. In some lymph nodes trabeculae are inconspicuous or absent.

The reticulin lattice constitutes the structural framework of the lymph node and consists of fine argyrophil fibres permeating the whole of the substance of the node. The form of the reticulin lattice is very variable in different regions of the lymph node, being open in the sinuses, more compact in the cortex, and concentrically arranged around the germinal centres (Diagram 4, p. 31).

The reticulin fibres are continuous with the connective tissue of the capsule and the trabeculae.

Lymphocyte 'homing' and 'retention'

Homing (ecotaxis, de Sousa, 1971, 1978) is the term generally used for the remarkable phenomenon of T- or B-lymphocytes localizing within particular parts of the peripheral lymphoid tissue. B-lymphocytes home to the cortex, while T-lymphocytes home to the paracortex (Hall et al, 1976, 1977). The mechanism is unknown.

Retention may be used to describe the factors 'holding' a population of lymphocytes within a particular part of the lymph node (e.g. retaining B-lymphocytes preferentially within the follicles), though, of course, a varying percentage of cells in any section are recirculating and are seen *en passant*. Parrott and de Sousa (1971) have suggested that B-lymphocytes may be retained preferentially within the follicular areas of lymph nodes and spleen as a direct consequent of the high density of immunoglobulin upon their surface. They visualise immunoglobulin bearing B-lymphocytes becoming entangled within the 'mesh' of processes of 'reticulocytes' (obviously meaning the dendritic reticular cells) within the follicles. It has been repeatedly demonstrated that the complex processes of these dendritic reticular cells bind immunoglobulins preferentially, and the mechanisms are discussed by Nossal and Ada (1971). T-lymphocytes with much less surface immunoglobulin would traverse these dendritic areas relatively freely. Similarly differentiating plasma cells, having lost their surface immunoglobulin, would not be retained, and would be free to pass into the medulla of the lymph node. More recently there have been suggestions that the surface density of lymphocyte C_3 receptors plays a role in retaining lymphocytes within follicle areas (Braylan et al, 1975; Taylor, 1977, 1978, 1979). Morris (1980) has presented an admirable review of the experimental and conceptual problems.

Diagram 5

Dynamics of Lymphocyte Circulation in the Lymph Node from Yoffey (1966)

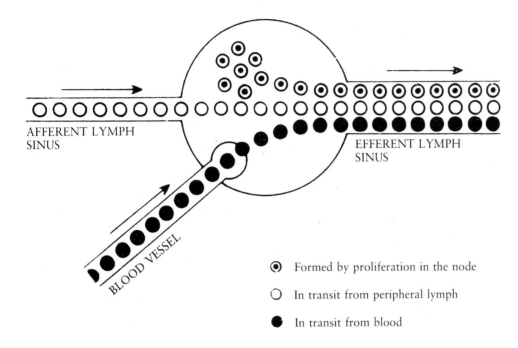

AFFERENT LYMPH
SINUS

EFFERENT LYMPH
SINUS

BLOOD VESSEL

◉ Formed by proliferation in the node

◯ In transit from peripheral lymph

● In transit from blood

Table 4

Response to antigenic stimulation in the sheep as an experimental model for cellular responses in circulating lymph

	Small Lymphocytes	Transformed[2] Lymphocytes	Histiocytes	Granulocytes
Afferent Lymph[1] Resting	85%	Rare	15%	Rare
Post-antigenic stimulation (3+ days)	85%	Small Number	15%	Variable
Efferent Lymph Resting	95%	Occasional	Occasional	Rare
Post-antigenic stimulation (3+ days)	50%	50%	Occasional	Variable

Percentage figures given are very approximate and represent merely the order of change occurring. Compiled from varions sources, principally Hall et al (1967), Yoffey and Courtice (1970), Nossal and Ada (1971), Bessis (1973).

[1] The number of lymphocytes in afferent lymph is only 10% of that in efferent lymph, thus 90% of the latter are derived from proliferation in the node or passage across the post-capillary venule.
[2] Transformed lymphocyte (large lymphocyte, pyroninophilic cells, lymphoblasts, immunoblasts etc.) A significant proportion of these transformed cells are shown to produce antibodies.

3. Patterns of Lymph Node Response

In experimental animals, in addition to the ordinary acute inflammatory reaction, three principal patterns of nodal response are recognisable: the humoral (B-cell) response; the cellular (T-cell) response; the histiocytic response.

It is probable that these basic types of response also occur in man. However, they are rarely observed in the form of 'pure type' responses, and the histological changes seen in human lymph nodes are usually composites of T- and B-cell reactions with histiocyte activity, though one or other type of response may predominate.

These basic responses will be considered in the animal models, as it is believed that an understanding of these responses may facilitate interpretation of the more complex changes in the reactive lymph nodes of man.

The Humoral Immune Response (B-cell mediated)

In the experimental animal the pattern of antigen distribution varies according to the route and site of antigen injection, in relation to the nature of the antigen itself, and with the presence or absence of existing specific circulating antibody. High molecular weight, or particulate, antigens are rapidly cleared from the lymph or blood by the phagocytic cells, including those in the lymph node sinuses and medulla, while low molecular weight antigens may circulate for several days, until the development of specific antibody facilitates clearance of the 'immune complexes' by phagocytic cells. Obviously, if specific antibody is present at the time of injection of antigen the 'antigen clearance' will be accelerated. Lymph nodes, for example, trap larger amounts of antigen in the presence of specific antibody, and reference has already been made to the antigen trapping mechanisms of the 'dendritic reticular cells' of the follicles.

Great variations occur in the mechanism of the response even under 'controlled conditions' in animals, and even more so in the reactive lymph nodes of man, where the nature and mode of entry of antigen are usually unknown. However, in the experimental animal the overall pattern of response is similar, whether the antigen is introduced by the intravenous or subcutaneous route, or following the more natural entry through the gastro-intestinal or respiratory tracts. It may, therefore, be profitable to consider a general account of the cellular responses of the lymph node following encounter with antigen, as an analogy for the probable sequence of changes in man.

The features of the primary immune response in the lymph node, following contact with antigen, may be summarised as follows:

(1) *Mobilisation of lymphocytes*, with little proliferation in the first twenty hours. There is a progressive increase in the number of lymphocytes in the efferent lymph, which appears to be the result of increased lymphocyte passage from the blood stream across the post-capillary venules (Brahim, Osmond, 1976).

(2) *Proliferation of lymphocytes* within the node increases dramatically and becomes very prominent after the second day. The products of this proliferative activity appear as large basophilic cells which are 'blast-like' in their morphology, and have been termed 'transitional cells' by Fagraeus (1948), activated reticulum cells by Marshall (1956), haemocytoblasts by André-Schwartz (1964) and others, or immunoblasts by Dameshek (1963). Here we have used 'transformed lymphocytes' to designate these cells (p. 20).

(3) *Proliferative activity in humoral immune responses* (B-cells) occurs principally, but not exclusively, in the lymph follicles (Craddock, 1972). The dense primary follicles enlarge to become characteristic reactive or germinal centres (secondary follicles). Also, some secondary follicles appear de novo. The newly formed 'transformed' lymphocytes (non-cleaved cells, centroblasts) are particularly obvious in the deeper part of the centre (Nossal and Ada, 1971), and are thought to emigrate rapidly from the region of the germinal centres to the area of the medullary cords. Some of these cells are still capable of division (plasmablasts), others show greater evidence of differentiation towards plasma cells, and contain demonstrable immunoglobulin.

(4) *Maturation of plasma cells* occurs within the medullary cords and antibody production is maximal from approximately the eighth day. Mature plasma cells remain within the node, and are found very rarely in the efferent lymph (Hall et al, 1967, 1976, 1977). Transformed lymphocytes (including many potential plasma cells) may, however, be numerous in the medullary sinuses and in efferent lymph (Hay et al, 1972) and mature into plasma cells at other sites. (Diagr. 5, Table 4).

(5) *In the primary response* the reactive (germinal) centres reach maximal development after approximately ten days, following which they gradually regress, unless re-stimulated. At the period of peak development they are found principally in the cortex, but some are also found in the paracortex and medullary cords. This effect may be exaggerated by cross cutting in smaller lymph nodes.

Tingible body macrophages are a feature of vigorously reacting centres. Proliferation of these cells precedes and accompanies lymphoid proliferation. They are distinct from the dendritic reticular cells (antigen trapping), which may be particularly concentrated in a 'cap' on the peripheral aspect of the germinal centre.

In the secondary immune response the primed or conditioned lymphocytes are stimulated. The sequential changes are similar to those described in the primary response, but are much more florid, and occur over a shorter span of time. In the early stages the predominant antibody forming cells are large transformed lymphocytes or immunoblasts, corresponding to the 'large blast cells' observed by Hay et al (1972) in the secondary response to horseradish peroxidase antigen. The follicle thus appears to consist largely of non-cleaved cells (centroblasts). The number of plasma cells developing is much larger, and they may expand the medullary cords to occupy a major part of the lymph node.

Any changes observed in the sinuses reflect the changes in afferent and efferent lymph, the variation in lymphocyte passage across the post-capillary venules, and the products of cellular proliferation within the node (Diagram 5). In the 'resting state' the majority of sinus lymphocytes are re-circulating; only a small proportion of sinus lymphocytes are labelled four hours after the injection of tritiated thymidine (Yoffey et al, 1961). In the reactive state up to sixty per cent of the total body lymphocytes may pass through a single reactive node in less than a week (Hay and Hobbs, 1977).

These aspects are well summarised in Diagram 5 (p. 41), and in the accompanying table of the relative proportions of cell types found in afferent and efferent lymph in the 'resting state', and following immunological stimulation.

The Cellular Immune Responses – T-cells – The Delayed Hypersensitivity Response, the Homograft Reaction

In practical terms the T-cell response is usually accompanied by a response of the B-cell series, which varies in degree but may be quite prominent in a 'homograft reaction'. However, B-cell stimulation is minimal in some of the experimental delayed hypersensitivity reactions where an almost pure T-cell response may be observed. For example, Turk (1967) induced a delayed type hypersensitivity response in the auricular node of the guinea pig by application of oxazolone.

The sequence of events described by Turk provides the dynamic basis of the following description, which has, however, been modified and expanded from other sources (Keuning, 1965), and integrated with the observations made by the authors, in studies of lymphoid reactions and lymphomas of the mouse.
The sequence of events may be summarised as follows:

(1) *Mobilisation phase*, in which lymphocytes leave the circulation to enter the lymph node, analogous to the B-cell response.

(2) *Appearance of transformed lymphocytes* (immunoblasts) within the para-cortex (deep cortical, or thymus dependent areas, Parrott et al, 1966). These cells actively synthesise DNA and label rapidly with tritiated thymidine. At two days the transformed lymphocytes are numerous, but do not appear to be associated with the primary follicles, or the few secondary follicles which are present. The proliferating cells appear to be of thymic origin (Davies et al, 1969), and in the mouse are immunoglobulin negative by immunoperoxidase methods.

(3) *The paracortical area is expanded* by the extensive proliferation of these cells and may develop a nodular or follicular appearance, constituting the tertiary follicles, or paracortical nodules, of other authors (Nossal and Ada, 1971).

(4) *The cortex and medulla are thereby reduced in extent*. In extreme hyperplasia of the paracortex, the proliferating cells appear to overrun the cortex, and the primary follicles become indistinct. The vigorously reacting lymph node of

glandular fever, in which the architecture may be entirely obscured, is probably an example of this phenomenon.

(5) *After six days the number of transformed lymphocytes falls*, and the predominant cell is again the small lymphocyte. However, the majority of these small lymphocytes are labelled by tritiated thymidine injected twenty-four hours earlier, indicating that they are, in all probability, the progeny of the proliferating transformed cells (maturing, primed, conditioned, or sensitised T-cells).

(6) *At about the same time some germinal centre activity may be seen*, and a few plasma cells appear in the medullary cords.

Homograft Reaction

The homograft reaction as described by Porter (1956); André et al (1962;) Billingham et al (1962); André-Schwartz (1964); and Davies et al (1969), also shows the features of the T-cell response as detailed above, but there is in addition an overlying B-cell reaction. Also, more florid responses have been described where the 'nodes showed many areas in which the normal architecture was replaced by a structureless mass of lymphocytic cells' (André et al, 1962). In these examples there was 'a marked increase in the number of primitive reticulum cells, which were seen in all areas of the lymph nodes', (germinal centres and medullary cords were particularly mentioned). The 'haemocytoblasts' and 'primitive reticulum cells' described by André appear to correspond to transformed lymphocytes (T-cell series, T-immunoblasts, see Diagram 3 p. 22), but include some cells with evidence of differentiation towards plasma cells (B-cell series, B-immunoblasts, immunoglobulin positive by immunoperoxidase methods).

In the secondary immune response these changes occur more rapidly, and B-cell responses particularly may be enhanced, with many plasma cells appearing in the medullary cords. In prolonged cellular hypersensitivity reactions features of a histiocytic response may become prominent.

Histiocytic Responses

Lymphocyte reactions are probably dependent upon macrophage processing of antigen (Nossal and Ada, 1971), and equally some of the primarily histiocytic responses occur in relation to lymphocyte activity (lymphokine production, Granger, 1972). Thus, the two types of response do not occur in isolation, but are concurrent, producing a composite lymph node reaction. In some circumstances the histiocyte response is dominant, and in others there is less evidence of histiocytic activity, and a predominantly lymphocytic response.

Histiocyte (macrophage) responses may be divided into two broad groups: those following phagocytosis of non-antigenic inert material, those following phagocytosis of antigenic material.

(1) *Phagocytosis of exogenous or endogenous materials* may be followed by complete degradation of the material, and minimal histological change. Alternatively, phagocytosed inert material may resist metabolism and so accumulate within the phagocytic cells of the reticulo-endothelial system (carbon, haemosiderin, lipoid material in foam cells). As a result there may be some hyperplasia of these elements leading to sinus histiocytosis.

In some circumstances the ingested material appears to induce giant cell formation, together with a transition in histiocyte morphology to form epithelioid cells (Lewis, 1925; Spector, 1969; Spector and Heesom, 1969; Papadimitriou and Wee, 1976). There is evidence that chronic inflammation, with lymphocyte infiltration and possibly fibrosis, occurs when the phagocytosed material is resistant to metabolic degradation, and also 'toxic' (e.g. beryllium, silica, lipoid materials). Similar morphological changes may also follow ingestion of antigenic material.

(2) *The histiocytic reactions following encounter with antigenic material* are complex and intimately involve the lymphatic system, including the production of 'opsonizing' antibody (Griffin et al, 1976).

The results of lymphocyte activity have a profound effect upon histiocytic behaviour and morphology, which is mediated to some extent by the 'lymphokines' which are released by transformed lymphocytes, and include factors effecting histiocyte function (e.g. macrophage inhibitory and activating factors p. 30). Thus, the histiocytes of previously sensitised animals are more actively phagocytic for a wide variety of organisms, and also display an enhanced bacteriocidal effect (Mackaness, 1968). Such histiocytes have been shown to possess changes in metabolism and morphology (Mackaness, 1964; Blanden, 1969), but these are not evident in histological sections. Identical histiocyte 'activation' has been observed during graft-versus-host reactions (Blanden, 1969). The cells of the histiocytic series are also particularly involved in delayed hypersensitivity reactions (Coombs Type IV hypersensitivity), as exemplified by the tuberculin reaction. The cellular infiltrate of delayed hypersensitivity (Mackaness, 1970) is similar to that occurring at the site of graft rejection, and the principal histiocytic cells appear to be derived from monocytes of bone marrow origin (Volkmann and Gowans, 1965; Volkmann, 1966; Spector and Ryan, 1970).

Granuloma formation is of particular interest, and occurs in many experimental and natural situations other than the classical tuberculin and sarcoid reactions; even hypersensitivity to sulphonamides (More et al, 1946). Glynn (1968) reported that sensitisation of rats to 'soluble protein' can convert an acute inflammatory response to a granuloma, and Spector and Ryan (1970) wrote that interference with the immune response can actually reduce granuloma formation, thus suggesting some role for the immune mechanisms in the pathogenesis of granuloma.

The role of immune complexes in granuloma formation has been extensively studied in animal models (Unanue and Dixon, 1967; Spector 1969). The proportion of antigen and antibody may be important. Complexes formed at antigen excess seem to produce an acute inflammatory reaction, while those at slight antibody excess are larger and are phagocytosed by the reticulo-endothelial cells. The antigen-antibody complexes may then be degraded (Sorkin and Boyden, 1959), though this does not always occur and may be incomplete, (especially at antibody excess, Spector, 1969). This interaction with immune complexes is believed to induce granuloma formation, with transition of histiocytes to epithelioid cells and giant cells. The process becomes chronic when the histiocytes prove incapable of metabolising the phagocytosed immune complex (Spector, 1969; Papadimitriou and Wee, 1976).

The precise stimulus to granuloma formation remains unclear, and certainly the mechanisms have not been elucidated in man.

However, granuloma formation is known to occur in the reaction to certain infective agents such as mycobacteria, brucella, fungi, toxoplasma and histoplasma; it is also seen on occasions in lymphoid tissue in Hodgkin's disease, regional ileitis, sarcoidosis and secondary neoplasms. These granulomatous reactions will be discussed in later chapters and there is an excellent review edited by Dhom (1980).

It must be appreciated that long before immunologists recognized that various areas in the lymph node were functionally distinct, and were related to different populations of lymphocytes, it had become apparent, by studying human lymph nodes in health and disease, that it was possible to identify three main zones of lymph node reactivity – follicles, equivalent to the modern humoral or B-cell response; medullary, equivalent to the paracortical, cellular or T-cell response; and the sinus reaction which was equivalent to the histiocytic response. Furthermore, in conformity with the modern concept of 'homing' (ecotaxis), it was shown that if there was a cellular reaction in one of these three zones, an analogous response would occur in the homologous area in other lymphoreticular organs (Robb-Smith, 1938, 1974).

The rest of this book will attempt to analyse lymph node histopathology on the basis of these concepts, whether derived from a pragmatic approach or the translocation of experimental observations.

4. Examination of a Lymph Node Biopsy – General Principles

Ideally the preliminary examination and diagnosis of any lymph node biopsy should be made without foreknowledge of the clinical history, thus avoiding any subliminal bias. Following the initial examination and preliminary diagnosis, or differential diagnosis, based upon histological features alone, the full clinical history should be studied, correlated with the histological findings, and confirmed by re-examination of the biopsy.

The first stage in histological examination of a lymph node should be a low power survey of the haematoxylin and eosin preparation in order to establish whether any lesion is present in localized or generalized form, and also to determine to what extent there is maintenance or loss of normal architectural features.

It is well worthwhile examining the section with the naked eye or a hand lens; for example it may then be possible to discern a pseudofollicular pattern which may not otherwise be apparent with the low power objective, and the relationship of the lymph node to any periadenoidal infiltrate may also be more clearly seen.

The capsule and pericapsular areas should be examined to determine whether there is fibrosis, and whether there is any extra-capsular proliferation of cells. The presence of fibrous spurs and bands extending in from the capsule are of particular significance in considering a diagnosis of nodular sclerosing Hodgkin's disease.

Next the presence or absence of follicular structures should be determined. If follicles are present they should be closely examined and their nature defined. Are they normally situated within the node, and are they composed of the various cell types found in normal follicles? Do they represent normal primary follicles, or secondary follicles with reactive centres, or nodular collections of abnormal cells having a 'pseudo-follicular' appearance? If characteristic reactive follicles are present are they abnormally large with features of severe reaction, or is there evidence of 'regressive' change or hyalinisation? Do the follicles have a normal relation to the surrounding cortical lymphocytes, and is there evidence of normal maturation of the products of follicular reaction (transformed lymphocytes) in the underlying paracortex or medullary cords?

The relative extent of cortex and paracortex and medulla should be determined, since precise delimitation of the cortical/paracortical junction is not possible in man. The cell types present in the cortex and paracortex should be noted, with particular reference to any increase in the proportion of transformed lymphocytes, plasma cells, histiocytes and acute inflammatory cells, or any abnormal predominance of one particular cell type, which might signify leukaemic infiltration or lymphomatous change. The post-capillary venules should be examined for evidence of endothelial swelling, lymphocyte emigration across the endothelium into the substance of the node, and inflammatory cell exudate.

Finally, the sinus system should be examined, with particular note of the types of cells contained within marginal and medullary sinuses. The presence of any abnormal cell types should be considered, for secondary neoplasms often appear first within the region of the marginal sinuses.

In making these assessments, use of the low power objective should be supplemented by detailed examination of cell types at higher magnification, including the use of oil immersion objective in some cases. Individual cell types should be identified according to the criteria given earlier, wherever this is possible, and any abnormalities of nuclear or cytoplasmic structure should be noted. It is unfortunate that some of the criteria generally in use for assessing malignancy, such as the frequency of mitoses and variation in cytoplasmic and nuclear morphology, are of limited value in examining lymphoid tissues, for mitoses are numerous in reactive nodes and the process of normal lymphocyte transformation involves radical morphological changes which may cause confusion with the pleomorphism of malignant neoplasia.

A provisional diagnosis may be reached as a result of the low power survey and categorisation of cell types. Armed with the provisional diagnosis, or possibly a number of differential diagnoses, the node should then be re-examined minutely for confirmatory diagnostic features. It is at this point that the pathologist should study and take heed of all the clinical features of the case, and especially of the peripheral blood picture, serum immunoglobulins, and any history of medication, vaccination or previous disease state.

The pattern of this book is designed to correspond to this approach – an initial low power survey coupled with a closer examination of cell types suggesting one or more provisional diagnoses – these diagnoses are then confirmed or refuted by reference to the histological features, and pertinent clinical details, of each suspect condition encountered during the preliminary assessment, and the lymph node is re-examined with particular attention to the fine histological criteria for differential diagnosis.

From the viewpoint of descriptive histology, it is much simpler, having adopted a particular classification, to enunciate the main features by which the various lymphadenopathies can be recognised, but this pre-supposes that the diagnosis has already been made, or else requires that the clinical histologist look at description after description until one is found that appears to match the node under examination. Following the notable seminar (Gall and Rappaport, 1958) on 'Diseases of Lymph Nodes and Spleen', held in New Orleans in 1958, Edward Gall (1964) wrote an essay 'The Enlarged Lymph Node: Differential Diagnosis'. More recently Butler (1969) and Dorfman and Warnke (1974) have also approached this problem, but in each case the assumption has been made that with the aid of some histological litmus paper or philosopher's stone, the diagnostic pathologist has been able to determine whether or not the node is affected by a 'malignant lymphoma', and if it is not so affected then an analysis can proceed to determine what type of lymphadenopathy is causing the lymph node enlargement. It is certainly true that it is of paramount importance to the patient and the physician to determine whether the illness is a manifestation of a malignant or a progressive lymphadenopathy or a more benign condition, yet this decision can be achieved only by experience and deductive reasoning. In some cases there is no difficulty; the microscope reveals at once that it is a sarcomatous or granulomatous lymph node disorder, but more commonly the initial examination may leave one in doubt and it is then necessary to assemble the various pieces of evidence, histological, haematological and clinical, before a considered opinion can be achieved. Naturally one hopes to recognise a condition of good prognosis, but it is difficult to know whether it is worse to diagnose a serious condition when it does not exist, exposing a young healthy individual to grave emotional

49

distress and to the very real hazards of modern oncotherapy, than to fail to make the correct diagnosis and so reduce the prospects of effective therapy. What is certain is that if the biopsy material does not allow a definite diagnosis, the pathologist should set this out quite clearly, recommending either a further biopsy forthwith, or, after a short period of careful clinical and haematological supervision.

Nevertheless the papers of Gall, Butler, and Dorfman and Warnke did give indications as to the features by which the reactive lymphadenopathies could be diagnosed, while Symmers (1978), consequent on his remarkable experience in this field, has provided a superb account of the whole range of infective lymphadenitis. A different approach was adopted by Cottier, Turk and Sobin (1972) in their proposal for a standardized system of reporting human lymph node morphology. These authors suggested that it would be possible, using an extremely complex protocol, to set down the changes observed in a lymph node in terms of immunological status. The cellular and topographical terminology they propose is gratifyingly simple and they rightly deplore the use of diagnostic terms such as 'lymph node hyperplasia' or 'non-specific lymphadenitis', but unhappily they restrict their abnormal lymph nodes to leprosy and the primary immune deficiency states, neither of which are likely to cause difficulty to the hospital pathologist, while their schema is too intricate and time consuming for general use.

In this book an attempt will be made to display the deductive analysis by which the diagnosis of a lymph node disorder may be achieved, following the principles set out a good number of years ago (Robb-Smith, 1947). In a normal lymph node the follicles are the structural units most easily recognized and so it is on their presence or absence that the initial analysis will be based. Subsequent chapters will discuss the significance of 'false follicles', sinus or paracortical proliferation. In this way it is hoped to render the diagnosis of lymph node disorders less complex than they are usually held to be.

CHAPTER II

The normal architecture of the node is maintained to a large extent, but with abnormal cellular proliferation in the paracortical region, while true follicles are present

ANALYTICAL
SUMMARY

1. **The follicles are large, with reactive centres**
   a) Nonspecific reactive hyperplasia: *immunodeficiencies; primary lymphadenopathies; metastases*
   b) Acute lymphadenitis
   c) Chronic lymphadenitis: *giant lymph node hyperplasia*
   d) Reactive hyperplasia associated with specific conditions: *rheumatoid arthritis; disseminate lupus erythematosus; Sjögren's Syndrome*

2. **Reactive follicles with clusters of epithelioid histiocytes:**

   Toxoplasmosis; leishmaniasis; syphilis; brucellosis; sarcoidosis; tuberculosis

3. **Reactive follicles with additional characteristic paracortical changes:**

   Vaccinia; herpes zoster; measles; infectious mononucleosis; T-zone lymphoma; dermatopathic lymphadenopathy; steatorrhoea lymphadenopathy

4. **Reactive follicles with focal necrosis or with granulomata**
   a) Necrotic foci: *salmonellosis; mesenteric adenitis; filariasis; eosinophilic granuloma; disseminated lupus erythematosus; cat scratch disease*
   b) Caseous foci: *tuberculosis; chronic granulomatous disease; coccidioidomycosis; histoplasmosis; brucellosis; rheumatoid arthritis*
   c) Focal giant cell granulomata with fibrosis: *foreign body granuloma; sarcoid reaction*
   d) Diffuse giant cell granulomata: *Hodgkin's disease; sarcoidosis; berylliosis; leprosy*
   e) Lymph node reactions in the lipidoses: *Gaucher's disease etc.*

5. **Normal follicles, with non-malignant epithelial inclusions in paracortex**

6. **Normal follicles and paracortex with vascular lesions:**

   polyarteritis nodosa etc.

THIS CHAPTER deals with lymph nodes, which may be enlarged, but on microscopical examination reveal that the normal anatomical features – follicles, sinuses, paracortical tissue, medulla – discussed in the first chapter, can be recognized. There may in addition be an infiltration of abnormal cells, often in the paracortical region. The majority of the lymphadenopathies that present these features are reactive, but as will be revealed later, such an appearance can also be found in the early stages of lymphoproliferative and malignant conditions.

In making a histological analysis of a lymph node, it is desirable to start by looking for the most obvious and striking feature in the normal node, namely the follicle; next it is necessary, if nodular collections of cells are present, to satisfy oneself as to their nature. If there are obvious nodular collections of cells, it is essential to know whether these are true follicles, as found normally in lymph nodes, or 'false' follicles formed of collections of cells arranged in a focal or circumscribed manner. (These are dealt with in chapter III):

Figs. I.2; I.3 If the low power survey reveals that the follicular structure have the architectural and cytological features of primary or secondary (reactive or germinal) follicles as described in chapter I, (pp. 35–8) then the analysis will proceed in the logical manner of a decision tree which may be summarized as follows:–

The nodular structures are true follicles and may be:

Reactive follicles

Reactive follicles together with epithelioid congeries

Reactive follicles with additional characteristic paracortical changes

Reactive follicles with focal areas of necrosis and/or histocytic granulomata in the paracortex

Normal follicles with non malignant epithelial inclusions in the paracortex

Normal follicles and paracortex with vascular lesions

1. The follicles are large and show reactive or germinal centres

The occurrence of follicular hyperplasia indicates a humoral (B-cell) response by analogy with animal models. The degree of hyperplasia may vary according to the intensity of the response, its duration, and the presence or absence of any associated paracortical (T-cell) or histiocytic responses, which may to some degree obscure the classical features of the humoral reaction. Thus, the occurrence of follicular hyperplasia in association with granulomata is not uncommon and varying degrees of follicular reaction may also be seen in association with sinus hyperplasia, and in responses which are believed to be predominantly of T-cell type. In man, B- and T-cell responses are not clearly separable, and pure B- or T- responses probably do not occur naturally, though some reactive conditions do show a marked predominance of B- or T-cell reaction.

1a. *General consideration of reactive hyperplasia*

Of the reactive hyperplasias, many have no characteristic features other than non-specific follicular hyperplasia, with paracortical reactions, swelling of the endothelium of post-capillary venules, and sinus catarrh. However, some conditions do display certain additional features which may allow the histologist to reach a diagnosis of a specific condition with some certainty. Those features of value in this respect are described and illustrated in the following pages.

The secondary follicles contain prominent reactive centres which are characterized by a predominance of large basophilic transformed type lymphocytes (non-cleaved cells or centroblasts), often in mitosis, and many tingible body macrophages with nuclear debris. The small lymphocyte cuff is usually well defined, and transformed cells and differentiating plasma cells can be seen around the secondary follicles, particularly upon their deep aspect, where these cell types extend into the medullary cords. The majority of follicles are within the peripheral cortex, but some appear at deeper levels within the node, even in the absence of cross cutting. Reactive secondary follicles are usually approximately spherical, but in acute florid reactions they may assume irregular shapes and lose the otherwise characteristic distinct lymphocyte cuff. Such reactive centres are possibly newly derived, and consist almost entirely of transformed type lymphocytes, with few of the 'cleaved' forms. 'Cleaved' cells are more prominent in reactive centres of nodes showing lesser degrees of reactivity, and in regressing or resting centres. Reactive follicles also show a quite characteristic circumferential arrangement of reticulin, and there is little apparent compression of the interfollicular lymphoid tissue.

The paracortex is often inconspicuous, and plasma cells do not ordinarily accumulate in the medullary cords. The sinus contents vary according to the phase of reaction, and there may be some 'sinus catarrh' – accumulation of histiocytes, macrophages, small and transformed lymphocytes, within the sinuses.

Reactive Hyperplasia is not a diagnosis, but rather a description of a tissue reaction, and its significance must be related to the age of the patient, the situation of the node, and the clinical condition. In children and young adults a moderate degree of reactive hyperplasia in cervical or mesenteric nodes can virtually be regarded as physiological, while the absence of this change, particularly in a patient with recurrent infections or pyrexial reactions, might raise the possibility of immunological impairment.

It is unlikely that a pathologist would be confident enough to make a diagnosis of immunodeficiency solely on the basis of a lymph node biopsy, but it could be that the morphological changes in the node in association with the clinical and family histories and the pattern of immunoglobulins would enable the particular disturbance of immune mechanism to be identified, so determining consequent treatment and prognosis (Fudenberg et al, 1971).

In the *immunodeficiencies*, there may or may not be preservation of the follicles, *Immuno-deficiencies* but there is invariably a paracortical deficiency of lymphoid cells; the former type will be discussed here, the latter in chapter V (p. 146).

In the first type, although the follicles are preserved and plasma cells are present, yet there is a deficiency of the follicular rim of lymphocytes while the lymphocytes in the paracortical zone are absent or greatly diminished; this is the reaction found in the Di George and Nezelof syndromes, in hereditary ataxia telangiectasia and in the familial lymphopenic thymic dysplasia with dysgamma-globulinaemia. In the Wiskott-Aldrich syndrome, the changes in the lymph nodes vary according to the age of the child, but in adolescents there may also be follicular preservation with deficiency of the paracortical lymphoid tissue (Bergsma, 1968).

The more usual problem that faces the pathologist is how one should determine what can be regarded as a 'moderate degree of reactive hyperplasia' which of course is a subjective impression based on experience. In a child a cervical lymph node up to 1cm in diameter, showing reactive hyperplasia, in which the germinal centres are less than 500 μm (approximately one high power field) in diameter, would not ordinarily be regarded as sinister; on the other hand large (2cm or more in diameter) fleshy, apparently hyperplastic nodes in the inguinal region of an adult warrant a careful investigation, even though the humoral response may simply be the consequence of inadequate pedal hygiene.

Before accepting that a node shows simple reactive hyperplasia, a careful survey should be made for any features which might suggest a more specific diagnosis.

A further point of cardinal importance is the realisation that a diagnosis of non-specific hyperplasia does not in any way exclude the presence of lymphoma in an adjacent lymph node, as was clearly shown by the block dissection studies of Slaughter et al (1958). In addition, a lymph node apparently showing an uncomplicated non-specific reactive hyperplasia may contain within it focal deposits of a *primary lymphadenopathy* such as Hodgkin's disease, or of carcinoma.

Primary lymphadenopathies; metastases Initial deposits of *carcinoma* are characteristically found within the marginal or cortical sinuses, while focal early Hodgkin's disease characteristically involves the deep cortex or paracortex. The problems in recognizing partial involvement of nodes in acute lymphoblastic leukaemias and kindred conditions is discussed in chapter V. Such focal involvement may be very difficult to detect, but should be considered wherever atypical transformed type cells are present locally within a node, rather than distributed diffusely throughout it, as occurs in phenytoin or post-vaccinial lymphadenopathy. Local concentrations of eosinophils, or condensations of reticulin (in silver preparations), or fibrosis, may also be valuable in alerting one to a possible diagnosis of focal Hodgkin's disease.

Some of the conditions in which there may be reactive hyperplasia with additional 'specific' features will be described in subsequent sections, but it is convenient first to consider the changes that may be characterised as acute and chronic lymphadenitis.

1b. Acute Lymphadenitis

Acute lymphadenitis designates an acute inflammatory response in a lymph node, normally associated with reactive changes in the follicles. The prominent feature is a dilatation of the sinuses, which are filled with neutrophils, histiocytes and a moderate admixture of red cells; in addition, there are often macrophages which have ingested red cells or neutrophils. The paracortical tissue is oedematous, and may contain collections of granulocytes, areas of fibrinous exudate, and occasionally small foci of necrosis. The post-capillary venules are prominent and also contain neutrophils. Variable numbers of transformed lymphocytes (immunoblasts) are present, and maturing plasma cells may be seen in the medullary area. The medulla and medullary sinuses show oedema and cellular infiltration similar to that observed in cortex and paracortex, but these changes are often more obvious, due to the looseness of the connective tissue in the medullary region. The inflammatory reaction may extend beyond the lymph node to involve the capsule and periadenoidal tissue.

1c. *Chronic Lymphadenitis*

Chronic lymphadenitis is a diagnosis which should be made with reserve, as in the past it was all too frequently a screen to conceal the pathologist's uncertainty as to the nature of the cellular proliferation present.

True chronic lymphadenitis does exist, and is to be seen in nodes draining areas of low grade persistent infection. It is characterised by a reactive hyperplasia in which the germinal centres are prominent, but not unduly large; tingible body macrophages are inconspicuous and there may be some degree of hyalinisation, particularly around capillaries. Large numbers of plasma cells may be present, and clumps of ill-defined multinucleate cells, some of which are clearly histiocytes, also occur. In the initial stages the paracortex may appear mottled due to the presence of many transformed lymphocytes, some of which contain immunoglobulin and are B-cells en route to the medulla, while others are presumptive T-cells and do not contain demonstrable immunoglobulin.

The sinuses may also show some hyalinisation, but the striking feature is the expansion of the medullary cords which are rich in plasma cells and plasmablasts. In later stages degrees of fibrosis are common, and a reticulin preparation will reveal increased fibre formation in the paracortex, as well as in the follicles and in the periadenoid tissue. However, in chronic lymphadenitis the basic structural pattern of the node is maintained in the residual cellular areas. When dense bands of collagen occur throughout the node the remaining cellular tissue should be examined critically for evidence of Hodgkin's disease, particularly of the nodular sclerosing type.

Many of the features of acute and chronic lymphadenitis may occur simultaneously in association with certain infective processes, such as yersiniosis (p. 77).

A particular variety of chronic lymphadenitis is the condition often known as the *plasma cell type of giant lymph node hyperplasia* (or follicular lymphoreticuloma etc., Keller et al, 1972). In essence, there is a large mass (10cm or more in diameter) of lymphoid tissue, most commonly in the mediastinum, but occasionally elsewhere, which on histological examination reveals a reactive hyperplasia with follicles scattered throughout, and large numbers of plasma cells

Giant lymph node hyperplasia

55

in the paracortical and medullary areas. This type of mediastinal lymphoid hyperplasia is often associated with chronic pyrexia, anaemia and hyperglobulin-aemia. Its relationship to the 'hyaline vascular' type of lymphoid hyperplasia, also termed lymph node hamartoma (p. 100), is unclear.

1d. *Reactive Hyperplasia associated with specific conditions*

Returning to the reactive hyperplasia proper, a generalised lymphadenopathy, often associated with splenomegally, in which the lymph nodes show many large secondary follicles distributed throughout the cortex, and sometimes within the *Rheumatoid* paracortex and medulla, is suggestive of a diagnosis of *rheumatoid arthritis*, *arthritis* including the Still-Felty syndrome.

Up to 75% of adults with rheumatoid arthritis may show clinical lymphade-*Fig. II.2* nopathy, and in such cases the enlarged lymph nodes reveal the presence of many secondary follicles distributed in the cortex, or throughout the node. The reactive centres are large (sometimes as much as 0.5mm in diameter) and irregular in size and shape. They contain many basophilic transformed type lymphocytes, together with much nuclear debris and many tingible body macrophages, which impart a classical 'starry sky' appearance to the follicle when examined at low magnification. The paracortex and medulla are reduced in area and may contain numerous plasma cells, often with prominent Russell body formation. A further feature is the presence of a general reactive response with swelling of the endothelium of post-capillary venules. In long standing disease some follicles may show regressive features and contain deposits of hyaline material resembling amyloid in haematoxylin-eosin preparations. However, amyloid stains are usually negative, though true amyloid may occur in rheumatoid arthritis.

It should be recognised that a generalised lymphadenopathy, showing reactive follicular hyperplasia, and associated with polyarthritis, may also occur in *dis-*
Disseminated lupus *erythematosus* *seminated lupus erythematosus* or *Sjögren's syndrome*, though a minority of *Sjögren's syndrome* patients suffering from these disorders may show other histological features to be described later (pp. 80, 216). A proportion of patients with the Still-Felty syndrome may present with generalised lymphadenopathy and splenomegally, before there is any evidence of arthritis, and in such cases the gross degree of *Fig. II.1* reactive hyperplasia is a valuable aid to diagnosis.

The most important differential diagnosis of reactive hyperplasia is follicular lymphoma which is described in detail in chapter III (p. 101). It is convenient to present at this point the morphological features distinguishing follicular lym-*Differentiation from* phoma from a reactive hyperplasia, such as that seen in rheumatoid arthritis *follicular lymphoma* (Table 5, opposite).

Fig. II.2 Provided the biopsy material is well prepared and the pathologist appreciates the importance of familiarity with the normal architecture of the lymph node and its range of variability, there should rarely be any risk of diagnosing a reactive hyperplasia as a follicular lymphoma. However, the converse is more difficult,

Table 5

Differential Diagnosis of Follicular Hyperplasia and Follicular Lymphoma

FOLLICULAR HYPERPLASIA – NON-SPECIFIC e.g. rheumatoid arthritis	FOLLICULAR LYMPHOMA
Follicles predominantly in cortex but may be distributed throughout the node as in rheumatoid arthritis.	Follicles throughout node.
Variation in size and shape of follicles is usual (Fig. II.2a).	Follicles relatively uniform in size and shape (Fig. II.3a).
Normal population of cells within follicles, including different morphological forms of the transformed lymphocyte (cleaved or non-cleaved cells) and tingible body macrophages, producing 'starry sky' appearance.	Follicles composed of relatively more uniform cell type (cleaved or non-cleaved), corresponding to the neoplastic cell line. Absence of macrophages.
Follicles show 'polarity' with transformed lymphocytes concentrated upon the deep aspect of the centre.	There is loss of polarity.
Products of follicular reaction (transformed lymphocytes and differentiating plasma cells) are seen outside the follicles. Plasma cells may be numerous in interfollicular areas and often contain Russell bodies.	Occasional transformed lymphocytes present within and without follicles, but plasma cells few in number.
Frequent normal mitoses in follicles.	Mitoses relatively uncommon in follicles, but may be seen in inter-follicular area in equal numbers.
Sharp distinction between types of cells in follicles and the cells found in interfollicular area (i.e. cleaved and non-cleaved cell types are confined to the follicles). Follicles are also clearly delineated with a cuff of small lymphocytes. Cracking artefact rare.	Little cytological distinction between follicular cells and cells of the interfollicular area (i.e. cleaved and non-cleaved cell types may be seen in intrafollicular areas) Follicle margins ill-defined and lymphocyte cuff absent. Cracking artefact common.
Other associated reactive features may be present including swelling of post capillary venules and neutrophils within sinuses.	Absence of associated inflammatory featutes.
Reticulin pattern shows lack of compression of reticulin and intact or dilated sinuses. (Fig. II.2b).	Reticulin preparation shows compression and collapse of sinused (Fig. II.3b).
Florid follicular hyperplasia may occur at any age, especially in the young, more rarely in the elderly.	Follicular lymphoma is rare before the age of 30. Has a peak incidence at 50+
In both conditions there may be infiltration of the node capsule by small lymphocytes, but the occurrence of follicles in the pericapsular area is uncommon except in follicular lymphoma.	

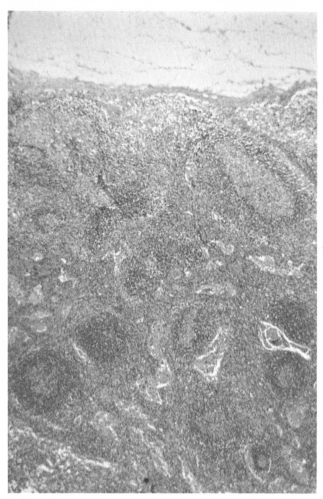

II.1a

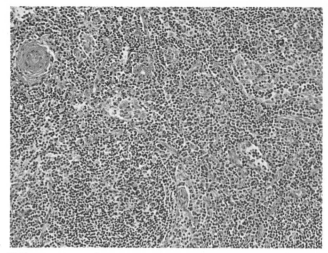

II.1b

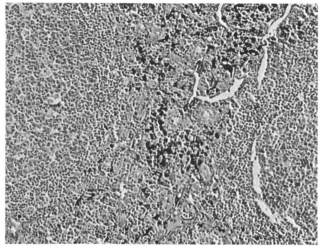

II.1c

II.1a-c Disseminated Lupus Erythematosus

II.1a Early lesion. Moderate reactive hyperplasia with prominent vessels in the paracortex.

II.1b Early lesion. Thickening and fibrinoid change in the arterioles with plasma cell proliferation and small clumps of haematoxyphil material in some of the sinuses. Unless the vascular changes were recognized, it would be difficult even to suggest the possibility of systemic lupus from this biopsy, as the haematoxyphile bodies are inconspicuous and the massive necrosis, which is characteristic, is absent.

II.1c Early Lesion with Reactive Change
Immunoperoxidase reveals many polytypic plasma cells in the paracortex.

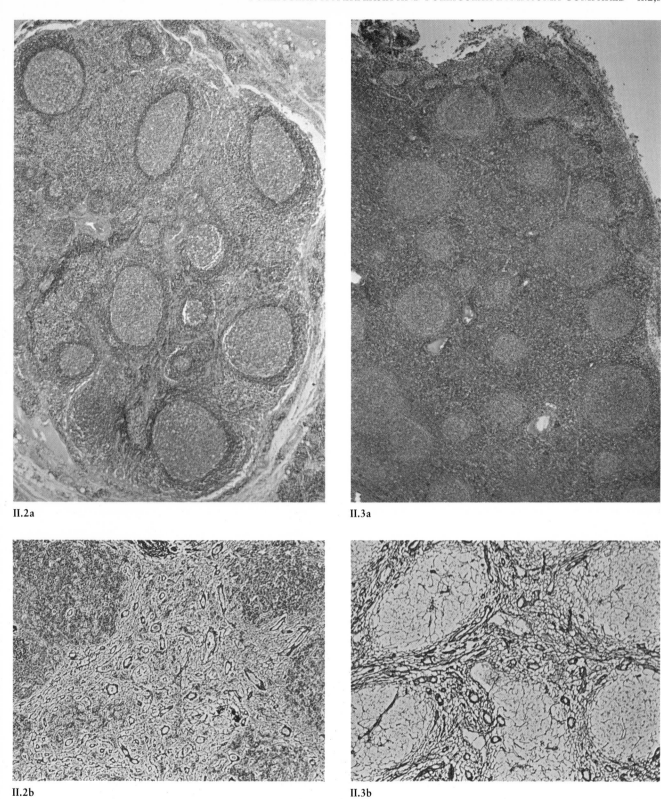

II.2a

II.3a

II.2b

II.3b

II.2a-b   Follicular Hyperplasia

    II.2a Haematoxylin-Eosin

    II.2b Reticulin impregnation.

II.3a-b   Follicular Lymphoma

    II.3a Haematoxylin-Eosin

    II.3b Reticulin impregnation.

and it may not be possible to distinguish an early follicular lymphoma from reactive hyperplasia. It is also true that sometimes, in a case of follicular lymphoma, the follicles near the cortex of the node show reactive features, while obvious neoplastic follicles are present in deeper parts of the node. Again such instances are usually clearly recognisable by following the criteria discussed, provided that the central parts of the lymph node have been adequately fixed. In large lymph nodes irregular fixation may cause follicles to vary markedly in appearance.

2. The follicles are large, reactive features are present, and in addition there are clusters of epithelioid histiocytes.

For many years histopathologists have recognised a characteristic appearance of lymph node reaction formerly designated as 'lympho-histiocytic medullary reticulosis', 'Piringer-Kuchinka lymphadenitis', etc., which is now known to be a pattern of reactive change peculiar to a number of infective agents, of which *Toxoplasmosis* the commonest is *toxoplasmosis*. In essence there is a reactive hyperplasia, in which there are small clusters of epithelioid histiocytes within the follicles and in the paracortical area.

There is usually evidence of follicular hyperplasia with the formation of secondary follicles, having prominent reactive centres. These secondary reactive follicles consist, characteristically, of large basophilic transformed lymphocytes, and tin-*Fig. II.4* gible body macrophages. The follicles are very irregular in size and shape, and whilst largely distributed within the cortex, a small number of newly formed centres may be seen in the deeper area of paracortex. Many transformed lymphocytes may be seen in relation to these reactive centres, and plasma cells are often numerous. However, the characteristic feature is the presence of a marked histiocyte response, manifested by variable numbers of pale pink epithelioid type histiocytes in the secondary follicles, and throughout the paracortex and cortex, occurring either singly or in small clusters of up to twenty cells (so-called 'congeries' of histiocytes). There is no true granuloma formation, no necrosis nor caseation, and giant cells are rarely seen. These are important features in the distinction from tuberculosis and sarcoidosis. In the paracortex there are numerous transformed lymphocytes and histiocytes, and on occasions the sinuses may be distended with similar cells. Often the post-capillary venules are prominent, and there may be evidence of capsular infiltration by lymphocytes and by plasma cells. The cuff of small lymphocytes usually present around the follicles may disappear, and some large irregular shaped follicles may appear to merge with the paracortex (Dorfman et al, 1973).

The sickle shaped toxoplasma has hardly ever been seen in histological sections, and only rarely observed in imprint preparations. Occasionally the cystic form of toxoplasma may be encountered in sections (Stansfeld, 1961). Calderon et al, (1973) have used an immuno-fluorescence technique for identifying the parasite.

It has been suggested that the histological picture may be confused with those forms of Hodgkin's disease associated with a marked histiocytic response, and that a valuable point of distinction is that histiocytes are not found within any persisting reactive centres in Hodgkin's disease (Rappaport, 1966).

In *leishmaniasis* the overall morphological picture is similar to that of toxoplasmosis, with the distinction that numerous Leishman-Donovan bodies may be seen within the epithelioid cells, in haematoxylin-eosin or Giemsa stained preparations. The Leishman-Donovan bodies are haematoxyphil and refractile, and may also be found in small giant cells, which occur more commonly than in toxoplasmosis. *Leishmaniasis*

Fig. II.5

A somewhat similar picture may be seen in *secondary syphilis*, but in this condition the epithelioid congeries are almost invariably restricted to the paracortex, and epithelioid giant cells are more often present. Furthermore, plasma cells are much more numerous in syphilis and zones of coagulative necrosis may occasionally be seen. The post-capillary venules are not unduly prominent but small arterioles in the paracortex may show endarteritis (Hartsock et al, 1970; Turner and Wright, 1973). While this form of reaction is that most commonly found in syphilis, other authors have reported significant follicular hyperplasia (Evans, 1944) or a more diffuse picture with prominent plasmacytosis. *Secondary syphilis*

Fig. II.6

It should be recognized that, although the appearance of reactive hyperplasia with epithelioid congeries is very characteristic, it is usually impossible (except in Leishmania) to make a specific diagnosis on histological grounds. In temperate countries, toxoplasmosis is the most likely aetiological agent to produce this change, and the Sabin-Feldman dye test, or the IgM immunofluorescent antibody test should be performed to confirm the diagnosis. Rarely brucellosis may present a similar appearance, but more commonly there is a coalescence of the epithelioid granulomata with necrosis (p. 85). Syphilis should also not be forgotten, particularly when plasmacytosis is a prominent feature. Finally, there will always be a number of young adults with enlarged, but otherwise symptomless, cervical nodes showing this change, in which a definite aetiological diagnosis cannot be made, while follow-up studies reveal no further illness.

The differential diagnosis, on histological grounds, from Hodgkin's disease with an epithelioid histiocyte component has already been mentioned, but should not, under ordinary circumstances, present any great difficulty, and the same is true for sarcoidosis, though for a different reason. In sarcoidosis (p. 89) the whole paracortex is replaced by rounded epithelioid congeries surrounded by lymphocytes and plasma cells, and the follicles are very small or non-existent. However, early involvement with tuberculosis may cause confusion, as it is usual at this stage for the normal anatomy of the node to be preserved, in addition to which the follicles may show reactive changes. However, in tuberculosis the epithelioid granulomata occur focally within the paracortex, whereas in toxoplasmosis, and related conditions, they are distributed diffusely throughout the node, including the follicles. Additional features favouring the diagnosis of *Differential diagnosis of toxoplasmosis*

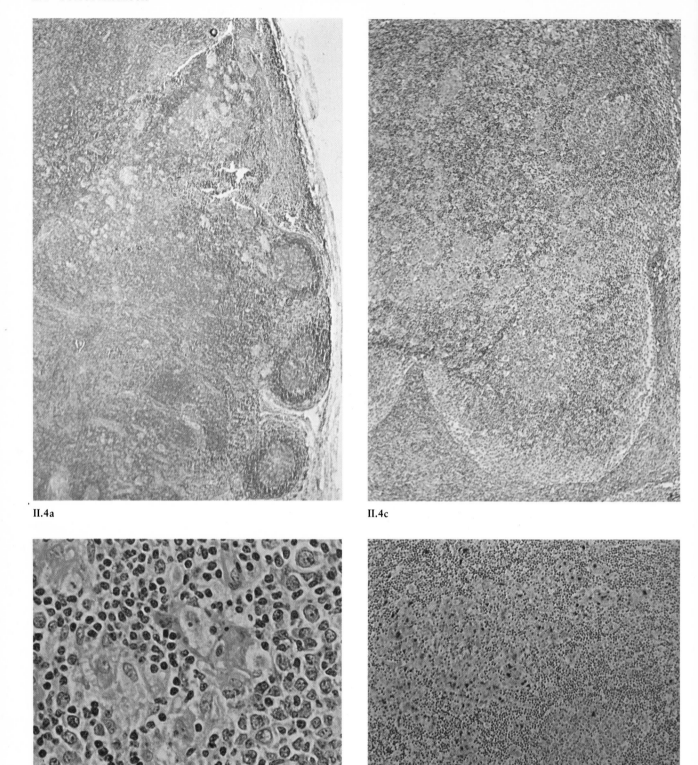

II.4a

II.4c

II.4b

II.4d

II.4a–d Toxoplasmosis

II.4a Reactive hyperplasia with pale foci of epithelioid cells both in the follicles and the paracortex.

II.4b Collections of epithelioid histiocytes with transformed lymphocytes and plasma cells.

II.4c The follicles are not so obvious but the epithelioid congeries in the loose paracortex are very clear.

II.4d Preparation stained by immunoperoxidase method for lysozyme (muramidase), showing positive reaction (brown) in the epithelioid histiocytes.

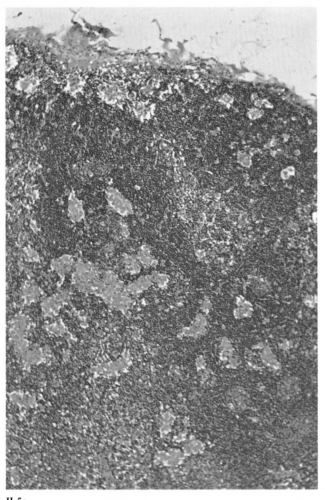

II.5a

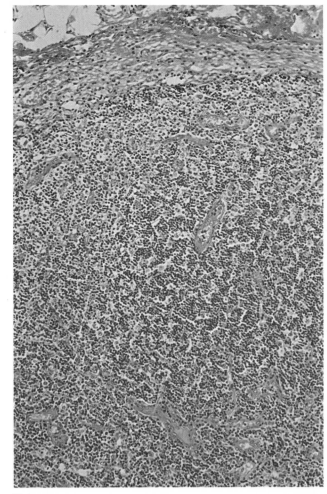

II.6a

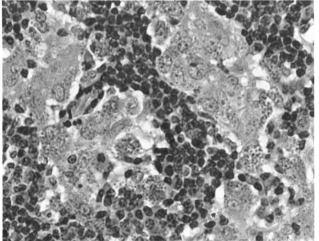

II.5b

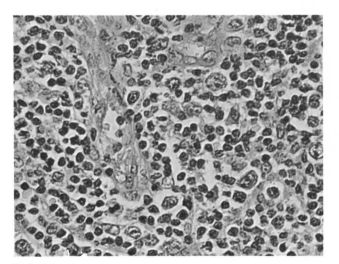

II.6b

II.5a-b   Leishmaniasis

II.5a   Epithelioid aggregates scattered throughout the follicles and the paracortex.

II.5b   Leishman-Donovan bodies clearly shown in the epithelioid histiocytes.

II.6a-b   Syphilitic Lymphadenitis

II.6a   Syphilitic Lymphadenitis. The follicles are inconspicuous but there is a marked paracortical cellular proliferation; postcapillary venules are prominent and thickened while there is considerable capsular thickening.

II.6b   The cellular proliferation consists of transformed lymphocytes, plasma cells and plasma cell precursors.

tuberculosis are the occurrence of significant numbers of giant cells, evidence of early caseous change, and coalescence of granulomata (see p. 81).

3. Reactive Follicles are prominent, together with additional characteristic paracortical changes

It is not unusual to encounter a lymph node in which there are reactive follicles, but between the follicles, there is a diffuse and striking paracortical cellular proliferation of varying character. These are an important group from a diagnostic aspect, for not only do they include reactive conditions, but nodes partially involved by progressive hyperplasias or malignant lymphomata may present a very similar appearance with consequent difficulties in interpretation.

Viral lymphadenitis   A particular form of reactive lymphadenopathy has been designated *viral lymphadenitis*, and though it is not usually possible to make a specific aetiological diagnosis, the appearances should be easily recognisable. In essence, reactive follicles are present but the striking change is in the paracortical area, where there is marked proliferation of transformed lymphocytes with numerous cells in mitosis, together with some histiocytes, and prominence of post-capillary venules, resulting in an overall mottled appearance.

Most commonly the follicles are clearly demarcated, but are not as large (up to 300 μm in diameter) as in a reaction to bacterial infection, and are more widely separate. Also, their margins may be blurred and encroached on by the *Fig. II.7* diffuse paracortical proliferation. This effect is enhanced by a variable degree of oedema and by the presence of some intercellular proteinaceous exudate. The paracortical cell population consists of lymphocytes of small and medium size with regular clumped nuclei, together with numerous larger transformed type cells with marked cytoplasmic basophilia and pyroninophilia, termed reticular lymphoblasts by Hartsock (1968). Only occasional cells show morphological evidence of plasmacytoid differentiation, and this is confirmed by the small proportion of cells containing immunoglobulin demonstrable by immunoperoxidase methods. There is often a high mitotic rate throughout the node, and the large vesicular nucleus, distinct nuclear membrane and prominent nucleolus of the transformed lymphoid cell has some resemblance to a mononuclear Hodgkin cell, which may lead to an erroneous diagnosis of Hodgkin's disease. Also there are moderate number of neutrophils and, on occasions, eosinophils and histiocytes may be seen scattered throughout the substance of the node. However, genuine tissue destruction with fibrosis does not occur. The post-capillary venules are prominent with marked endothelial swelling, indeed the lumen may be obscured and only be recognisable by the accumulation of neutrophils and lymphocytes; if seen in transverse section these venules may simulate epithelial cell collections, while if they are cut in the long axis, they give the impression of a sinus endothelial proliferation throughout the node. The lymph sinuses are inconspicuous, being compressed by the cellular proliferation, while the capsular tissue is oedematous and may contain small aggregates of lymphoid cells.

This viral lymphadenitis picture is seen frequently in enlarged cervical or axillary lymph nodes from young adults following vaccination against smallpox, and closely similar changes may occur following other viral infections such as herpes zoster, where the intranuclear inclusion bodies can often be found. In *measles* the multinucleate Warthin-Finkeldy giant cells may be found in the *Measles* paracortical area and on occasions, when an abdominal lymph node has been *Fig. II.8* excised from a child with the prodromal 'pseudo appendicitis' syndrome (Corbett, 1945), it is possible for the pathologist to make the diagnosis before the rash has appeared.

It would seem from Hartsock's (1968) paper that half his cases of viral lym- *Differentiation from* phadenitis had been misdiagnosed as Hodgkin's disease or as sarcoma. Although *Hodgkin's disease* it is probable that there is now greater familiarity with the vagaries of lymph node histology than there was ten or more years ago, it might be desirable to emphasise the distinguishing features. Leaving on one side the difficulties that will arise if the material to be examined is inadequately stained and fixed, a diagnosis of a primary lymphadenopathy should not be seriously considered if the reactive follicles are generally distributed throughout the node, separated by a mixed cellular paracortical proliferation; the features by which one can recognize a reactive lymph node partially infiltrated by Hodgkin's disease will be dealt with subsequently (p. 205).

Real difficulties can arise when the margins of the reactive follicles are blurred, *Differentiation from* and the reactive centres appear to blend with the paracortical proliferation, giving *immunoblastic* a false impression of a diffuse infiltration of atypical lymphoid cells, some of *sarcoma* which show nuclear lobulation (cleaved cells) while others possess prominent nucleoli (non-cleaved cells). A sarcoma (such as large cell sarcoma or immunoblastic sarcoma, p. 169) can usually be excluded, for though there may be cellular pleomorphism in a sarcoma, the malignant cells are of a single type. Also, one should not be mislead by the high mitotic rate in viral lymphadenitis, for mitoses may be frequent in reactive hyperplasias.

Another differentiating feature is the presence of the swollen post-capillary venules. It is extremely uncommon to find such endothelial reaction in a primary lymphadenopathy and a pathologist should have very good reasons for making a diagnosis of Hodgkin's disease or malignant lymphoma if this change is prominent. However, where these features are less obvious the question as to Hodgkin's disease, either of the lymphocyte predominant or mixed cellular type, may arise. In these circumstances the diffuse pattern of the cellular distribution, and the absence of any diffuse increase in reticulin are against a diagnosis of Hodgkin's disease of mixed cellular type. The differentiation from lymphocyte predominant Hodgkin's disease can be more difficult, as in this form of lymphadenopathy there is no increase in reticulin. However, in lymphocyte predominant Hodgkin's disease there is a curious monotonous appearance, with sheets of

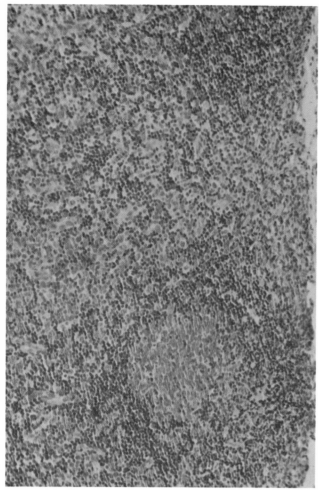

II.7a

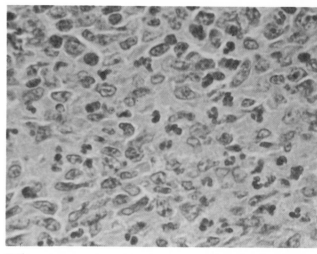

II.7b

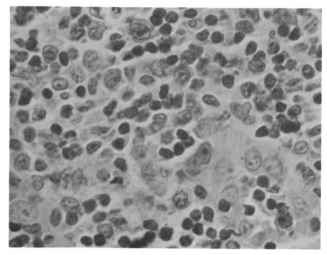

II.7c

II.7a-c   Viral Lymphadenitis

II.7a   The diffuse mottled appearance of the paracortical proliferation separating the reactive follicles is well seen.

II.7b   Sheets of transformed lymphocytes, small lymphocytes,
and plasma cells, there are also scattered neutrophils and
eosinophils.

II.7c   There are two post-capillary venules containing lymphocytes and red cells. The morphological similarity of the swollen
endothelial cells and the transformed lymphocytes is apparent.

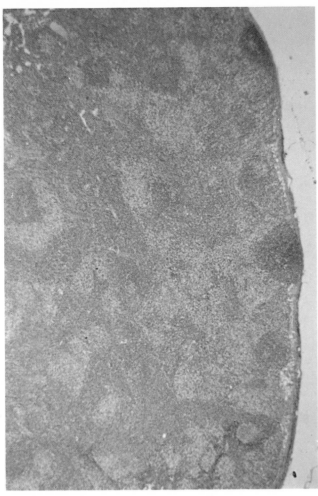

II.7d

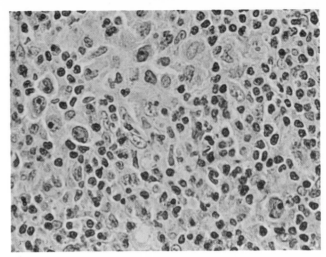

II.7e

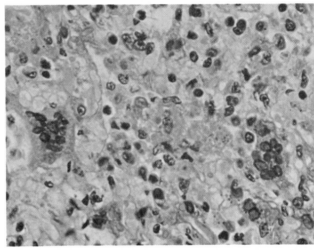

II.8

II.7d-e   Viral Lymphadenitis

II.7d   The follicles are less obvious while the paracortical pro-liferation has resulted in pale irregular zones in close relationship to the finger-like projections of the medullary tissue.

II.7e   There is considerable eosinophilic infiltrate in the para-cortical area and many of the large transformed lymphocytes with prominent nucleoli have a resemblance to the mononuclear Reed-Sternberg cell variant of Hodgkin's disease.

II.8   Measles

The multinucleate Warthin-Finkeldy giant cells in the para-cortical region.

closely set small lymphocytes interspersed with isolated mononuclear Hodgkin cells (chapter V, p. 150) and transformed type lymphocytes are decidedly rare. This contrasts with the polymorphic cellular infiltrate already described as characteristic of viral lymphadenitis. Finally, the reticulin preparation is also of value in demonstrating the extent of maintenance of normal architecture in viral lymphadenitis.

There appears to be considerable overlap between some forms of immunoblastic lymphadenopathy (see chapter V, p. 201) and certain forms of viral lymphadenitis.

Infectious mononucleosis A variant of viral lymphadenitis is seen in the lymph nodes in *infectious mononucleosis*. In this condition the number of large transformed type cells (infectious mononucleosis cells, glandular fever cells, virocytes), is often greater, and the degree of cellular atypia more pronounced, than in most other forms of *Fig. II.9* viral lymphadenitis. Large irregularly shaped reactive centres may be present in the cortex or deep within the node, and consist of large transformed type cells, morphologically indistinguishable from many of the cells comprising the diffuse infiltrate. Some active follicles have no lymphocyte cuff, and almost appear to merge into the diffuse structure of the node. In addition, tingible body macrophages and nuclear debris, although prominent in some follicles, are often absent in others, which therefore simply appear as irregular clusters of basophilic transformed type cells. Mitoses are frequent both within follicles and within the diffuse substance of the node.

The 'infectious mononucleosis' cells are characterised by a large nucleus, distinct nuclear membrane, one or more prominent nucleoli, and an irregular or complex folded nuclear outline. There is also considerable variation in cell size *Differentiation from* and in the extent of the basophilic cytoplasm. For these reasons the cellular *Hodgkin's disease* infiltrate appears quite pleomorphic and a diagnosis of malignancy may be made in error (as in the case reported by Rappaport, 1966). When they are available imprint preparations can be of considerable value, as the proliferating cells can be seen to be very similar to the atypical mononuclear cells present in the peripheral blood. Tindle et al (1972) have pointed out that multinucleate cells closely resembling Reed-Sternberg cells may be found in the paracortex in infectious mononucleosis. Other writers believe that these 'reactive' multinucleate immunoblasts (Dorfman and Warnke, 1974) have special cytological features; however, the operative point is that the presence of Reed-Sternberg cells, true or 'pseudo', in a lymph node does not of itself justify a diagnosis of Hodgkin's disease. Indeed, the histological features of infectious mononucleosis (less precisely termed glandular fever) have always proved difficult to interpret, and have been confused with leukaemic infiltration, or with forms of Hodgkin's disease. These aspects of the earlier literature were reviewed in some detail by Gall and Stout (1940), who cited the diagnostic problem encountered by MacCallum, Longcope, Fox, Downey and Stasney and others. The principal histological features were clearly described by Downey and Stasney (1936) and Gall and Stout

(1940). The significance of Gall and Stout's contribution was in recognizing a relatively characteristic morphological pattern in their cases, as opposed to the more variable responses described by earlier authors.

Thus Gall and Stout reported three features which served to distinguish infec- *Infectious* *mononucleosis* tious mononucleosis from ordinary hyperplasias.

First was the proliferative activity in the 'pulp' which served to obscure the margins of the follicles.

Second was an extensive, but distinctly focal, proliferative activity of histiocytes (termed clasmatocytes), the cytoplasm of which became progressively more abundant and acidophilic until the appearance of epithelioid cells was simulated.

The final and most nearly pathognomonic feature was the appearance throughout the pulp, on the edges of the germinal centres, and in the sinuses, of large numbers of specific infectious mononucleosis cells. The infectious mononucleosis cells were large with 'abundant basophilic, either granular or relatively coarsely vacuolated, sharply delimited cytoplasm. . . ', and the nuclei were vesicular, round or slightly indented, and eccentric in position' (Gall and Stout, 1940). These same cells have been variously termed activated reticulum cells (Marshall, 1956), atypical histiocytes (Rapapport, 1966), or immunoblasts (Tindle et al, 1972), and are probably the products of both B- and T-lymphocyte transformation in response to viral antigens (Carter, 1975; Gowing, 1975).

The majority of these transformed lymphocytes or infectious mononucleosis cells do not contain demonstrable immunoglobulin, and are believed to be of T-cell origin. There is however some evidence of an associated B-cell response in the form of irregular follicular hyperplasia, particularly in the early stages of the reaction. Secondary centres may appear within the cortex and also in the deeper regions of the node. These centres, consisting almost entirely of basophilic transformed type cells (non-cleaved cells and immunoblasts), sometimes retain a lymphocyte cuff, but are characteristically irregular in shape and ill-defined. In the later stages of the reaction there are increasing numbers of transformed lymphocytes in the paracortical area, and these eventually become the predominant cell type over-running and obscuring the follicles, medullary cords and sinuses. However, these structures persist and may be identified by reticulin methods. In fact, on careful examination, the sinuses may be seen to be distended and packed with large transformed type cells, a finding emphasised by Lennert in 1961. The large transformed type cells, or infectious mononucleosis cells, correspond to the atypical mononuclear cells, or virocytes, of the peripheral blood, and just as the blood picture of infectious mononucleosis may be mimicked by other viral infections, so also may the lymph node picture. Thus, the changes are not dissimilar from those already described for post-vaccinial lymphadenitis, and identical changes may be seen in other circumstances where there is no evidence of either infectious mononucleosis or vaccination, presumably the result of unidentified viral infection. There are also a number of non-viral conditions which may induce a marked paracortical cellular proliferation in association with reactive follicles, of which

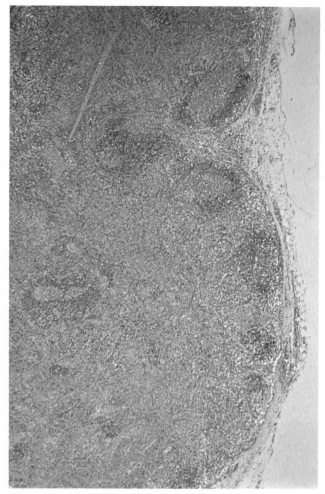

II.9a

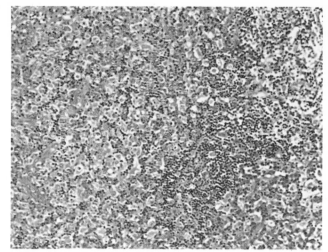

II.9b

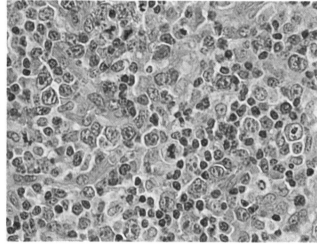

II.9c

II.9a-c Infectious Mononucleosis

   II.9a The reactive follicles are apparent but are blurred, and to some extent invaded by the diffuse paracortical proliferation.

   II.9b The paracortex is largely replaced by sheets of infectious mononuclear cells.

   II.9c The character of the infectious mononuclear cell is well shown:- a large bizarre transformed lymphocyte (immunoblast) with a prominent nucleolus, having a superficial resemblance to mononuclear Hodgkin cells.

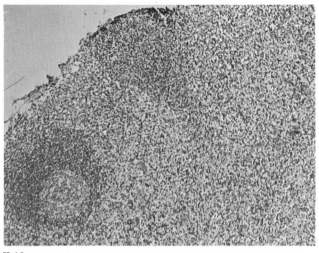

II.10a

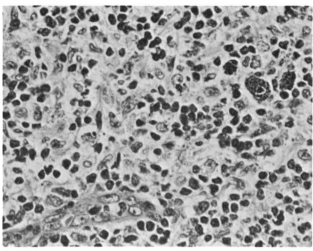

II.10b

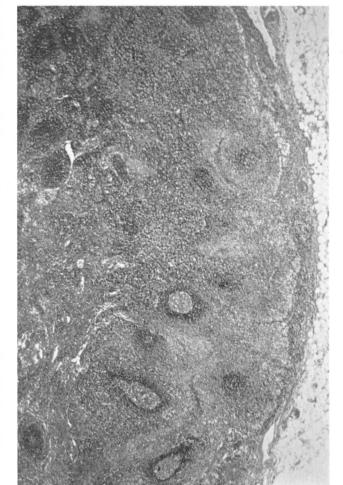

II.11a

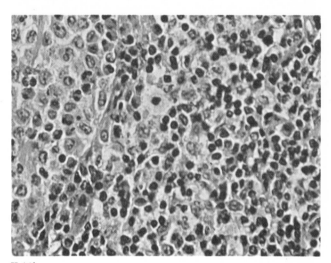

II.11b

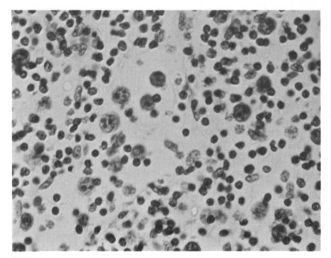

II.11c

II.10a-b Dermatopathic Lymphadenopathy

II.10a The reactive follicles have been preserved and the paracortical tissue consists of pale histiocytes, eosinophils and lymphocytes.

II.10b The paracortical area is replaced to a large extent by histiocytes, many containing melanin, eosinophils and lymphocytes.

II.11a-c Steatorrhoea Lymphadenopathy

II.11a The reactive follicles have been preserved but the paracortical and interfollicular proliferation is apparent.

II.11b The marked histiocytic proliferation in the sinuses and paracortical area is apparent as well as the eosinophilia.

II.11c An early stage showing the abnormal histiocytes in the sinuses and paracortical tissue.

71

the most important are the dermatopathic and steatorrhoea lymphadenopathies.

T-zone lymphoma   Prior to considering these, it would be convenient to refer briefly to the *T-zone lymphoma* which Lennert (1976, 1978) has characterized.

The nodes are moderately enlarged and in the low power view of the haematoxylin-eosin preparation, the follicles stand out as dark blue areas widely separated, consequent on the widened paracortical zone, which has a uniform faintly eosinophilic hue, while numerous pre-capillary venules are easily made out. The predominant cells are T-lymphocyte, whose nature can be confirmed by marker studies and histochemistry; they are larger than B-lymphocytes, with an oval nucleus having an irregular outline, often convoluted, while mitoses are not infrequent. Although the cytoplasm cannot easily be made out, the cells are much more loosely packed than B-lymphocytes and though there may be a few immature cells, plasma cells and eosinophils, the striking feature is the cellular monotony of the paracortical zone. This, together with the persistance of the follicles, distinguishes the T-zone lymphoma from the angio-immunoblastic lymphadenopathy (p. 201), though in the past it would probably have been included under the diffuse Hodgkin group. From Lennert's small series and the report by Waldron et al (1978), it seems that the condition mainly affects patients in the higher age groups, with generalised lymphadenopathy and splenomegaly and an indifferent prognosis. Symmers (1978) has mentioned the condition briefly and it would appear to have affinities with the monomorphic adult T-cell leukaemia of Japanese authors (Hanaika et al, 1979; Suchi et al, 1979) though Lennert's cases only showed a terminal leukaemia.

Dermatopathic lymphadenopathy   The histological appearances in *dermatopathic lymphadenopathy (lipomelanic reticulosis)* are distinct from those described for the viral forms of lymphadenitis, in that in the early stages the increase in cell numbers may be largely confined to the sinuses. However, subsequently the sinus pattern becomes obscured, particularly around the marginal sinus, extending down between the lymphoid follicles *Fig. II.10* of the cortex. There is thus an increasing area of infiltration of the cortex and paracortex by pale eosinophilic histiocytes with delicate ovoid or reniform nuclei. These cells may show a foamy cytoplasm due to lipoid or may contain brown granular inclusions of melanin. The concomitant presence of haemosiderin may confuse the diagnosis and in some instances the presence of melanin is not obvious in haematoxylin-eosin preparations, but is revealed by silver stains (such as Fontana's method).

The histiocytic reaction may become very intense and may obscure many of the normal architectural features. Persisting follicles often show marked reactive centre formation and plasma cells and transformed cells are then prominent. The presence throughout the node of such a mixed cell population of small lymphocytes, large transformed type cells, plasma cells, histiocytes and on occasions eosinophils, with some apparent loss of normal architecture, may be confused with those types of Hodgkin's disease having a marked histiocytic component. The distinction from Hodgkin's disease may be made by the lack of nuclear pleomorphism, the complete absence of Reed-Sternberg cells, and the inconspicuous fibrosis in dermatopathic lymphadenitis. In addition there is no necrosis and no true destruction of nodal architecture, the reticulin pattern being intact, though often distended and distorted by the cellular infiltrate. The coexistence of *Hodgkin's disease* a chronic skin disease is a valuable diagnostic pointer, but it should be remembered that Hodgkin's disease and other lymphomas do occur in association with a variety of skin reactions. Nevertheless many of the earlier accounts of diffuse Hodgkin's disease of the skin were in reality instances of exfoliative erythrodermia with dermatopathic lymphadenopathy (Randerath and Ullbricht, 1952).

Steatorrhoea lymphadenopathy was the term proposed by Whitehead (1968) *Steatorrhoea lymphadenopathy* to describe a peculiar form of lymphadenopathy, associated with chronic malabsorption, with a liability to undergo sarcomatous change; the condition had originally been described by Robb-Smith (1938, 1964) as 'prohistiocytic fibrillary reticulosis'. Although other authors recognized the association between lymphoid malignancy and steatorrhoea (Harrison, 1975), the initial lympho-proliferative *Fig. II.11* condition had not been identified, but was sometimes interpreted as Hodgkin's disease. Freeman et al (1977) recognized the lymphoproliferative character of the intestinal lesions in sprue which have been designated 'ulcerative non-granulomatous jejuno-ileitis', while Isaacson et al (1978, 1979) emphasized the histiocytic origin of the proliferation, but classed it as a malignant histiocytosis, a viewpoint to be discussed in a later chapter.

In the early stages the lymph nodes show follicular hyperplasia with prominent *Fig. IV.2a* reactive centres, together with expansion and dilatation of the sinuses. The sinus lining histiocytes are markedly prominent and have quite extensive eosinophilic cytoplasm. Cells of similar morphology and others with large nuclei and prominent nucleolus, appear free in the sinuses and occasionally also within the paracortex of the node. Varying numbers of eosinophils may also be present, particularly within the sinuses. Transformed lymphocytes are present in relation to the cortical follicles and in the paracortex and medullary cords. In the latter site plasma cells are especially numerous.

In later stages there is increasing sinus hyperplasia with extension of the cellular proliferation from the medullary area into the paracortex and cortex. There are large numbers of pink histiocytic-type cells, including many forms resembling monocytes, with a more rounded vesicular nucleus and often a small distinct nucleolus; giant cell forms are not uncommon. Intermingled with these histiocytes may be numerous eosinophils. The remnants of cortex and paracortex show continuing evidence of general hyperplasia with transformed lymphocytes and scattered histiocytes, but the follicles become inconspicuous. Ultimately there may be a sarcomatous change which will be dealt with in a later chapter (p. 177).

It will also be more suitable in a subsequent chapter to discuss the recognition of the early stages of involvement of lymph nodes in Hodgkin's disease and malignant lymphomas etc, where there has been preservation of normal or reactive follicles and partial infiltration of the paracortical tissue (p. 205).

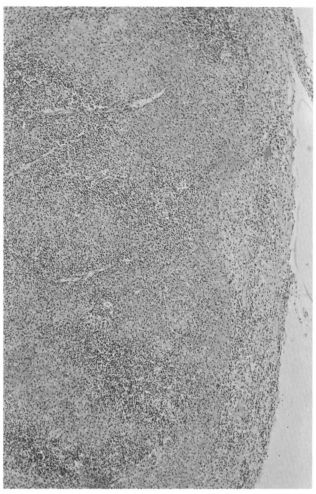

II.12a

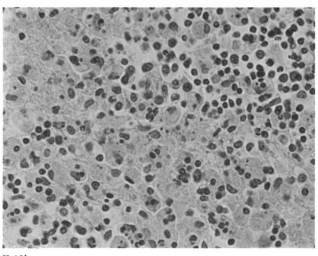

II.12b

II.12a-b   Typhoid Lymphadenitis

II.12a   The paracortical tissue is replaced by ill-defined histiocytic nodules.

II.12b   The paracortical tissue consists of macrophages. Many have ingested lymphocytes and erythrocytes and undergone coagulative necrosis. In addition there are foci of transformed lymphocytes.

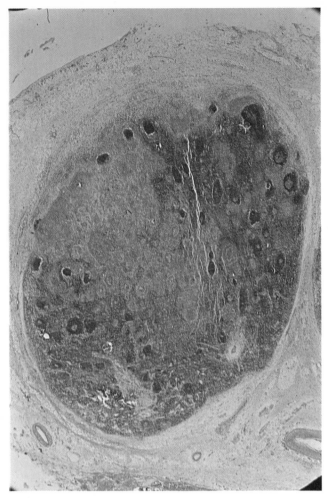

II.13a

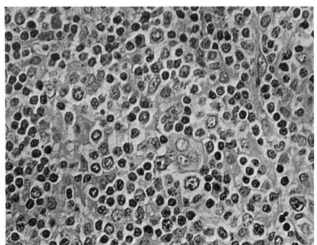

II.13b

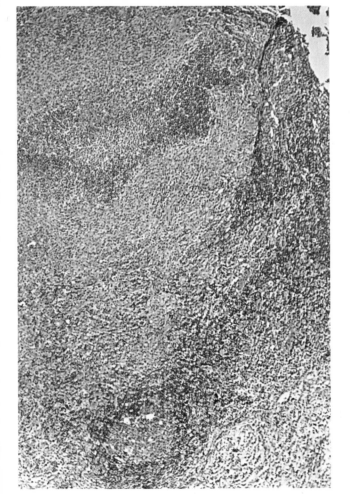

II.13c

II.13d

II.13a-d Mesenteric Adenitis

II.13a It can be seen that a large portion of the node has been infarcted; in addition there are smaller foci of necrosis elsewhere in the node.

II.13b The reactive follicles have been preserved but there are large areas of focal necrosis in the paracortex.

II.13c A closer view of the massive necrosis consisting of histiocytes and neutrophils.

II.13d The paracortex around an area of necrosis showing transformed lymphocytes and histiocytes.

4. Granulomatous lymphadenitis – reactive follicles are present together with focal area of necrosis and/or histiocytic granulomata in the paracortex

There are a number of conditions, the majority being of infective origin, in which in addition to a reactive hyperplasia there are focal histiocytic granulomata within the paracortex. These range from necrotic foci to fibrotic nodules in which multinucleate giant cells may be associated with an identifiable aetiological agent; small foci of epithelioid histiocytes occurring both within follicles and paracortex may be associated with toxoplasmosis and have already been discussed. Sometimes the granulomatous process, instead of remaining focal, may, as is usually the case in sarcoidosis, involve the whole substance of the node and render the follicles relatively inconspicuous. (Dhom, 1980).

This review of granulomatous lymphadenitis will follow this progression, but it is necessary to recognize that although there may be a typical reaction to a particular agent, the range of tissue response, influenced by the proportion and type of antigen and antibody, is wide. Therefore, it is desirable in searching for an infective agent to use a battery of stains, which can reveal micro-organisms, fungi or parasites, and it should not be forgotten that a metachromatic stain will sometimes display infective agents which have been difficult to demonstrate by more specific methods. Unhappily it is seldom possible to anticipate a granulomatous lymphadenitis, and have material available for culture or animal innoculation. On occasion a second biopsy may be justified to provide this. It is also necessary to recognize that epithelioid granulomata may be found in association with non-infective processes such as Hodgkin's disease or metastatic carcinoma.

4a. *Necrotic foci*

It is unusual to excise lymph nodes involved in acute pyogenic infections, but in such cases small abcesses will be found in the paracortex while the reactive follicles show an infiltration of neutrophils.

Salmonellosis　It might seem unlikely that a lymph node biopsy would be needed to make a diagnosis of *typhoid fever* or *salmonella infection* yet we, like Lennert (1961) have on several occasions suggested such a diagnosis after examining an abdominal lymph node removed at laparotomy from a patient with suspected acute
Fig. II.12　appendicitis; the diagnosis was subsequently confirmed bacteriologically.

Significant lymphadenopathy may occur in salmonella infection, particularly in the mesenteric and para-aortic lymph node areas. At low magnification the nodes appear very cellular, but the normal architectural features are largely obscured by ill-defined nodular collections of pale pink cells. On closer examination these cells are seen to be relatively small rounded histiocytes (or monocytes) with delicate nuclear membranes and small nucleoli, while the cytoplasm often contains cellular debris. They occur in great numbers, first in the sinuses, and later as nodules throughout the substance of the node. These collections of histiocytes form the so-called typhoid nodules, the characteristic feature of the disease in lymph node and spleen. The nodules may undergo necrosis and auto-lytic softening, but there is no neutrophil reaction. There may be marked follicular hyperplasia and transformed lymphocytes can be seen in moderate numbers in paracortex and medulla, while plasma cells become more prominent in later stages. The normal architecture, although obscured, is not destroyed as evidenced by reticulin preparations.

It is unlikely, on morphological grounds, that salmonella lymphadenopathy would be confused with *mesenteric lymphadenitis*, a diagnosis to be considered in children having symptoms suggestive of acute or subacute abdominal inflam-mation, usually associated with infection by *Yersinia enterocolitica, Yersinia (Pasteurella) pseudo-tuberculosis* etc. In this condition there are large areas of necrosis containing numerous degenerate neutrophils. The foci merge with the surrounding paracortex which is rich in histiocytes, and there is no sharp zone of demarcation of the histiocytes around the necrotic foci. It is unusual to identify the organism in sections, though culture of suitable material is often positive, as are serological agglutinations. Granulomatous lymphadenitis due to this group of gram negative coccobacilli may not be restricted to abdominal nodes, and on occasion the node may be converted to a breaking down abscess or an area of necrosis. It should not be forgotten that a somewhat similar appearance to that found in mesenteric adenitis can occur in *non-reactive tuberculosis*, in which there are zones of necrosis without caseation and with minimal cellular reaction; usually there are very large numbers of acid-fast bacilli in the necrotic areas.

Mesenteric lymphadenitis

Fig. II.13

Necrotic foci surrounded and infiltrated by eosinophils inside a histiocytic zone may be seen in eosinophilic granuloma (histiocytosis X) or filariasis. In *filariasis* the histiocytes are small and pale, and have regular uniform nuclei with small inconspicuous nucleoli. Also the cytoplasm appears of uniform consistency and is weakly eosinophilic. The central area frequently has the appearance of a frank abscess, containing degenerating eosinophils, histiocytes and debris. The remain-der of the node may show features of reactive hyperplasia and acute inflammatory infiltration. In persistent cases there are broad bands of fibrosis, giving a nodular appearance, which with the presence of eosinophils, histiocytes and plasma cells, may be confused with a nodular sclerotic form of Hodgkin's disease. However, in filariasis there are no atypical cells and no Reed-Sternberg cells. In addition, serial sections through the node should reveal the presence of parasites, often calcified and staining deeply with haematoxylin.

Filariasis

Fig. II.14

Eosinophilic granuloma should also be distinguishable from filariasis on the basis of the more variable histiocyte morphology in this condition. Firstly the histiocytes of eosinophilic granuloma are large, with ill-defined boundaries. The cytoplasm is characteristically eosinophilic and foamy and there may be variation in nuclear size and form, together with some degree of hyperchromatism. In addition, small giant cells may be present with similar foamy or vacuolated cytoplasm, and three or four nuclei. Electron microscopy reveals the presence of

Eosinophilic granuloma

Fig. II.15

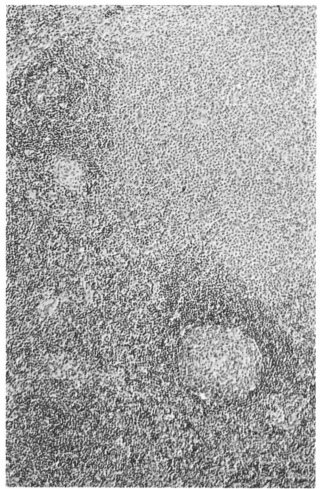

II.14a

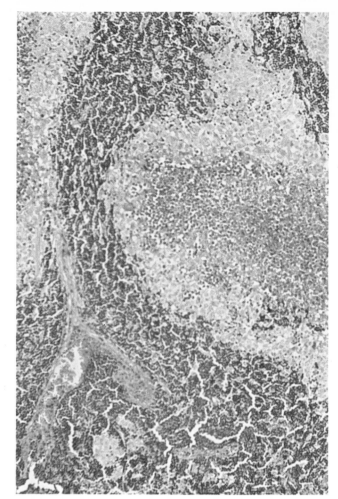

II.15a

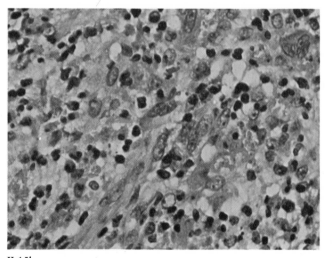

II.14b

II.15b

II.14a-b   Filariasis

II.14a   This shows the eosinophilic abscess with very little re-action around it.

II.14b   A fibrotic lesion in which the worm is embedded. The cellular reaction is for the most part plasma cell.

II.15a-b   Eosinophilic Granuloma

II.15a   The eosinophil 'abscess' in the paracortex is surrounded by histiocytes.

II.15b   Edge of the 'abscess' showing masses of eosinophils, histiocytes and histiocytic giant cells.

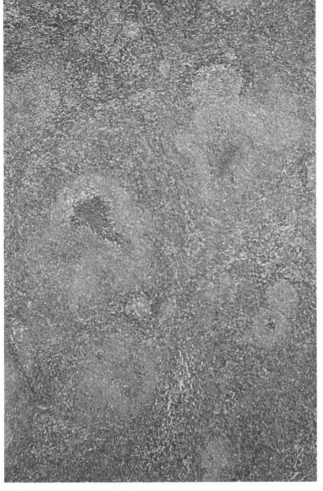

II.16a

II.16b

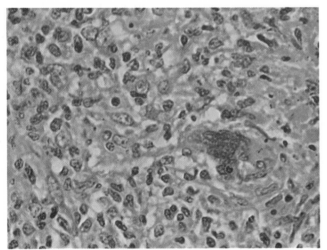

II.16c

II.16a-c 'Cat-Scratch' Disease

II.16a The areas of focal necrosis are clearly seen.

II.16b The central area of necrosis surrounded by histiocytes some of which are multinucleate and beyond this a zone of neutrophils.

II.16c Wall of the abscess showing the histiocytic giant cells surrounded by small histiocytes and transformed lymphocytes.

intracytoplasmic rods similar to those normally present in the epidermic Langerhans cells. Eosinophils are numerous and may show degenerative features. In addition lymphocytes and plasma cells will be present within the granulomata, and plasma cells may occur throughout the node. Quite often the lymph sinuses are distended with histiocytes and eosinophils. The rest of the lymph node does not show specific reactive features and there is no vasculitis, a point of distinction from some of the granulomatous hypersensitivity responses. Fibrosis is less of a feature than in filariasis. Generally only the diffuse, ill-defined forms show any resemblance to Hodgkin's disease, and again the distinction may be made by the complete absence of Reed-Sternberg cells in eosinophilic granuloma, and by the foamy appearance of the histiocytes which is not a feature of the histiocytes in Hodgkin's disease.

Disseminate lupus erythematosus

Necrotic foci of characteristic type may be seen in *disseminate lupus erythematosis (DLE)*. There are zones of cellular necrosis in the paracortical tissue with no sharp zone of demarcation, but a gradual change from normal lymphocytes to cells with varying degree of nuclear dissolution. In the necrotic zone, in addition to pyknotic cells and small fragments of nuclear debris, there will be large irregular masses of deeply basophilic material ('haematoxyphile bodies'). In DLE the degree of reactive change in the follicles is much less than is seen in the lymph nodes in rheumatoid arthritis (see p. 56), but in addition to the necrotic zone, haematoxyphil material is often deposited on the walls of the blood vessels and lymph sinuses. (Moore et al, 1956; Symmers, 1958).

Cat-scratch disease

Fig. II.16

There are a number of conditions such as *cat-scratch disease, lymphogranuloma inguinale*, etc. in which there are necrotic foci or micro-abscesses surrounded by a palisade of histiocytes. They cannot be distinguished one from another histologically, and in addition they show serological cross reactivity.

Naji et al (1962) described the early stages of cat scratch disease as 'reticulum cell hyperplasia' and emphasised 'the predominance of the same kind of cell (reticulum cell) within the germinal centres and in the lymphoid tissue around the follicles'. These cells, termed reticulum cells by Naji et al, possessed a large vesicular nucleus with distinct nuclear membrane and one or two prominent nucleoli, and appear to us to correspond to transformed lymphocytes occurring in the reactive centres or in the diffuse tissue of the cortex, paracortex or medulla. Many of these cells in the medulla show some plasmacytoid features and a high proportion contain demonstrable immunoglobulin indicative of their B-cell origin. A number of distinct pale histiocytes are also present and have a more delicate nuclear structure. In the 'intermediate stage' recognised by Naji et al, definite granulomata occur at random throughout the node, but are rarely associated with giant cells. Finally Naji and colleagues distinguished a 'late stage' in which the lesions took the form of micro- or macro-abscesses. This is the stage at which the histological features are quite characteristic of cat scratch/LGV (lymphogranuloma venereum disease), for the abscesses are typically large and irregular, often having a distinct stellate or Y shape in section. The walls are composed of necrotic debris, neutrophils and an outer zone of pale histiocytes, which are to some degree regimented and may appear as a palisade. At this stage Langhans' type giant cells may be present. A further feature is the presence of small developing granulomata alongside large well formed abscesses, together with irregular fibrosis and scarring during the later stages. Capsular infiltration and fibrosis may also occur. The condition should be easily distinguishable from tuberculosis or sarcoidosis by the acute nature of the lesions, and from Hodgkin's disease with focal necrosis by the complete absence of either pleomorphic mononuclear Hodgkin cells or of true Reed-Sternberg cells.

The characteristic histological picture correlates quite well with a positive complement fixation test to psittacosis–lymphogranuloma–trachoma (PLT) antigen and to a positive skin test (Frei test) against a preparation of pus from either a known cat scratch or lymphogranuloma inguinale (venereum) node as appropriate.

Although it is impossible to distinguish histologically between cat scratch disease and lymphogranuloma inguinale (venereum), nevertheless an axillary lymph node is more likely to be affected by the former, and an inguinal lymph node by the latter; furthermore there is a greater tendency for the nodes in LGV to break down and form sinuses. Another form of granulomatous lymphadenitis with pallisading of histiocytes around the micro-abscess is *tularaemia*. The foci *Tularaemia* are smaller and do not usually show a tendency to coalesce.

4b. *Caseous foci*

Partial replacement of the foci by coalescent epithelioid tubercles with caseation epitomises the histological appearance of *tuberculous lymphadenitis,* but the *Tuberculosis* manifestations are protean and can on occasions simulate or be simulated by a whole range of other conditions.

A lymph node containing tuberculous granulomata often shows moderate *Fig. II.17* hyperplasia of residual follicles, together with evidence of T-cell reactivity, in an expanded paracortical zone containing many immunoglobulin negative transformed type cells, and often also some degree of sinus histiocytosis. Tuberculous granulomata may appear as small collections of spindle shaped histiocytes with characteristic epithelioid appearance and little central necrosis, or they may be larger with extensive central caseous necrosis. Caseation is characterised by its granular pink staining reaction and its structureless appearance. Reticulin preparations show a general loss of reticulin fibres within caseous areas. The granulomata may be small, discrete and numerous, or large, confluent and few. Giant cells may be scarce or they may be numerous, and of foreign body or of Langhans' type.

The granulomata characteristically contain some lymphocytes among the histiocytes. This is particularly evident at the periphery of the granulomata, which are thus not distinctly defined, as the lymphocytes and histiocytes intermingle. In

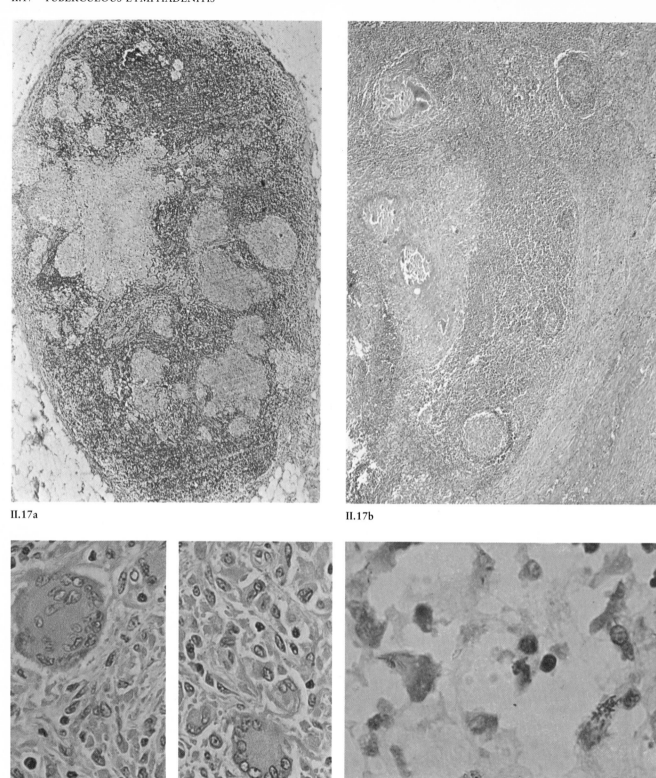

II.17a

II.17b

II.17c

II.17d

II.17e

II.17a–e Tuberculous Lymphadenitis

> **II.17a** Multiple granulomata of varying size showing coalescence and early caseation.
>
> **II.17b** Fibrocaseous foci.
>
> **II.17c,d** Langhans' giant cells and epithelioid histiocytes.
>
> **II.17e** Acid-fast mycobacteria in histiocytes.

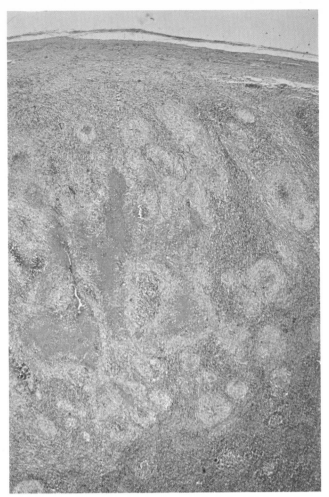

II.18a

II.19a

II.18b

II.19b

II.18a-b Coccidioidomycosis

II.18a There are multiple granulomata with some tendency to coalescence and consequent necrosis. There is a fibrotic reaction at the edge of the granuloma.

II.18b The edge of a granuloma showing a giant cell and histiocytic reaction. Fungal bodies can be seen and in the lower right hand corner is a mature sporangium of *Coccidiodes immitis* filled with endospores.

II.19a-b Histoplasmosis

II.19a Focal epithelioid granulomata are scattered throughout the paracortex.

II.19b Detail of an epithelioid granuloma. Fungal bodies are present but are not well displayed in an ordinary stained preparation.

chronic cases irregular fibrosis may occur, involving capsule, trabeculae and the substance of the node, where granulomatous lesions are replaced by dense hyaline fibrous tissue. Lymphocytes and plasma cells are often present bordering and infiltrating this fibrous tissue, and calcification is not uncommon.

The diagnosis of tuberculosis may be confirmed by the demonstration of acid-fast bacilli using the Ziehl-Neelsen stain. However acid-fast bacilli are only present in small numbers in most cases, and failure to identify them by no means excludes a diagnosis of tuberculosis. In some cases of tuberculosis, where the granulomata appear more acute and florid in form, numerous acid-fast bacilli may be found, and this constitutes the atypical response to tuberculosis often observed in the elderly or immunoparetic. There are no specific histological features to enable identification of infection by the so-called 'atypical acid-fast bacilli'.

Differential diagnosis of caseous granulomata The chief differential diagnosis of tuberculosis is from other caseous granulomata and from sarcoidosis. The presence of caseation is distinctive for tuberculosis, although central necrosis occurs in other conditions and may give a superficial resemblance to caseous material. The differential diagnosis from sarcoidosis is considered later and in addition it should be remembered that syphilitic gummata may rarely occur in lymph nodes and then closely resemble caseous tuberculosis. However in syphilis the central necrotic tissues retain some vestiges of structure, which are best appreciated by reticulin stains, plasma cells are more prominent, and there is often vasculitis and endarteritis obliterans. Historically an important differential diagnosis of tuberculosis was from Hodgkin's disease and this was complicated by the frequent coexistence of tuberculosis and Hodgkin's disease – 'Tuberculosis follows Hodgkin's disease like a shadow'. This differential diagnosis should not be difficult if rigorous criteria are applied for the recognition of mononuclear Hodgkin cells and for Reed-Sternberg cells.

Chronic granulomatous disease *Chronic granulomatous disease* closely simulates caseating tuberculosis, but no acid-fast bacilli will be found, though other organisms may be present. The most significant distinguishing feature is the presence of 'sea-blue histiocytes', ceroid-containing macrophages whose cytoplasm is either diffusely pigmented or contains coarse particles of varying size. In unstained sections or sections stained with haematoxylin alone, the particles appear brown, though haematoxylin and eosin renders the colour less obvious. The granules are acid-fast, and give a positive reaction with PAS and lipid stains in paraffin sections, while with Romanowsky stains the pigment appears sea-blue or sea-green. These pigmented histiocytes are not peculiar to chronic granulomatous disease, but found in association with a necrotizing tuberculoid granuloma are highly suggestive of the condition. In an affected node they are usually easily seen, not in relation to the necrotic foci, but in clusters in the paracortical tissue and sinuses which may in addition contain macrophages with ingested neutrophils.

Fungal granuloma Certain *fungal granulomata*, particularly coccidioidomycosis and histoplasmosis can simulate caseous tuberculosis quite closely, as they may present with a necrotic centre surrounded by epithelioid histiocytes and lymphocytes. In some *Figs. II.18,19* cases the fungi may be present in giant cells, in others in the necrotic material. Apart from the detection of fungal bodies recognition can only be achieved on a suspicion that the appearances are unusual and justify more careful inspection and the use of special stains.

Brucella lymphadenitis may simulate early involvement of the lymph node by *Brucellosis* tuberculosis. In brucellosis, there are epithelioid granulomata in the paracortical tissues, together with well marked reactive follicles. The granulomata are seldom of any size and tend to coalesce with central areas of necrosis, in which there are fragments of nuclear material and neutrophil leucocytes, but true caseation does not occur. Accordingly brucellosis should be suspected in a granulomatous lymphadenitis if there are epithelioid granulomata and central areas of necrosis infiltrated with granulocytes. Sometimes the epithelioid granulomata are less obvious, while throughout the paracortical tissue there are transformed lymphocytes often binucleate, and in these cases there is a possibility of confusion with Hodgkin's disease.

Finally massive fibrinoid necrosis of collagen within a lymph node, with a surrounding well formed palisade of histiocytes, may occur in *rheumatoid ar-* *Rheumatoid* *thritis*, giving a superficial resemblance to some of the granulomatous conditions *arthritis* already described. The distinctive features of the rheumatoid nodule are in the *Fig. II.20* nature and appearance of the fibrinoid change (with the tinctorial properties of fibrin in trichrome stains) and the distinct palisade of histiocytes. The surrounding inflammatory response is generally of a chronic type, with numerous plasma cells, but occasionally significant numbers of acute inflammatory cells are present. There is no vasculitis, and the co-existence of follicular hyperplasia and plasmacytosis in the residual parts of the lymph node serves as another pointer to the diagnosis of rheumatoid arthritis.

Micro-abscesses may occur in certain forms of *fungal lymphadenitis* (nocar- *Fungal* diosis, candidosis, blastomycosis, sporotrichosis) but fungal bodies are usually *lymphadenitis* readily identifiable with ordinary staining procedures and the more precise morphological identification can be achieved by the use of specific stains. Furthermore, micro-abscesses may be found in breaking down *secondary deposits of* *Metastases* *neoplasm* in lymph nodes and simulate some of the other conditions that have *Fig. II.21* already been described.

4c. *Focal giant cell granulomata with fibrosis*

There are a number of conditions in which the lymph node is distorted to a greater or lesser extent by fibrous tissue in which there are giant cell granulomata, while the rest of the node, apart from reactive follicles and an increase of plasma cells in the paracortex and medulla, shows little abnormality. It is convenient to divide this group of granulomata according to the predominant giant cell type

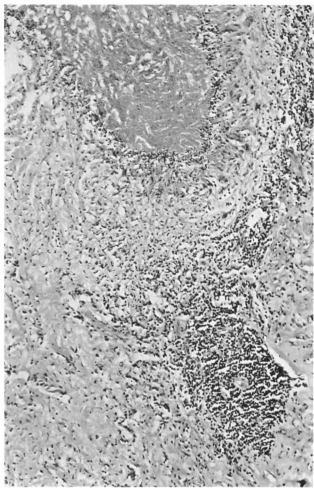

II.20

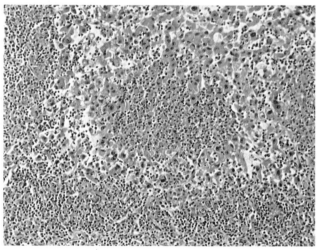

II.21a

II.20 Rheumatoid Nodule

There is a large area of fibrinoid necrosis surrounded by a palisade of histiocytes while the node as a whole is fibrotic and scarred with small surviving foci of lymphoid tissue.

II.21a-b Carcinomatous Micro-abscesses

II.21a The low power view would suggest a fibrotic granuloma with necrotic foci replacing a large part of the node.

II.21b It can now be seen that the cellular foci consist of carcinomatous metastases with central areas of cellular necrosis which are infiltrated by neutrophils.

II.21b

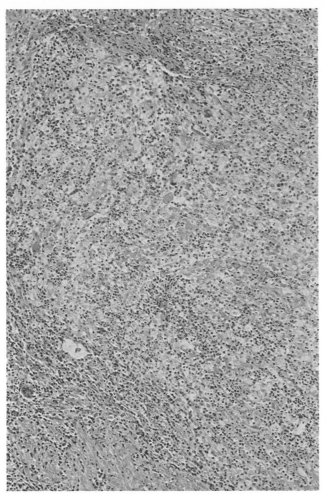

II.22a

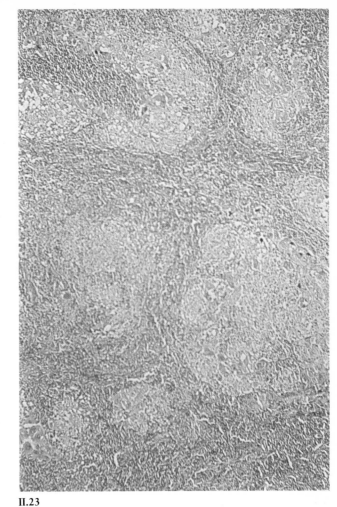

II.23

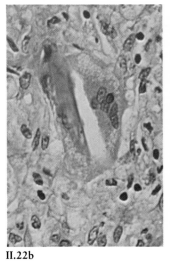

II.22b

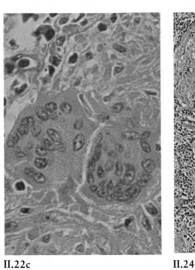

II.22c

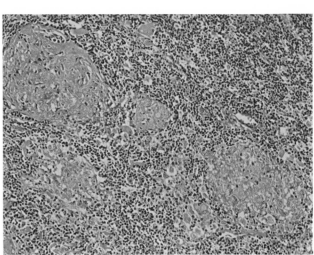

II.24

II.22a-c   Granulomatous Foreign Body Reaction

II.22a   An extensive ill-defined granulomatous reaction in the paracortex, consisting for the most part of vacuolated macrophages, some of which are multi-nucleate with foci of lymphoid cells.

II.22b-c   Foreign body giant cells; that on the left showing a lipoid cleft in the cytoplasm.

II.23   Sarcoid Reaction

These are typical sarcoid granulomata in a lymph node involved by secondary carcinoma; the photo-micrograph does not show any neoplastic tissue.

II.24   Sarcoid Reaction

These epithelioid granulomata occurred in a node from a patient with Hodgkin's disease. Adjacent nodes were involved with Hodgkin's tissue but this node after serial section failed to reveal any lymphadenomatous involvement.

– foreign body or epithelioid – although almost invariably there is an overlap. In the foreign body type of granuloma, giant cells tend to be discrete surrounded by loose connective tissue, while there may be small areas of necrosis or micro-abscesses. In the epithelioid or sarcoid-like granuloma, the giant cells usually form small congeries, which on occasions may show tiny zones of hyaline necrosis, but there is never the enlarging coalescence of the granulomata with areas of caseous necrosis such as in seen in tuberculosis. The epithelioid granulomata are surrounded by sheets of small lymphocytes in which the follicles can be made out. In certain conditions the granulomata will be surrounded by fibrous tissue and in the end may be replaced by hyaline material in which an occasional giant cell survives.

Focal giant cell
The foreign body type granulomata is typically seen in fungal granulomata, and less commonly as a reaction to a foreign body. In the fungal granulomata the fungal bodies may be contained within the giant cells or may lie loose connective tissue surrounded by giant cells. Cryptococcosis, coccidioidomycosis, blastomycosis, histoplasmosis and paracoccidioidomycosis may all induce this *Fungal granulomata* type of reaction and can be distinguished on the morphological characters of the *Figs. II.18, 19* organism, more clearly displayed by specific stains (e.g. Gridley, Grocott-Gomori, PAS etc). In general the fungal bodies are easily detected and if not obvious it is unlikely that proof of a fungal aetiology will be achieved. An exception to this statement is a fibrotic granuloma in which there are vacuoles within the giant cells. They may just be fat but equally well they may be scant fungal infestation and special stains may well clarify the situation. This type of granuloma should always be examined under polarised light. They may be due to a foreign body but it should not be forgotten that the capsule of *Histoplasma duboisii* (the large or African type of histoplasma) and the spherule of *Coccidioides immitis* is doubly refractile. Symmers (1978) provides an admirable account of the whole range of fungal granulomata.

Foreign body granulomata
Granulomatous reactions to foreign bodies are not frequent in lymph nodes and generally there is a history of accidental trauma or surgical intervention related to the site of the lymphadenopathy, though the time interval may be quite long. The typical appearance is of collections of foreign body type giant cells, *Fig. II.22* and smaller numbers of Langhans' type cells, scattered diffusely, in association with large histiocytes, plasma cells, lymphocytes and sometimes acute inflammatory cells. Distinctive nodular granulomata like those of tuberculosis and sarcoidosis do not occur commonly, instead there is an ill-defined granulomatous reaction which appears to spread quite extensively. In addition there may be areas of necrosis with acute inflammatory change or there may be fibrosis of irregular distribution. The presence of foreign material can often be detected by polarised light microscopy, either present as large aggregates surrounded by histiocytes and foreign body giant cells, or occurring finely dispersed within histiocytes and giant cells. Not infrequently giant cells may be seen with clefts in the cytoplasm where some foreign body crystalline material has been lost during

processing or sectioning. Typical epithelioid cells are not usually present in foreign body reactions, except where the foreign material has a lipoid nature or where there is chronic necrosis of tissue liberating endogenous complex lipids.

Epithelioid or sarcoidal granulomata have already been considered (toxoplasmosis, p. 60 syphilis, p. 61) in relation to a subacute lymphadenitis, but they may be the only abnormal histological feature of an enlarged lymph node and the pathologist is required to assess their significance. This appraisal will be greatly influenced by the anatomical situation of the node, whether there is a generalised or localised lymphadenopathy and whether the granulomatous involvement is focal or generalised, replacing the whole substance of the node. It is important to recognise that the characteristic sarcoid reaction is not representative of a disease entity, but is a response to several different agents, some unknown. The histological appearances in these cases are indistinguishable from those observed in the lymph node in *generalised sarcoidosis*. The granulomata are typically quite small and cellular. Occasionally central necrosis may occur but this has a peculiar hyaline appearance and should not be confused with caseation. The epithelioid cells are plump, have a distinctly eosinophilic granular cytoplasm and are arranged concentrically. Like all epithelioid cells (including those of tuberculosis and other granulomata) these cells contain large amounts of lysozyme (muramidase) demonstrable by immunoperoxidase methods. Within the granulomatous nodules, lymphocytes are relatively uncommon and the margins of the sarcoid nodules are thus clearly defined. Also confluence of granulomata is uncommon in sarcoidosis and these features are of considerable value in making the distinction from tuberculosis.

Giant cells may be numerous and of foreign body or Langhans' type. Concentrically laminated Schaumann bodies, crystals and asteroid inclusions were once thought to be pathognomonic of sarcoidosis, but they also occur in tuberculosis and other conditions and are thus of limited diagnostic value.

Sarcoid nodules may undergo hyaline acellular fibrosis or diffuse hyalinization may occur throughout the node. The dense coarse fibrosis with plasmacytic and lymphocytic infiltration and calcification often seen in tuberculosis is not a feature of sarcoidosis.

Focal epithelioid granulomata are seldom seen in sarcoidosis proper, but, apart from the infective conditions which have already been dealt with (p. 60 et seq), may be found in mesenteric nodes in Crohn's disease and sometimes in enlarged nodes in the region of the gall bladder ('lipogranulomatous pseudo-sarcoid') (Spain, 1957). The curious condition of cheilitis granulomatosa (Melkerson-Rosenthal syndrome) may be associated with enlarged upper cervical lymph nodes in which there are non-caseating epithelioid granulomata in the follicles and immediately around them. Epithelioid granulomata in these sites do not usually present any difficulties, but it is a different matter when occurring in cervical or axillary nodes. There is always the possibility of association with metastatic carcinoma or Hodgkin's disease. It is well in such cases to take sections at several

Sarcoidal granulomata

Fig. II.25

Sarcoidal granuloma in neoplasia

Figs. II.23,24

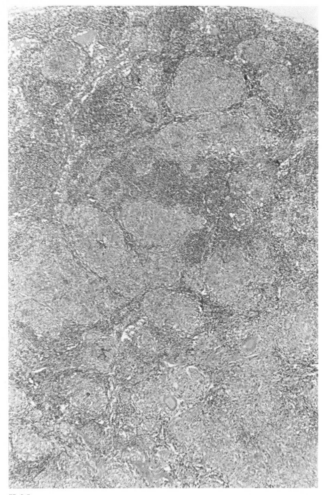

II.25a

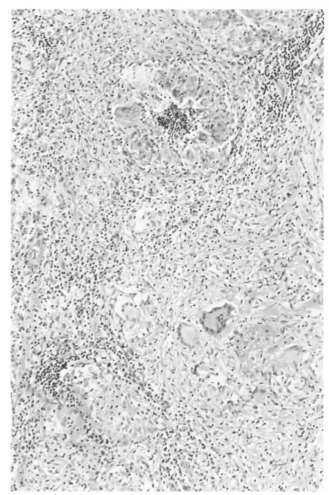

II.25b

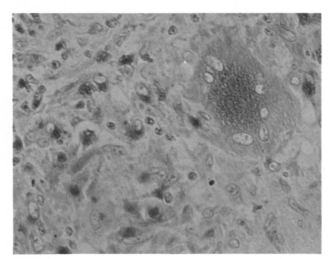

II.25c

II.25a-c Sarcoidosis

    II.25a The node has been almost entirely replaced by epithelioid granulomata, discrete and of uniform size with limited islets of surviving lymphoid tissue.

    II.25b The fibroepithelioid granulomata are well-defined and there is no caseation but there may be fibrinoid change, seen in the lower right, or else an area of necrosis rich in neutrophils and surrounded by epithelioid cells which is well shown in the upper part of the field.

    II.25c Sarcoid granuloma stained by anti-lysozyme (muramidase) showing a positive reaction in the giant cells and certain of the histiocytes (immunoperoxidase method).

II.26a-c Leprous Lymphadenitis ▶

    II.26a The follicles and cortex have been preserved, but the paracortex has been replaced by vacuolated histiocytes.

    II.26b The higher power shows that many of the vacuoles contain faintly haematoxyphil masses (bacillary clusters or globi) typical of the Virchow cell, but some of the cells have a foamy cytoplasm.

    II.26c The Ziehl-Neelsen preparations show that the 'globi' are masses of acid-fast bacilli while in addition, individual bacilli are scattered through the cytoplasm of the histiocytes.

II.27a-b Adenolymphoma ▶

    II.27a Follicles and paracortical tissues form a background to the epithelial tubules.

    II.27b The double layer of acidophil epithelial cells is apparent.

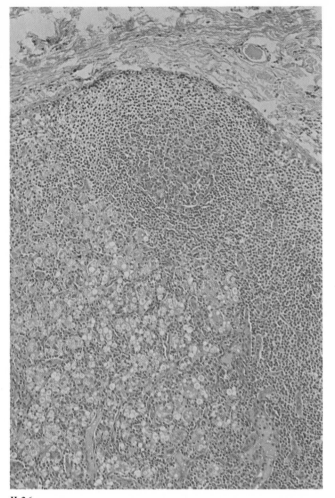

II.26a

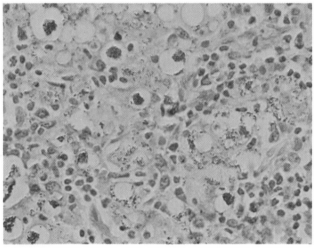

II.26b

II.26c

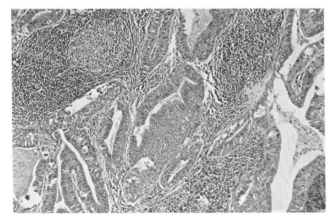

II.27a

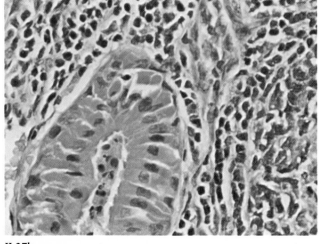

II.27b

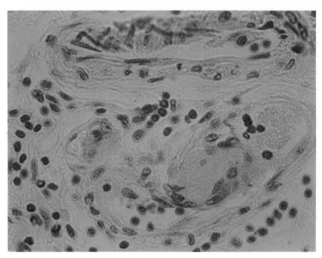

II.28

II.28 Microangiopathy

Portion of hilum of lymph node showing platelet thrombi occluding the lumen of vessels with changes in the walls.

levels. This may reveal a small secondary deposit or early involvement by Hodgkin's disease.

4d. *Diffuse giant cell granulomata*

Sarcoidosis

Fig. II.25

In *sarcoidosis*, as against a sarcoidal reaction, the characteristic feature is that the whole node is replaced by epithelioid granulomata, clearly demarcated from the background of small lymphocytes in which the follicles can sometimes be recognised. It is the monotonous uniformity that is so characteristic, and even when the nodes are becoming scarred and hyalinised there is the same impression of monotony.

Differentiation from diffuse epithelioid Hodgkin's Disease

Fig. III.14

Fig. V.39

Again it is the lack of uniformity which should enable one to distinguish the so-called *diffuse epithelioid type of Hodgkin's disease* from sarcoidosis. In this variant of the lymphocytic predominant type of Hodgkin's disease, follicles cannot be identified and the normal architecture is replaced by a background of small lymphocytes and scattered transformed lymphocytes together with mononuclear or binucleate Hodgkin cells, but seldom true Reed-Sternberg cells. Amongst these are small clusters of epithelioid macrophages which may on occasions be surrounded by eosinophils. In sarcoidosis, the low power impression is of diffuse epithelioid granulomata in a background of lymphocytes, while in this variant of Hodgkin's disease the low power impression is of a lymphocytic background in which are scattered small groups of epithelioid cells and transformed lymphocytes. There is no doubt that this form of Hodgkin's disease corresponds in part to Lennert's lymphoepithelioid lymphoma (Lennert and Mestdagh, 1968), which Dorfman and Warnke (1974) have suggested should be equated with one form of immunoblastic lymphadenopathy (see p. 201).

The exact status of these interrelated conditions can only be determined when more precise information is available as to their morphological characters and natural history. However, this diffuse epithelioid type of Hodgkin's disease (known eponymically in Oxford as Peedell's disease) has been recognized both morphologically and clinically for over thirty years and has a characteristic natural history (Robb-Smith 1976).

Noel, Helbron and Lennert (1979) have reviewed a series of 114 cases diagnosed as epithelioid cell lymphogranulomatosis between 1952 and 1976. They decided that 51 of these were a variant form of Hodgkin's desease – lymphoepithelioid (Peedell-Lennert) lymphoma; 37 conformed to Lennert's 'lymphogranulomatosis X' (angio-immunoblastic lymphadenopathy), while of the remaining 26, half were reclassified to other lymphadenopathies, the residium being unclassifiable. Burke and Butler (1976) identified a group of nodes in which there was a diffuse lymphoepithelioid proliferation. The lymphocytes were somewhat larger with more irregular nuclear outlines than normal small lymphocytes; this was confirmed by Klein et al (1977), who suggested that the lymphoid cells might be of T-cell origin and this has been endorsed in other laboratories (Delsol et al,

1978; Palutke et al, 1978). Lennert and his colleagues (1979) recognized the special cytological character of the lymphoid cells in this condition but as yet lack material to confirm the presence of T-cell receptors. Accordingly, in agreement with Robb-Smith, they maintain their original view that this lymphadenopathy is best regarded as a special variant of Hodgkin's disease, provided critical diagnostic criteria are adopted to exclude angio-immunoblastic lymphadenopathy, etc. It has been reported that a small proportion of cases evolve to a more aggressive large cell malignant neoplasm, classed as a T-cell immunoblastic sarcoma, just as may occur in other variants of lympho-histiocytic predominant Hodgkin's disease (Robb-Smith, 1947). Kim et al (1978) and Mann et al (1979) have likened some cases to the category of diffuse mixed lymphocytic-histiocytic malignant lymphoma of the original Rappaport classification, where they may well have been concealed.

Reverting to the epithelioid granulomata, it can be difficult to distinguish sarcoidosis from *berylliosis* although under ordinary circumstances one would *Berylliosis* anticipate that the clinical history should provide a guide. Nevertheless berylliosis has certain specific features over or above a diffuse involvement of the node with non-caseating epithelioid granulomata. In *berylliosis* one does not see circumscribed epithelioid granulomata surrounded by lymphocytes, but instead there are sheets of epithelioid cells, with a higher proportion of giant cells and conchoidal bodies. The epithelioid cells are more loosely arranged and the lymphoid cells are restricted to small foci, usually in relation to the blood vessels. It is said that in contrast to sarcoidosis, the conchoidal or Schauman bodies do not react with elastin stains and that naphthochrom green is a specific stain for the beryllium granulomata.

The granulomatous reaction in *leprosy* is variable, determined to a large extent *Leprosy* by the immune response of the host (Turk and Waters, 1971). Rarely in the early stages of the disease there may be a generalised lymph node enlargement in which there is preservation of follicles and diffuse paracortical proliferation of vacuo- *Fig. II.26* lated epithelioid cells and Langhans' giant cells without caseation or necrosis but large numbers of acid-fast bacilli can be displayed (Symmers, 1970).

In chronic leprous lymphadenitis, one can distinguish the lepromatous and the tuberculoid reaction. The lepra cell is a large pale histiocyte with small delicate nucleus and eosinophilic foamy cytoplasm, which in some cases progresses to the formation of large intracellular vacuoles. Small foreign body type giant cells are present and show similar cytoplasmic features. These cell types clearly contrast with the normal lymphocyte population, and occur initially within the sinuses. At this stage there is preservation of follicles, but no marked follicular reaction. Later the histiocytes extend into the paracortex and medulla of the node, often obliterating normal architectural features. The organisms are usually abundant and the characteristic clusters or globi are apparent. In the tuberculoid type of reaction the diagnosis is much more difficult, and unless considered, may be mistaken for sarcoidosis as there is no caseation and organisms are very scanty and difficult to identify. However the proportion of giant cells is higher in tuberculoid leprosy, the granulomata are not so discrete and eosinophils are often present. In the late stages scarring and hyalinisation may occur.

4e. *Lymph node reactions in the lipidoses*

Although not a granulomatous reaction, it is convenient at this point to mention *Lipidoses* the lymph node reactions in the *lipidoses*. In these metabolic disorders, which are included in the large group of lysosomal diseases, there is a preservation of follicles and a proliferation of abnormal histiocytes in the paracortical tissues *Gaucher's disease* (Hers and van Hoff, 1973). In *Gaucher's disease* there are clumps of 15 to 20 of the characteristic cells surrounded by lymphocytes giving a superficial resem-*Fig. IV.3* blance to a sarcoidal reaction. It is usually possible to make out the brownish discolouration of the littoral cells due to the presence of haemosiderin.

The typical Gaucher cell has a small vesicular nucleus with a distinct nuclear membrane; binucleate forms are not uncommon and occasionally there may be cells with as many as ten nuclei. The extensive pale eosinophilic cytoplasm has a ground glass appearance which in thin sections may be seen to possess an irregular fibrillary appearance. The definition of such fibrils is accentuated in a PAS preparation and may then be considered diagnostic for this disorder, as the accumulated substance is a PAS positive cerebroside staining weakly with oil red O in unprocessed tissue.

Niemann-Pick In *Niemann-Pick disease* sphingomyelin accumulates in cells of all types and *disease* one does not see haemosiderosis in the littoral cells of the sinuses. The histiocyte is somewhat smaller than the Gaucher cell, and there are never more than two nuclei. The foamy faintly eosinophilic cytoplasm lacks striae and is diffusely PAS positive. The phospholipid can be identified by histochemical methods.

There is good evidence that adult Niemann-Pick disease and the familial sea-blue histiocyte syndrome (ceroid storage disease) are a single clinical entity and it is possible to identify the pigmented histiocytes in the sinuses of the lymph nodes (Wegmann et al, 1976; Quattrin et al, 1978).

Histiocytosis X The eosinophilic granulomatous variant of *histiocytosis X* has already been discussed (p. 77) but on occasions lymph nodes may be involved in a more diffuse histiocytic proliferation in the paracortical zone while the follicles have been *Fig. V.26* preserved (p. 188). The presence of eosinophils scattered in the interstitium may increase the difficulty of distinguishing this condition from Hodgkin's disease particularly the epithelioid type (p. 92). In histiocytosis X there are no Reed-Sternberg cells or transformed lymphocytes, follicles are preserved although they may be difficult to make out, and the majority of the histiocytes are not of the epithelioid type and are distributed irregularly and unevenly through the para-*Distinction from* cortex. Nevertheless a firm histological differential diagnosis from Hodgkin's *Hodgkin's disease* disease can be difficult and the clinical history and manifestations may influence the conclusions. If material is available for electron microscopy the presence or absence of the Langerhans-like bodies in the cytoplasm of the histiocytes is a significant factor.

5. The Preservation of Normal Follicles with non-malignant epithelial inclusions in the paracortex

The occurrence of secondary deposits of malignant neoplasms in a lymph node *Fig. III.11* in which the follicles can still be identified will be considered in a later chapter, but there are one or two 'catches' that can mislead the less experienced histologist.

Pre-parotid lymph nodes and less commonly, nodes in other sites (sub-maxillary and axillary regions) on occasions may have inclusions of columnar or rarely squamous epithelium in tubular or cystic form; the cystic zones may contain proteinageous material. The epithelium is well differentiated and often they are basal cells with a water clear cytoplasm which can be shown to be myoepethelium, but there is nothing to suggest a malignant process. It is generally believed that there are embryonic inclusions from the salivary glands (Garrett and Ada 1957), though there is some similarity to Cruikshank's (1965) benign lymphoepithelial eosin. There is also the possibility that one may see inclusions of epithelial cells associated with an adeno-lymphomatous proliferation in which the adenoid element is very minor.

Much more rarely endometrial tubules and associated stroma may be found in inguinal and pelvic lymph nodes (Lange, 1955), but whether arising from nectafolasia or lymphatic permeation is uncertain, as in many of the cases reported the eosin was a chance finding unassociated with peritoneal endometriosis; however, epithelial tubules somewhat resembling non-secretory endometrium but without any stroma-like tissue, are also occasionally found in the iliac and inguinal regions.

There may be confusion when a nodule of non-lymphoid tissue, containing lymph follicles and epithelial tubules is submitted as a lymph node for histological examination.

For example, a thyroid nodule in Hashimoto's disease with prominent reactive follicles intermingled with thyroid glandular tissue may be misinterpreted as a secondary deposit of a moderately differentiated adeno-carcinoma in a reactive lymph node; a similar difficulty may arise in a salivary gland containing a papillary cystadenoma lymphomatosum (adeno-lymphoma) with its granular eosin- *Adeno-lymphoma* ophilic epithelium. However, confusion should not occur if the detailed double *Fig. II.27* layered structure of the epithelium is recognized, or if it is realised that there is no basic nodal structure present, but simply a collection of follicles with reactive centres in relation to the papillary epithelium of the cystadenoma.

Finally there is the problem of thyroid inclusions in cervical lymph nodes (Roth, 1965). If the inclusion has a papillary or mixed papillary and follicular pattern, the eosin must be assumed to be a metastasis from a papillary carcinoma of the thyroid, but the matter is more complex if the inclusion has a follicular pattern. It has been shown that small inclusions of normal follicular thyroid tissue may rarely be found in lymph nodes; these nodules are usually small, usually consisting of less than a dozen follicles, and are found in the cortical portion of the node. In contrast metastases of a well differentiated follicular carcinoma usually replace the whole node and are associated with an overt thyroid swelling; furthermore, there are invariably some solid areas, atypical cell forms, a sinusoidal blood supply and, on occasions, renous invasion.

6. The Preservation of Normal Follicles and Paracortex with vascular lesions

In the examination of a lymph node, it should not be forgotten that examination of the hilum or the capsule may provide a diagnosis even where the rest of the node appears normal. Polyarteritis nodosa or giant cell arteritis can be recognized and on occasions thrombotic microangiopathy may be revealed. The characteristic lesion is a platelet thrombus, which has a hyaline appearance, occluding the lumena of the small blood vessels, which may develop microaneurysms.

Microangiopathy

Fig. II.28

Of rather different vascular lesion are the cortical glomana which have recently been identified (Van den Berg, Kaiserling and Lennert (1976). Initially these groups of closely packed cells in the cortex of nodes were described as 'naevus cells', and it has not yet been proved that some of these masses are not of this nature, but histology and electron microscopy has made it clear that the majority of such eosins are in fact hamartomatous glomangiomata.

In this chapter some of the lymph nodes changes have been discussed in which the follicles have been preserved and easily identified. In a later chapter there will be consideration of those conditions in which the alterations are predominantly in the sinuses though there is usually some preservation of the follicles as well and so it might appear that these should also be considered here; however from a visual point of view it will be the sinus proliferation which is the striking feature in the conditions to be considered in the fourth chapter, whereas in this chapter it is the preservation of the usually reactive follicle which is noticeable. The next chapter will consider those conditions in which abnormal follicular structures (pseudo or false follicles) are the predominant feature.

CHAPTER III

The normal architecture of the node is obliterated, completely or in part, and abnormal follicular structures, or pseudo-follicles, are present

ANALYTICAL
SUMMARY

1. **The pseudo-follicles consist of relatively normal lymphoid tissue:**

   Lymphoid nodules in a scarred node; amyloidosis; angio-follicular lymph node hyperplasia; accessory spleen

2. **The pseudo-follicles consist of monomorphic neoplastic lymphoid cells:**

   Follicular lymphoma; centroblastic sarcoma; chronic lymphocytic leukaemia; myeloid leukaemia; nodular sclerotic lymphosarcoma

3. **The pseudo-follicles consist of non-lymphoid neoplastic cells:**

   Metastatic carcinoma; melanoma

4. **The pseudo-follicles consist of polymorphic lympho-reticular cells:**

   Follicular lymphoma of mixed cellularity; nodular lymphocyte predominant Hodgkin's disease; nodular sclerotic Hodgkin's disease

IN THIS CHAPTER lymphadenopathies will be considered in which there is partial or total loss of the normal architectural features of the lymph node, and replacement by a cellular infiltrate having an intrinsic nodular or pseudo-follicular pattern. In all cases the structure of any nodule is distinct from that seen in primary and secondary follicles. The conditions to be described include a small number involving relatively normal lymphoid tissue, and several neoplastic processes. The former will be dealt with first, because these may show residual features of normal secondary follicles as a part of the disease process.

1. The pseudo-follicles consist of relatively normal lymphoid tissue

Extensive irregular fibrosis with the persistence of focal, ill-defined, collections of lymphocytes, plasma cells and histiocytes, may occur in *scarred* or *hyalinised* *lymph nodes* consequent on chronic inflammatory disease; some recognisable reactive centres remain and usually show regressive features or partial or complete hyalinisation. There may be fibrosis and hyaline sclerosis of the residual diffuse lymphoid tissue, in addition to the coarse bands of well formed collagen. Such appearances are entirely non-specific and may follow any of the chronic infective conditions already described in the previous chapter. It is essential to distinguish

Lymphoid nodules in a scarred node

Figs. III.1,2

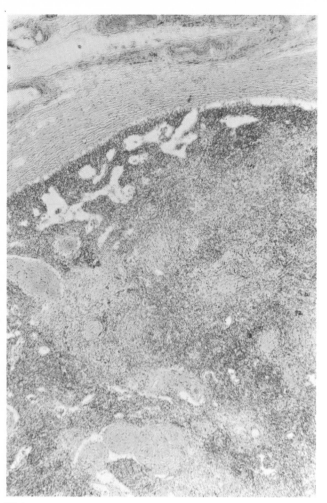

III.1

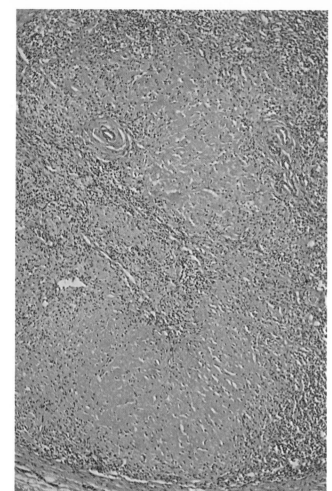

III.2

III.1-2   Scarred and Hyalinized Lymph Nodes

III.1   The normal architecture is not easily discerned as some of the nodules are residual lymphoid tissue, others hyaline masses. It is possible to recognise the hyaline masses in the medullary sinuses which should not be confused with trabecular thickening. The cortical sinuses are dilated and there is marked capsular thickening and obliterative arteritis.

III.2   In this example there are widespread hyaline nodules with considerable reduction of lymphoid tissue; the appearances can be confused with amyloid.

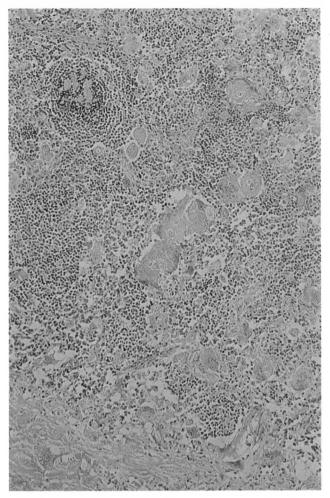

III.3a

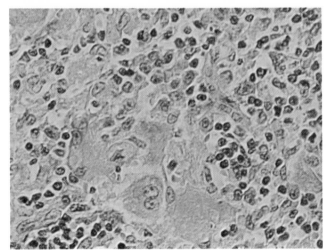

III.3b

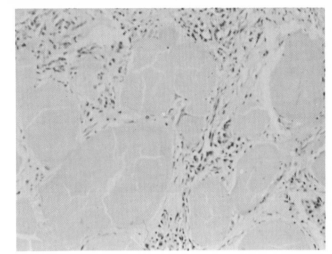

III.3c

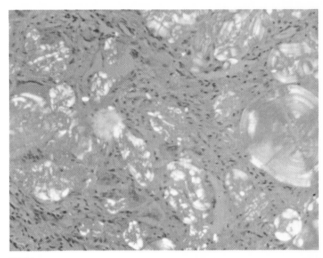

III.3d

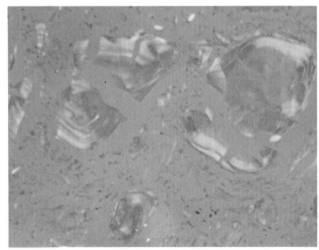

III.3e

III.3a-e   Amyloid Lymphadenopathy

III.3a   A follicle can be recognized but the main features are the nodules of amorphous acidophil material in the paracortical region.

III.3b   Amyloid masses, lymphocytes and plasma cells with some histiocytes; some are binucleate and require to be distinguished from Reed-Sternberg cells.

III.3c   Amyloid masses stained with congo-red.

III.3d   Amyloid masses stained with Thioflavin-T viewed under ultra-violet light.

III.3e   Amyloid masses stained with congo-red viewed under ultra-violet light.

this type of scarred lymph node from nodular sclerotic Hodgkin's disease and this will be discussed in relation to the latter condition (p. 116).

Amyloidosis

Amyloidosis may present as a lymphadenopathy but the microscopical appearances are very variable. On occasions the deposits may be restricted to the blood vessels in the follicles. In other cases it may occur in a much more diffuse

Fig. II.3 form, almost completely obliterating the lymph node architecture, only leaving some residual nodules of cells, mainly small lymphocytes, histiocytes and plasma cells. The latter are particularly numerous and are of value in distinguishing this 'amyloid tumour' (Isobe and Osserman, 1974) from simple hyaline fibrosis. Tissue immunoglobulin typing shows that the plasma cells are polyclonal and reactive in type, and so distinct from the amyloid deposits which may occur in multiple myeloma. The amyloid material itself does not stain consistently with the standard anti-immunoglobulin antisera but can be revealed by specific stains of which thioflavin T is the most valuable (Baker, de Nevasquez and MacLean, 1949; Mackenzie, 1963).

In the section dealing with the plasma cell type of giant lymph node hyperplasia, (p. 55) it was mentioned that there was a tendency to link this condition with

Angiofollicular lymph node hyperplasia another form of lymph node hyperplasia commonly known as *lymph nodal hamartoma, angiofollicular or hyaline-vascular lymph node hyperplasia etc.*, but the nomenclature of these two conditions has also been confused. In a typical

Fig. III.4 example of the hyaline vascular lymphoid hyperplasia, there is a considerably enlarged lymphoid nodule or mass of lymphoid tissue most often in the mediastinum but occasionally in the cervical or axillary region; in contrast to the plasma cell lymphoid hyperplasia, one does not usually find a group of nodes matted together, nor is there the very close relationship to the bronchi that can be seen in the plasma cell form. Sections usually reveal absence of normal follicles, but scattered through the mass of lymphoid tissue are small false follicles or nodules. At the centre of these nodules the cells are arranged concentrically (so-called 'onion skin' effect) and sometimes have a squamoid appearance, that may be confused with Hassall's corpuscles; often there is also a considerable deposit of hyaline material which may form quite large nodular masses. Between the nodules the lymphoid stroma is extensively vascularised, but lymph sinuses cannot usually be recognized. Around the large vessels there are concentric fibrohyaline masses which may undergo calcification.

Although the matter is still under discussion, it seems probable that this hyaline vascular lesion is of hamartomatous nature, though some authorities still support the view that it represents a burnt out chronic lymphadenitis. In any event the hyaline vascular condition should be distinguished both morphologically and clinically from the plasma cell lesion which is clearly a chronic inflammatory lymphadenopathy. Rarely chronic inflammatory changes may be found in the hyaline vascular variety of hyperplasia (Keller et al, 1972).

Infective granulomata, discussed in chapter II, may on occasions present a pseudo-follicular appearance, but usually normal, often reactive, follicles have been preserved while the granulomata themselves are so irregular in size and shape that they are unlikely to be regarded as 'pseudo-follicles'.

Finally a *small accessory spleen* or splenunculus may be confused with a splenic hilar lymph node, especially if the Malpighian nodules are hyperplastic and contain prominent reactive centres, with tingible body macrophages and 'fibrin' deposits centrally. In these circumstances the red pulp between the nodules may be reduced in extent or compressed, and therefore not obviously recognizable at low magnification. However detailed examination reveals features distinctive of splenic architecture, with thick walled arterioles in the centre of the lymphoid nodules (thus showing them to be splenic Malpighian nodules) and the system of sinuses with plump eosinophilic sinus lining cells, red cells and leucocytes comprising the red pulp. An accessory spleen may of course be involved by the same pathological processes as a lymph node, and when extensively involved by Hodgkin's disease the distinction from hilar lymph nodes may be more difficult.

Accessory spleen

Fig. III.5

2. The pseudo-follicles consist of monomorphic neoplastic lymphoid cells

Some of the difficulties of diagnosis of those lymphomas having an intrinsic nodular pattern have already been described and tabulated (Table 5, p. 57), to assist the differential diagnosis from reactive follicular hyperplasia.

*Follicular lymphomas**, at present more often termed *nodular lymphomas*, have a spectrum of cytological forms, and while the diagnosis of neoplasm from reactive hyperplasia may be simple in some cases, it can be extremely difficult; the relationship of nodular lymphomas to other lymphomas is reviewed in the section on classification in Appendix I, and only the features of diagnostic import will be considered here. It commonly presents as a generalised lymphadenopathy. The individual lymph nodes may be considerably enlarged and though a group of nodes may be involved, they are not usually matted together. The capsule may be infiltrated by lymphoid cells having cytological identity with those comprising the tumour nodules, and in many cases there is pericapsular infiltration with definite nodule formation by the tumour cells.

Follicular lymphoma

Fig. III.6

Within the lymph node as demarcated by the capsule (which is often slightly thickened), there is usually complete loss of normal architecture and reactive type follicles and sinuses cannot be discerned, even with the aid of reticulin preparations. The abnormal tumour follicles are distributed randomly throughout the node, and characteristically are all rounded in shape and relatively uniform in

---

* Synonyms: Centroblastic-centrocytic follicular lymphoma (Kiel); Prolymphocytic-lymphoblastic nodular lymphosarcoma (WHO); Well or poorly differentiated nodular lymphocytic lymphoma (Rappaport); Small or large follicle cell follicular lymphoma (NLI) (National Lymphoma Investigation); Follicular type of follicular centre cell lymphoma (Lukes and Collins); Small or large lymphoid follicular lymphoma (Dorfman); Lymphoid follicular reticulosis (Robb-Smith, 1938); Brill-Symmers' disease (Craver, 1934): Follicular lymphoblastoma (Baehr, 1932). The initial bracketed designations indicate the six classifications assessed in the U.S. National Cancer Institute's retrospective review (1978) and the nomenclature is that submitted by the authors for the review documents; details of these classifications are to be found in Appendix I.

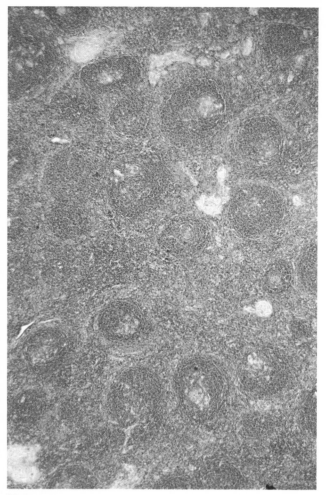

III.4a

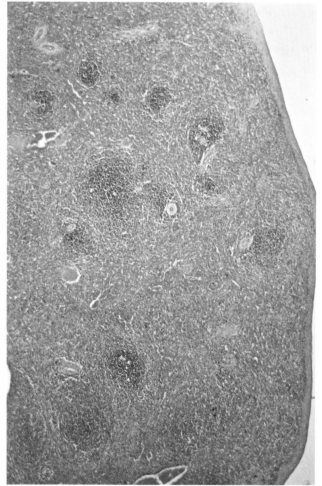

III.4b

III.4a-b Angiofollicular Lymph Node Hyperplasia

III.4a The nodules have a superficial resemblance to germinal centres, but it soon becomes apparent that the pale central area is formed of a complex vascular hyaline structure lacking macrophages and what would appear to be paracortical tissue lacks sinuses.

III.4b The pattern of the hyaline vascular structure at the centre of the nodules can be recognised and has a superficial resemblance to a Hassall's corpuscle.

III.5 Splenunculus

Apart from the engorgement of the red pulp, critical examination reveals the structural features of the Malpighian bodies and the littoral cells of the venous sinuses.

III.5

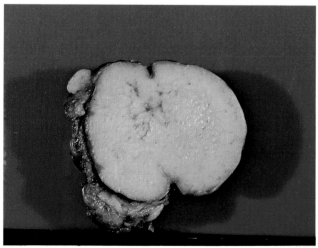

III.6a

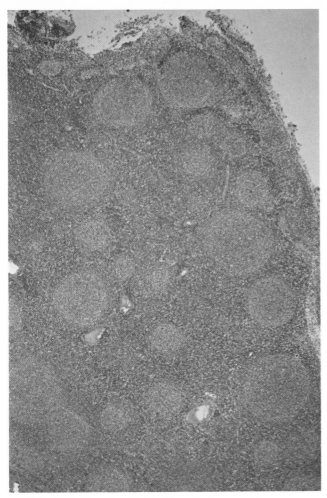

III.6b

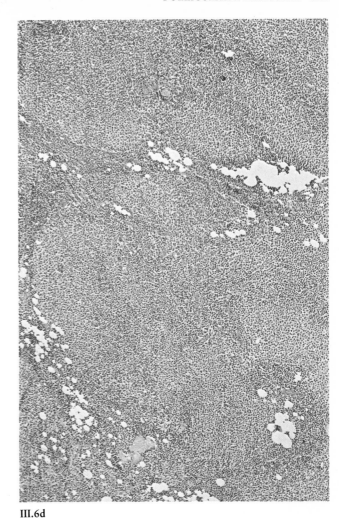

III.6d

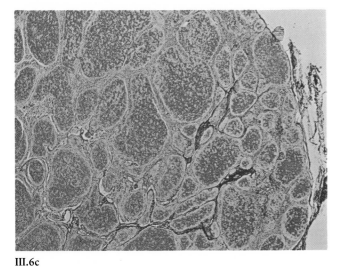

III.6c

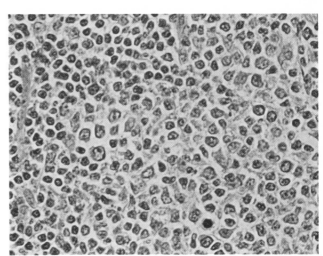

III.6e

III.6a-e Follicular Lymphoma

◀ **III.6a** Lymph node (actual size). Multiple small nodules can be discerned on the cut surface.

III.6b The neoplastic follicles are relatively uniform and though clearly demarcated from the stroma, lack a cuff of small lymphocytes or macrophages.

III.6c Reticulin impregnation. The demarcation between the false follicles and the stroma is more easily recognized than in the ordinary stained preparations. There is a lack of vascular pattern in the nodules while the compressed reticulin of the stroma is easily seen.

III.6d The follicular pattern in the periadenoid tissue can be easily seen although the demarcation between the false follicles and the stroma is not so clear, while destruction of reticulin and coalescence of follicles indicates more rapidly progressive disease.

III.6e Margin of follicle from section III.6d. Small and large non-cleaved cells (centroblasts) predominate though a minority of cleaved cells (centrocytes) are also present. There is in addition some mitotic activity. This cytological pattern confirms the low power impression of rapidly progressive disease.

103

size. However, the size of the follicles may vary greatly between different cases, with small follicular, intermediate and giant follicular forms. The latter is the classical Brill-Symmers disease or giant follicular lymphoma. Occasionally the neoplastic nodules are falsely demarcated by peripheral 'cracking' due to a fixation shrinkage artefact, which rarely affects normal follicles having an intact reticulin framework.

Follicular lymphoma   The tumour nodules ('false follicles') differ from normal reactive centres in several respects. Firstly they are not limited to the cortex, and they do not contain the usual proportions of the varieties of cell present in reactive centres, namely tingible body macrophages, and the various phases of B-lymphocyte transformation (cleaved and non-cleaved type cells). Instead neoplastic follicles are comprised predominently of one cell type, corresponding morphologically to a narrow phase of B-lymphocyte transformation, either the cleaved or non-cleaved cell (centrocyte or centroblast of Lennert). The cells in the interfollicular zone may be normal small lymphocytes in the early phase of the disease where the process is confined to the follicles or may be of the same cytological type as in the tumour follicles, making it difficult to distinguish follicles from interfollicular areas. Apart from the value of reticulin impregnations which will be considered shortly, it is ordinarily quite easy to recognize a follicular lymphoma by examining a stained slide with the naked eye or hand lens.

The lack of clear demarcation of follicles is aggravated by the complete absence of the small lymphocyte cuff, which occurs around reactive follicles. Mitoses may be present within and without the follicles, but are not numerous. However, just as between different cases there may be marked differences in the standard size of the neoplastic follicles, so also there may be marked differences between the principal cells comprising the follicles in different cases.

As has already been mentioned, in the majority of cases the predominant neoplastic cell is of the small cleaved type (centrocytes), less often the small non-cleaved cells (centroblasts) predominate. However, even in these cases variable numbers of cleaved or folded type cells are present, both small and large, together with some larger forms of the non-cleaved cell, having more basophilic cytoplasm and a more prominent nucleolus (large transformed type − large non-cleaved cell). In fact all four types of cells (small and large cleaved and non-cleaved) are always present, but in an individual case any of these different morphological forms of the B-lymphocyte may predominate, and thus alter the overall cytological features of the nodular lymphoma quite radically. For example nodules may be *Figs. III.6e–h* comprised mainly of small cleaved type cells, or of large complexly folded cells or of small or large transformed type cells. Those tumours in which the follicles consist of large cells (centroblasts), often with prominent nucleoli, were once described as nodular reticulum cell sarcomas (malignant lymphoma, histiocytic, nodular), and it is recognized that the classical forms, composed of small lymphocytes, may over the years progress to this more aggressive large cell form. Of this group, the most aggressive tumours appear to be those composed of large non-cleaved cells, the large cleaved cell follicular centre cell lymphomas running a relatively more benign course. (Butler et al, 1975).

Characteristically those neoplasms composed of small cells retain their follic- *Sarcomatous change in follicular lymphomas* ular pattern and have a good prognosis. The appearance of larger cells with an increased mitotic rate is normally associated with loss of follicular pattern and a bad prognosis, thus constituting the so-called 'sarcomatous change'. Loss of the distinct nodular appearance, with blurring and fusion of the neoplastic nodules, may also occur in the absence of progression to this large 'sarcoma cell type'. This usually occurs in follicles consisting of small transformed type cells, but also having some significant components of cleaved cells and large transformed types (Galton et al, 1978). However, malignant tumours of these cell types may initially be diffuse (chapter V, p. 181).

The diagnosis and recognition of the phase of development of follicular lymphoma is greatly facilitated by the use of a reticulin impregnation. It will at once be apparent that the neoplastic follicles are free from reticulin fibres except immediately around blood vessels, but these follicles are sharply outlined by the compressed paracortical tissue rich in blood vessels. When a follicular lymphoma is changing to the more aggressive 'sarcomatous' form, there is destruction of this paracortical reticulin background and the follicles merge one with another; *Fig. III.6d* this may be mistaken for a diffuse infiltration. In the aggressive form in which there is a change in cell type from the cleaved cell to the large darkly staining cells, it may appear on ordinary staining preparation that the follicular pattern has been maintained but reticulin impregnations will reveal that there has been a destruction of argyrophil fibres.

On occasions the tumour cells may show cytoplasmic vacuolation with nuclear *Signet-ring variant* distortion recalling the mucin-secreting 'signet-ring' carcinoma; it has been shown that this appearance is associated with immunoglobulin accumulation in the *Fig. III.6l* cytoplasm (Kim et al, 1978; Van den Tweel et al, 1978; Lennert, 1978).

The retention of follicular pattern may be associated with the phase of transformation cycle 'arrest' of the majority of the neoplastic cells, for normal B-lymphocytes, after entry into reactive follicles are retained only to a certain stage of transformation, beyond which those destined to become plasma cells leave the follicles. A possible mechanism for follicular retention, based upon surface immunoglobulin or surface complement receptors, has been suggested (Taylor, 1976), while Lennert et al (1978) believe that a mantle of dendritic reticulum cells determines the nodularity.

Thus in the classical case the diagnosis may not be difficult, and the prognosis should be related both to the predominant cell types, comprising the neoplastic follicles and to the retention of a follicular pattern or the occurrence of 'diffuse change'. Generally a poor prognosis is indicated by (a) the loss of a follicular pattern throughout the node, (b) the evolution of an increased proportion of transformed type cells (small and large non-cleaved centroblasts).

Nevertheless, the diagnosis in early cases remains difficult. Tingible body

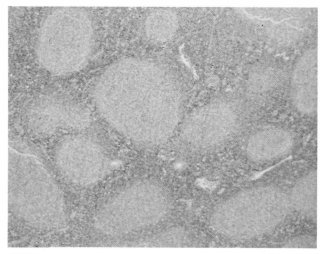

III.6f

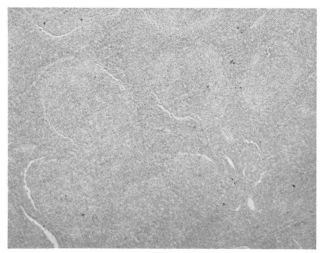

III.6g

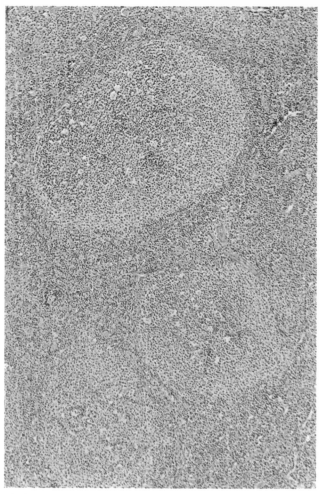

III.6i

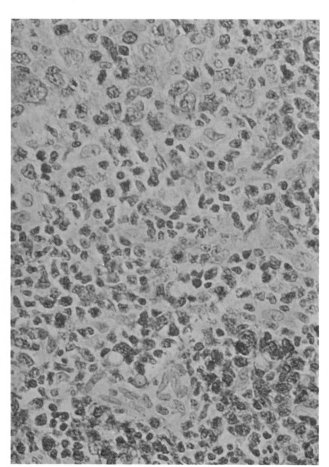

III.6h

III.6f-i   Immunoglobulin in Follicular Lymphoma

III.6f,g   Sequential sections have been stained by immunoperoxidase for anti-λ (6f) and anti-K (6g). The upper section (6f) shows that many of the interfollicular cells are anti-λ positive whereas there are no cells stained for anti-K, thus indicating a monotypic (monoclonal) pattern. The artifactual cracking of the follicle is well seen in Fig. III.6g.

III.6h   High-power view of section 6f. stained for anti-λ. The bottom right-hand corner shows the interfollicular plasmacytoid cells strongly stained, whereas in the neoplastic follicles, only a few large cells are stained.

III.6i   This section shows a follicular pattern in which there is little evidence of lymphocytic cuffing but tingible body macrophages are present in the follicles which are made up largely of small transformed type lymphocytes with a limited number of cleaved cells (centrocytes). Accordingly there could be doubt as to whether this is a follicular lymphoma or a reactive condition.

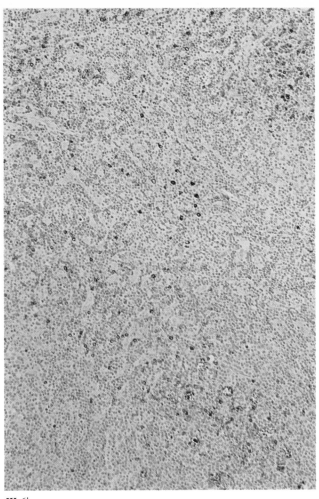

III.6j

III.6k

III.6j-l   Immunoglobulin in Follicular Lymphoma

III.6j-k   Sequential sections of case 6i stained for anti-K (6j) and anti-λ (6k) shows that it is a monotypic staining pattern, positive anti-K cells are present both in the follicles and stromal area while there is no evidence of any anti-λ staining. Accordingly this would indicate a follicular lymphoma rather than a reactive hyperplasia and the subsequent progress of the case confirmed this.

III.6l   'Signet cell change' in Follicular Lymphoma. Portion of a follicle showing large cleaved cells (centrocytes) with cytoplasmic vacuoles and nuclear displacement resulting in a 'signet ring' effect; these cells are interspersed with cleaved cells and lymphocytes. This is an immunoperoxidase preparation stained for anti-λ and the cytoplasm around the vacuoles is positive.

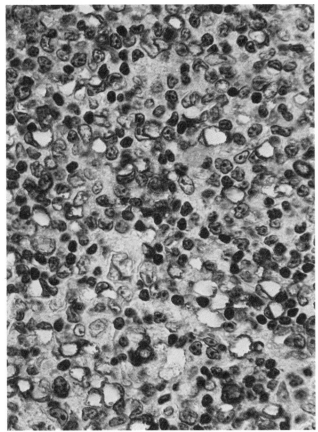

III.6l

107

Figs. III.6i–k macrophages are present in small numbers in most cases, but may be quite numerous, so producing real difficulty in making the distinction from vigorously reacting centres. However, if the lymphocyte cuff is present and if there appears to be evidence of normal production of transformed lymphocytes and plasma cells around the follicles then the condition is a reactive one, and not a follicular lymphoma, even though in extreme hyperplasia there may be reactive follicles in paracortex and medulla as well as in cortex. Immunoglobulin studies can be of great help.

Fig. III.7 Continuing with the monomorphic nodular lymphomas, it is necessary to recognize that a highly malignant type of follicular lymphoma may arise de novo, as opposed to developing from a pre-existing less aggressive form of follicular lymphoma. This tumour, *a follicular centroblastic sarcoma*, corresponds histologically to Lennert's primary centroblastic (germinoblastic) malignant lymphoma or Lukes and Collins' large non-cleaved follicle centre cell (FCC) lymphoma. It occurs in the elderly, usually presenting initially as a mass of rapidly enlarging nodes in a single site (often inguinal) and a short history with no indication of previous lymphadenopathy suggestive of follicular lymphoma. The nodular pattern may be difficult to make out, even on low power, when the whole node is replaced by neoplastic cells, though a reticulin impregnation may reveal the follicles. However, in contrast to the ordinary cleaved cell follicular lymphoma, one does not see a reticulin free follicle surrounded by a compressed vascularised reticulin stroma. Instead there are scattered reticulin fibres in the nodule, and there is coalescence of the follicles with stromal destruction. The cell type corresponds to a malignant transformed lymphocyte, (lymphoblasts of old fashioned terminology) with a narrow basophilic rim of cytoplasm and a large leptochromatic nucleus with medium sized nucleoli near the nuclear membrane. There is considerable mitotic activity and it is not uncommon to see scattered histiocytes, sometime epithelioid, resulting in a superficial resemblance to the Burkitt type. In fact this lymphoma may be more closely related to classical Burkitt's lymphoma than previously supposed, for Mann et al (1976) have demonstrated follicle formation in the early phases of Burkitt's lymphoma.

Pseudo follicles in leukaemia *Leukaemic involvement of a lymph node* is ordinarily diffuse and will be dealt with in chapter V, but can on occasions simulate a follicular proliferation. In *lymphocytic leukaemia* there can be a marked infiltration of leukaemia cells into the capsule, trabeculae and perivascular tissue, which are separated from the paracortical tissue by empty lymph sinuses; the paracortical area may be mistaken for a follicle but a reticulin impregnation will reveal the true state of affairs.

Chronic lymphocytic leukaemia Occasionally in *chronic lymphocytic leukaemia*, pseudofollicular proliferation centres may be seen and are of two types – either the small lymphocytes are more closely set together in darker zones, or there are lighter zones formed of prolymphocytes and lymphoblasts (large non-cleaved cells) in which the individual cells are more widely separated one from another than in the rest of the paracortex. These nodules are seldom more than 500 μm in diameter and a reticulin im-

Fig. III.9

pregnation shows that there is no perifollicular compression of the fibrils as in follicular lymphoma, and cleaved cells are not present. Lennert (1975) who first called attention to these proliferation centres, said that they could be seen in most biopsy cases, but this is not our experience.

Another feature of diffusely infiltrating leukaemia that can cause confusion is that residual pockets of the normal cell population of the node often remain and appear in sections as isolated 'follicles' of lymphocytes. In these circumstances the normal architectural features of the node are not visible and the greater part of the node is completely replaced by a monomorphic population of cells of the leukaemia type. The leukaemic process is usually an *acute myeloid leukaemia, or myelomonocytic leukaemia* and the residual follicles of small dark lymphocytes contrast clearly with the diffuse 'sheets' of leukaemic cells; less commonly this may be found in chronic lymphocytic leukaemia. A similar picture may be seen in *acute reticulosis of infancy (Letterer-Siwe syndrome)* and certain *diffusely infiltrating malignant neoplasms,* either *anaplastic carcinoma* or *sarcoma.* *Myeloid leukaemia*

Fig. III.10

Fig. III.11

Broad bands of fibrosis, not confined to capsular or trabecular thickening, may be seen in the so-called '*nodular sclerotic lymphosarcoma*' as described by Bennett and Millet (1969) and Bennett (1975). This variety of lymphoma, which it would be better to designate as nodular sclerotic malignant lymphoma, does not form cellular neoplastic nodules (follicles) as does classical follicular lymphoma, but instead develops a coarser nodular pattern due to the occurrence of broad bands of fibrosis, some of which run circumferentially around enclosed 'nodules' of malignant lymphoma cells. This scirrhous reaction has been observed in malignant lymphomas of all types and is associated with an improved prognosis. The differential diagnosis from classical follicular lymphoma is not difficult, for the neoplastic cells are diffusely distributed within the confines of the fibrous tissue, and usually show no tendency to intrinsic follicle formation. However, in most of these tumours the cytology of the lymphoma cells places them in the follicle centre cell group (cleaved and non-cleaved) as defined by Lukes and Collins (1975), while Lennert (1978) suggests that the majority should be regarded as follicular lymphomas. The diagnosis from nodular sclerotic Hodgkin's disease is also not difficult for Reed-Sternberg cells and eosinophils are not present in nodular sclerotic 'lymphosarcoma' which has a characteristic quite uniform cellular appearance. *Nodular sclerotic lymphosarcoma*

Fig. III.8

3. The pseudo-follicles consist of non-lymphoid neoplastic cells

The so-called *lympho-epithelioma,* which ordinarily represents a secondary deposit of an anaplastic carcinoma, often of nasopharyngeal origin, may in a lymph node produces the type of appearance in which there are nodules of neoplastic cells lying in the lymphoid stroma. Such neoplasms should be readily recognized on critical cytological examination, as the nuclei do not closely resemble those of the true lymphoma group, particularly the immunoblastic sarcoma group *Metastatic carcinoma*

Fig. III.11

Fig. V.13c

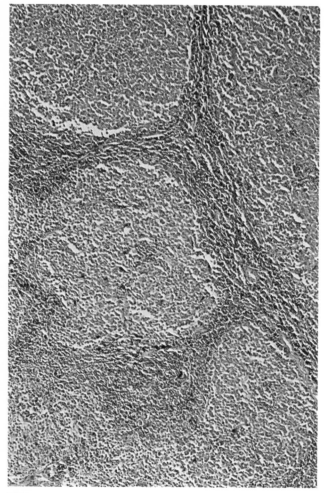

III.7a

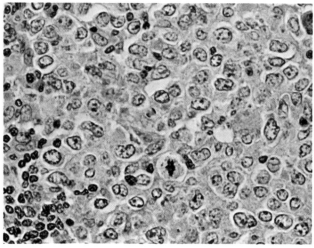

III.7b

III.7a-b   Follicular centroblastic sarcoma (large non-cleaved)

III.7a   The nodular pattern is more easily discerned than is often the case, but the demarcation is less well shown in the right-hand side of the field.

III.7b   The false follicles consist of bizarre large non-cleaved cells (centroblasts) and very few cleaved cells (centrocytes). Mitoses and cellular atypia is marked.

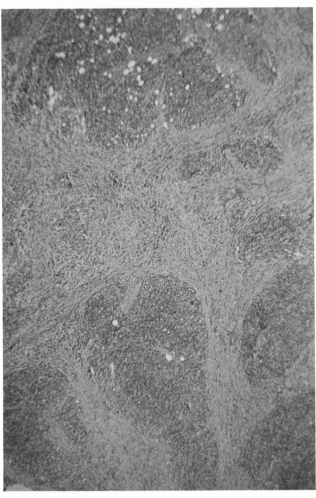

III.8a

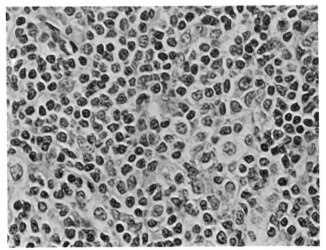

III.8b

III.8a-b   Nodular Sclerotic Malignant Lymphoma

III.8a   The characteristic features are foci of monomorphic malignant lymphomatous tissue separated by coarse septa of fibrous tissue. In this example the foci of malignant tissue have extended beyond the lymph nodes to the periadenoid tissue.

III.8b   The nodular sclerotic variant is not associated with any particular cell type; in this example the majority of the neoplastic cells are of the small cleaved cell type (poorly differentiated lymphocytic).

(formerly malignant lymphoma, histiocytic; reticulum cell sarcoma). The nuclei of the anaplastic carcinoma are more obviously hyperchromatic and pleomorphic with very variable nuclear outline and much variation in the number and size of any nucleoli present.

Metastatic neoplasms in lymph nodes may also produce a nodular appearance in other ways. Firstly by inciting a sarcoid response as described (p. 89) but also when occurring as relatively well defined nodular deposits of tumour within a lymph node. The residual part of the node often shows follicular and, paracortical hyperplasia and usually sinus histiocytosis. The cytological appearances of metastatic nodules are obviously as variable as the number of possible primary *Melanoma* tumours. Malignant melanoma is particularly important in the differential diag-*Fig. III.12* nosis of lymph node biopsies, for it may occur in nodular or diffuse form and have a carcinomatous appearance, or alternatively appear as a spindle cell sarcoma, or as a wildly pleomorphic tumour with giant cells and frequent mitoses.

4. The pseudo-follicles consist of polymorphic lympho-reticular cells

Follicular
lymphoma of mixed Although it has been stressed that the various nodular lymphadenopathies so far
cellularity considered are monomorphic, yet it must be recognized that this is a relative term and that there is often an admixture of various types of histiocytes and lymphocytes of cleaved and non-cleaved types. The nodular lymphomas of mixed (lymphocytic/histiocytic) types according to Rappaport's classification, are now considered to be follicular lymphomas, the mixed appearance being due to the presence of large and small cleaved and non-cleaved forms.

It remains to consider nodular lymphadenopathies in which there is a true mixed cell population. With few exceptions these are manifestations of Hodgkin's disease. However, it should not be assumed that this makes diagnosis easy for the nodular character may not be obvious and there is the possibility of confusion with the scarred lymph node mentioned at the beginning of this chapter.

These forms of *nodular Hodgkin's disease* fall into the lymphocyte/histiocyte predominant group and are distinct from nodular sclerosing Hodgkin's disease in which the nodules are demarcated partly or entirely by dense fibrous bands.

The different histological sub-types of Hodgkin's disease are reviewed in a later chapter (p. 209). Lukes and Butler (1966) distinguished several sub-varieties of lymphocyte/histiocyte predominant Hodgkin's disease (often simply termed lymphocyte predominant Hodgkin's disease – LP-HD), according to whether the major cell types was the small lymphocyte, or whether there were a significant number of definite histiocytes, or whether the cell population occurred diffusely or in a distinctly nodular form. The nodular form had already been characterised by Harrison (1952) and others as benign or nodular Hodgkin's disease. In the Rye conference condensation of the classification of Hodgkin's disease (see Appendix I), the designation 'LP–HD' (lymphocyte predominant) was used to include even those forms with many histiocytes. Poppema et al's (1979) suggestion that this should be regarded as a distinct entity is mentioned briefly in the Appendix (p. 236).

Both the pure lymphocyte predominant and the mixed lymphocyte/histiocyte predominant varieties occur either in nodular or diffuse forms. In each type the nodules are of relatively uniform size, are rounded or wedge-shaped and are usually only demarcated from the surrounding cells by their concentric arrangement, though there may be fine septa of fibrous tissue. There is no lymphocytic cuff, and the cell population of the nodules does not differ markedly from the cell population in the remainder of the diseased lymph node.

Nodular lymphocytic predominant Hodgkin's disease

Such nodules may occur throughout the enlarged lymph node or only in parts, the remainder being occupied by an identical cell population distributed diffusely. The normal architecture of the node is usually destroyed, but persisting sinuses or reactive follicles may be seen at the periphery. These reactive follicles are clearly distinct from the nodules of Hodgkin's disease.

In the pure lymphocyte, and the lymphocyte/histiocyte form, true Reed-Sternberg cells are uncommon and it may be necessary to search several sections for a diagnostic cell. However, mononuclear Hodgkin cells occur somewhat more frequently, though they are still much less numerous than in the mixed cellular form of Hodgkin's disease. Lukes and Butler (1966) described in lymphocyte/histiocyte predominant Hodgkin's disease a special form of giant cell as 'peculiar and abnormal reticulum cells ... with folded overlapping lobes, with delicate lacy chromatin and small nucleoli'. They reported that these cells were quite numerous, but they lacked the distinct prominent nucleoli and thick nuclear membrane of the true Reed-Sternberg cell. The relation of these cells to Reed-Sternberg cells remains uncertain. Histiocytes are usually present in small numbers even in the pure lymphocyte form but in lymphocyte/histiocyte predominant disease they may be so numerous as to dominate the histological pictures. Some of these histiocytes have pale granular cytoplasm and may be termed epithelioid cells. The size of these cells varies according to the amount of cytoplasm which may be extensive. The nucleus is oval and regular with delicate nuclear membrane and a small nucleolus. However, binucleate forms occur, but the nuclei are also small and delicate and should not be mistaken for true Reed-Sternberg cells.

The differential diagnosis is from those reactive hyperplasias in which histiocytes occur singly or in clusters, particularly toxoplasmosis, dermatopathic lymphadenitis, and some of the granulomatous conditions (chapter II).

The pure lymphocyte predominant form, occurring in nodular pattern, may be difficult to distinguish from follicular lymphoma. It is said that this diagnostic problem may be encountered in children, but almost all such cases prove to be Hodgkin's disease, for one should never consider making a diagnosis of follicular lymphoma in a patient under the age of twenty, unless all the histological features of follicular lymphoma are present. The ultimate criterion for the diagnosis of lymphocyte predominant Hodgkin's disease is the admixture of normal and abnormal cells of which the Reed-Sternberg cell is the classic example.

113

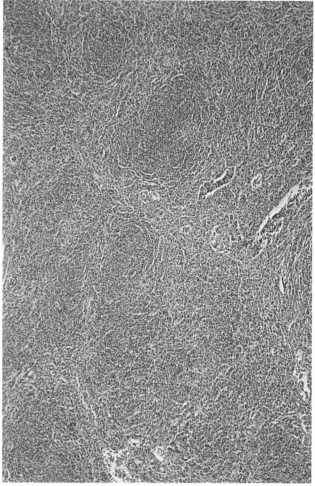

III.9

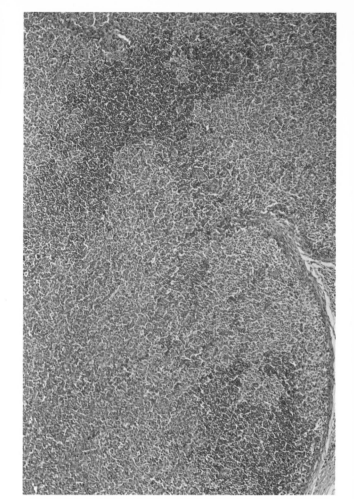

III.10a

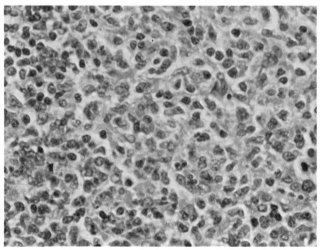

III.10b

III.9 Pseudo Follicular Pattern in Chronic Lymphocytic Leukaemia

Chronic lymphocytic leukaemia. There is a diffuse paracortical infiltration with small lymphocytes and the sinuses are also distended; the surviving paracortical tissue consists of closely packed lymphocytes normal and transformed, giving an impression of a follicular pattern but a reticulin impregnation would reveal that this is paracortex and the true follicles are compressed and inconspicuous (cf. also Figs V.1 and V.2).

III.10a-b Pseudo Follicular Pattern in Acute Myeloid Leukaemia

III.10a Acute myeloid leukaemia. Once again there is paracortical infiltration but the contrast between the irregular false follicle of surviving paracortical lymphoid tissue and the sheets of myeloid cells is more obvious.

III.10b It is possible to recognize the cellular range of the infiltrate from the delicate myeloblasts to the segmented promyelocytes and myelocytes (including eosinophilic forms). The chloroacetate esterase staining technique is of value in confirming the diagnosis (cf. Fig. V.24).

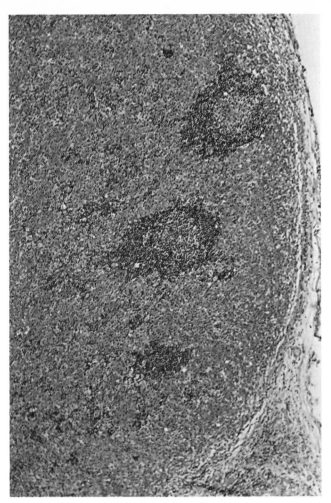

III.11a

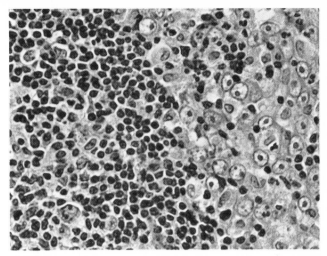

III.11b

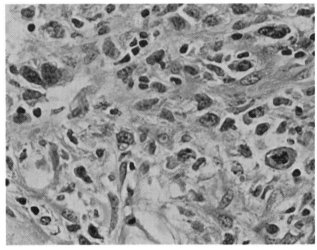

III.11c

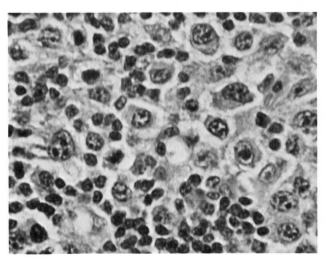

III.11d

III.11a-d   Pseudo Follicles of Residual Lymphoid Tissue in Metastatic Infiltration of Nodes

III.11a   Lymph node showing a diffuse infiltration of the para-cortical tissue and sinuses by an anaplastic carcinoma – so called lympho-epithelioma – with surviving islands of lymphoid tissue consisting of follicles with the peri-follicular paracortical tissue. This appearance may be seen in a whole range of metastatic neoplasms diffusely infiltrating a lymph node.

III.11b   High power view of lympho-epitheliomatous invasion of lymph node showing the characteristic acidophil cytoplasm of the cells with a pachychromatic nucleus, having a prominent nucleolus and dense nuclear membrane.

III.11c   High power view of secondary carcinoma of bronchus resulting in a diffuse infiltration of a lymph node.

III.11d   High power view of metastatic infiltration of a lymph node by a poorly differentiated malignant lymphoma, in this case a plasma cell sarcoma. It is possible to recognize a range of cell types from some resembling a plasma cell to multi-nucleate types and cells whose identity it would be difficult to determine but for the related plasma cell differentiated forms.

The *nodular sclerotic form of Hodgkin's disease* was distinguished by Lukes in 1963 (Hanson, 1964; Lukes and Butler, 1966) and shown to have a more favourable prognosis than the mixed cellular form of Hodgkin's disease. The criteria for the diagnosis of nodular sclerosing Hodgkin's disease were laid down by Lukes and Butler, but have since been modified to some extent by different centres in different ways. This had led to considerable variation in the reported frequency of nodular sclerosing Hodgkin's disease, probably partly due to differing histological criteria as well as to some true variation in the incidence of different types of Hodgkin's disease.

Figs. III.15a–c The diagnostic criteria given by Lukes and Butler and by Hanson included bands of connective tissue, composed of mature collagen and of fibroblasts, that circumscribe nodules of abnormal lymphoid tissue. Lukes stressed the value of polarised light birefringence in distinguishing these mature collagen bands from the more diffuse 'immature fibrosis' of other forms of Hodgkin's disease. The diagnostic difficulties arise in relation to the fact that only part of a diseased lymph node may show this characteristic nodular fibrosis, the remainder having a more diffuse pattern. It can be imagined that a diagnosis of nodular sclerosing Hodgkin's disease would be difficult if the section did not include a definite nodular area. In such circumstances the presence of a thickened capsule with fibrous spurs extending inwards obliquely, helps to make a diagnosis of nodular sclerosis – though others would consider this to represent nothing more than trabecular fibrosis, thus placing the lesion in the mixed cellular group where such changes do occur.

Figs. III.15m–o Some authors have stressed the presence of peculiar variants of the Reed-Sternberg cell – so-called 'lacunar cells' as diagnostic of the nodular sclerosing type of Hodgkin's disease. Lacunar cells have abundant pale clear cytoplasm with sharply defined borders and are often situated in a clear space separating the individual cells from the surrounding lymphocytes. This clear lacuna is a result of artefactual shrinkage collapse of the extensive lacunar cell cytoplasm, and is particularly apparent in formalin fixed tissue. In Zenker fixed tissue this change is less obvious. The nucleus is often multilobulate, characteristically delicate in type, with thin nuclear membrane, lacy chromatin, and small but distinct nucleoli within each of the nuclear lobules (Anagnostou et al, 1977). These cells are seen most characteristically in classical nodular sclerosis. Some authors believe them to be pathognomonic of the nodular sclerosing type of Hodgkin's disease and if they are present, are prepared to make the diagnosis even when there is absence of capsular fibrous spurs or of distinct fibrous bands. This appearance has often been termed the cellular phase of nodular sclerosis and may progress to the classical fibrotic form. But not everyone accepts this interpretation with the result that some cases with this appearance are classified as nodular sclerosis while in other centres they would be classified as mixed cellular Hodgkin's disease.

For a diagnosis of nodular sclerotic Hodgkin's disease, we believe that definite collagenous bands must be present at least in part of the tissue and that in doubtful cases, multiple sections or blocks should be examined. Lymph node biopsies in which there are only occasional fibrous spurs or some trabecular fibrosis together with cells showing cytoplasmic collapse resembling classical lacunar cells, should be regarded as suspicious of nodular sclerosis particularly in young female patients with mediastinal disease.

The diagnosis of nodular sclerosing Hodgkin's disease is further complicated by the occurrence of cases in which the fibrotic bands are ill-formed and the nodules thus ill-defined. These cases are often associated with central necrosis, though necrosis occurs more rarely in nodular sclerosis than in mixed cellular Hodgkin's disease. The overall appearances are suggestive of a granulomatous *Figs. III.15i–k* reaction and bordering the necrotic areas are large polypoid cells, which, though *Fig. V.19* atypical, are not diagnostic of Hodgkin's disease for they often lack prominent nucleoli. They have indistinct clear or pale eosinophilic cytoplasm and indistinct cell boundaries. With numerous eosinphils present there may be a resemblance to eosinophilic granuloma. In addition these cells show nuclear degeneration and eosinophilic cytoplasmic degeneration – a form of the cellular necrobiosis which is believed by some to be of value in the diagnosis of Hodgkin's disease generally (Cross, 1969). However, the diagnosis of Hodgkin's disease may be made by careful high power examination when occasional Reed-Sternberg type cells may be found, with thick nuclear membranes, prominent nucleoli and often lobulated nuclei.

Lacunar cells may also be difficult to identify when they occur in large numbers packed close together, for their characteristic appearance is in part due to the contrast between an isolated lacunar cell and the surrounding dark lymphocytes. Lacunar cells occurring together appear as large clumped clear cells, with or without cytoplasmic collapse, but they may be identified by the characteristic polylobulated nucleus. Finally sheets of lacunar type cells may occur throughout a lymph node with little semblance of any fibrosis or nodular pattern. These appearances may suggest lymphocyte depleted Hodgkin's disease but such cases often show distinct fibrous bands at other levels in the node, or in an adjacent lymph node. Such a case is illustrated in Figs. III. 15 and V. 19, which are sections from the same case, thus showing the value of several sections or repeat biopsies in cases where diagnosis and categorisation is uncertain.

The most difficult differential diagnosis in nodular sclerosis is the scarred lymph node mentioned at the beginning of the chapter. Here the node is largely replaced by fibrous hyaline material in which are small islands of lymphoid tissue which consist of small lymphocytes, occasionally transformed lymphocytes, plasma cells and histiocytes, sometimes multinucleate. It is the histiocytes that will cause the trouble and must be distinguished from lacunar cells. A helpful feature of the scarred node is the presence of post-capillary venules which are seldom seen in Hodgkin's disease, and the absence of concentric hyaline around the partially obliterated blood vessels in the sclerotic area, which is a valuable diagnostic point in Hodgkin's disease. The presence or absence of eosinophils or

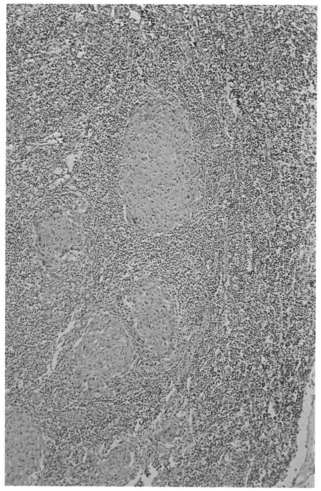

III.12a

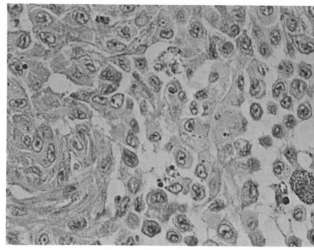

III.12b

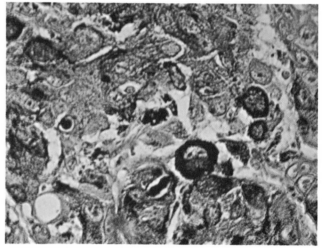

III.12c

III.12a-c   Pseudo Follicles Formed of Metastatic Neoplastic Tissue

III.12a   The nodules in the paracortical area in a focal deposit of neoplastic cells – in this case a secondary melanoma, while the true follicles have largely disappeared.

III.12b   The high-power view shows the squamous-like character of the metastatic cells but on the extreme right a cell containing brown pigment reveals the true nature of the neoplasm.

III.12c   A similar section stained for melanin by the silver impregnation method reveals that many more of the cells contain pigment in their cytoplasm.

III.13a-b   Nodular Form of Lymphocytic Predominant Hodgkin's Disease ▶

III.13a   The nodular pattern is not easily seen and does not become more apparent in a reticulin impregnation; at a low power view the impression is of a monotonous lymphoid proliferation and larger cells are not easily seen.

III.13b   At the high power it is possible to recognize the histiocytes and mononuclear Hodgkin cells lying between the lymphoid cells, but true Reed-Sternberg cells, plasma cells and eosinophils are scanty and there is little increase of fibrosis. A particular variant of the Reed-Sternberg cell is said to occur (Lukes, 1969). This has a delicate polylobulated nucleus and somewhat smaller nucleoli than the classical Reed-Sternberg cell.

III.14a-b   Nodular Form of Lymphocytic Histiocytic Predominant Type of Hodgkin's Disease ▶

III.14a   The nodules are apparent by reason of the foci of epithelioid histiocytes within them but there is no real outline to the individual nodules.

III.14b   The foci consist of epithelioid histiocytes and lymphocytes with occasional mononuclear Hodgkin's cells but typical Reed-Sternberg cells are seldom seen.

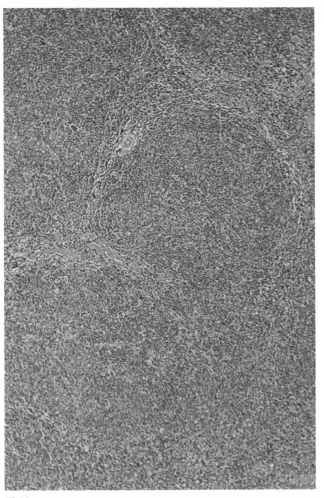

III.13a

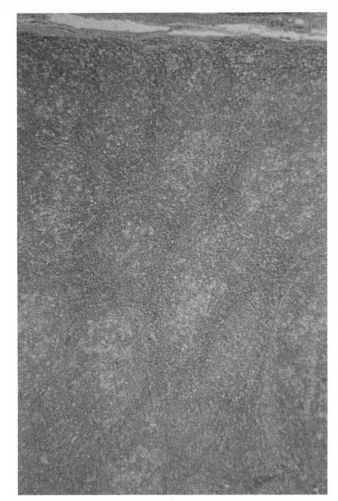

III.14a

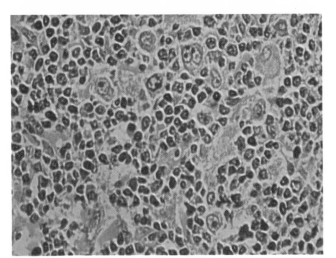

III.13b

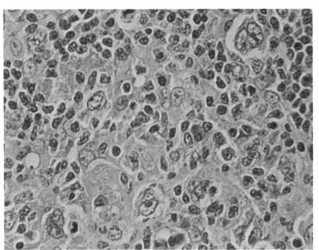

III.14b

plasma cells is of no value. In the end one comes back to the basic feature that if one can recognise all the cells in the nodules as normal reactive cells, one is not justified in making a diagnosis of Hodgkin's disease, but if there are atypical cells suggestive of lacunar, Reed-Sternberg or mononuclear Hodgkin cells, then a decision must be taken; it is not only the nodular sclerotic but also the lymphocyte depleted type of Hodgkin's disease that can cause difficulty in that type of histological picture; less commonly a similar type of confusion can arise in a scarred tubercular or fungal granulomatous node. Difficulties may also arise in an extremely scarred node associated with a secondary carcinoma. Once again there are small cellular islands lying in sheets of fibrous tissue and once again the islands consist of lymphoid cells in which lie isolated carcinoma cells, and of course the problem here is that these cells are abnormal and may simulate lacunar or mononuclear Hodgkin cells quite closely.

In these difficult cases there is no simple solution. In the future histochemical or histo-immunological methods of diagnostic significance may be available but at the present time the chief aids to decision making are well stained sections of high quality and critical experience.

In this chapter consideration has been given to lymphadenopathies in which there is a nodular pattern formed of hyperplastic or neoplastic lymphoid cells or non-lymphoid cells. Emphasis has been placed on the diagnostic features enabling one to distinguish these nodules or pseudo-follicles from the normal primary or secondary follicles, whether hyperplastic or undergoing involution.

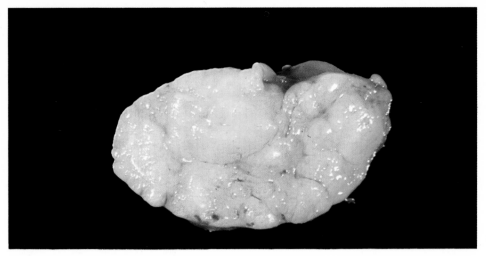

III.15a

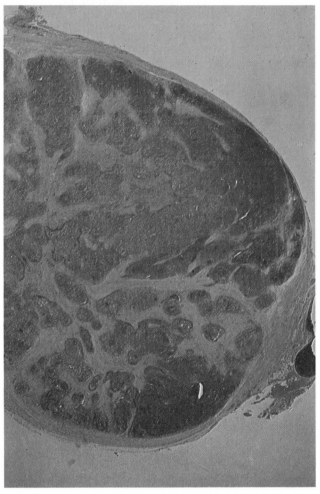

III.15b

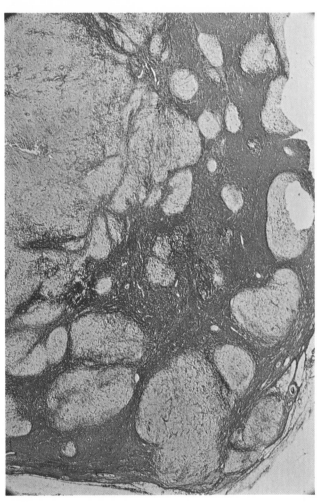

III.15c

III.15a-c   Nodular Sclerotic Hodgkin's Disease

    III.15a   Bissected lymph node (X2). The nodules are easily seen.

    III.15b   This shows very clearly the capsular thickening and the trabecular thickening resulting in the wedge-shaped areas of abnormal lymphoid tissue.

    III.15c   The reticulin impregnation emphasizes the broad bands of collagen derived from the trabeculae and isolating the foci of abnormal cellular tissue.

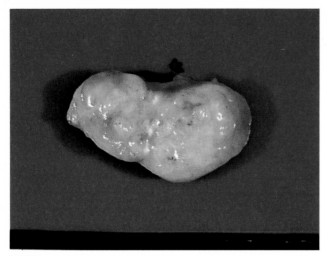

III.15d

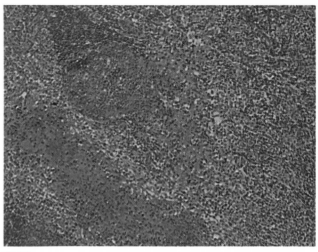

III.15e

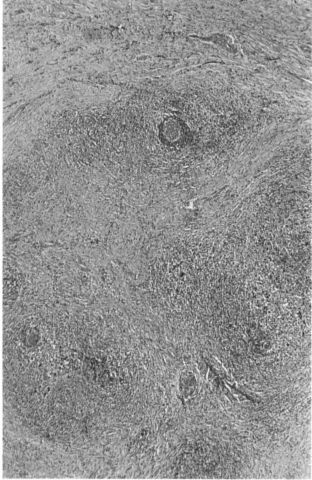

III.15f

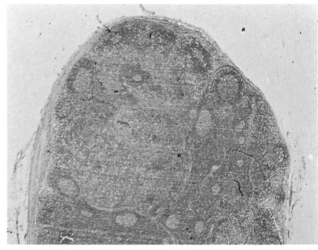

III.15g

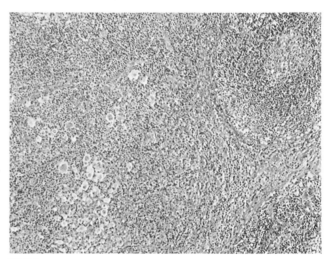

III.15h

III.15d-h Nodular Sclerotic Hodgkin's Disease

III.15d Bissected lymph node (X2) showing foci of necrosis with tissue liquifaction.

III.15e Around the zones of focal necrosis, lacunar cells can be recognized which with the other features, determine the diagnosis of Hodgkin's disease.

III.15f The foci of cellularity merge with the zones of fibrous tissue revealing that the fibrosis is not a stromal scirrhous reaction but an integral part of the lymphadenomatous process. A residual focus of reactive lymphoid tissue is apparent deep to the capsule; this is an unusual feature.

III.15g Focus of Hodgkin's Disease in the paracortex. The normal pattern of the rest of the node is apparent.

III.15h The margin of the focus of Hodgkin's tissue shows the complete disorganization of the lymphoid tissue with clumps of lacunar cells and polymorphic cellular infiltrate evolving towards fibrosis and beyond this an uninvolved reactive centre.

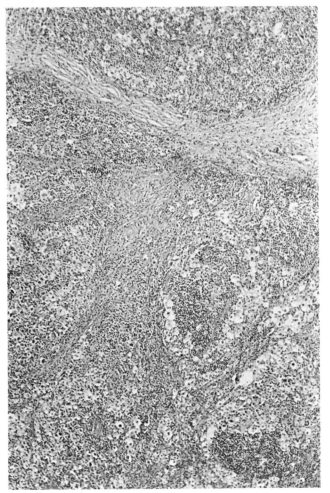

III.15i

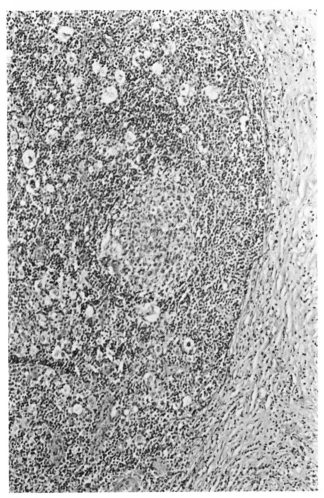

III.15j

III.15i-j   Nodular Sclerotic Hodgkin's Disease

III.15i   The fibrous strands, the polymorphic cellular infiltrate and the clumps of lacunar cells are well shown.

III.15j   The thickened capsule and a residual reactive centre being invaded by the Hodgkin's tissue in the paracortex.

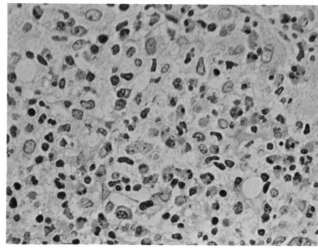

III.15l

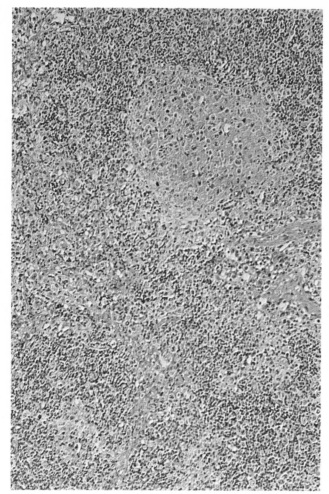

III.15k

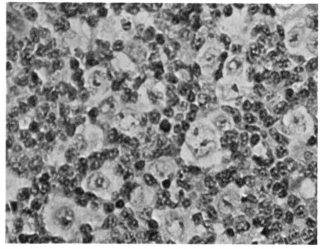

III.15m

III.15k-m   Nodular Sclerotic Hodgkin's Disease

III.15k   In this particular field the characteristic features of nodular sclerotic Hodgkin's Disease are not very obvious, although
lacunar cells are present. It emphasizes the foci of necrosis and
early fibrosis.

III.15l   Granulomatous area with mononuclear Hodgkin cells.
It may be necessary to search for classic Reed-Sternberg or lacunar cells.

III.15m   Mononuclear Hodgkin cells with a watery cytoplasm,
vesicular nucleus with a distinct nuclear membrane, and a prominent nucleolus. These resemble fully formed lacunar cells.

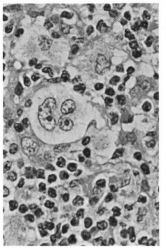

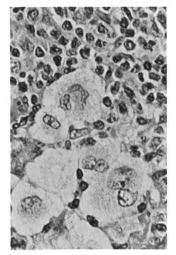

III.15n

III.15o

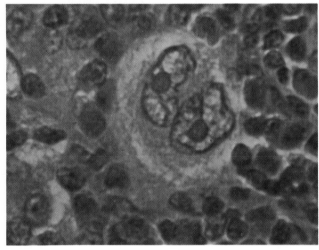

III.15p

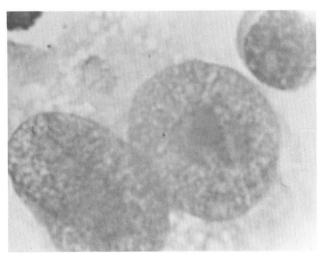

III.15q

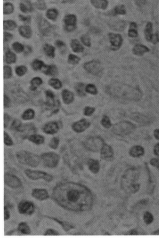

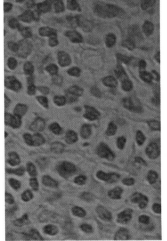

III.15r

III.15s

III.15n-s   Nodular Sclerotic Hodgkin's Disease

III.15n   Multi-nuclear lacunar cell with a pale cytoplasm and lobulated nucleus.

III.15o   Typical lacunar cells.

III.15p   A classical Reed-Sternberg cell, eosinophilic nucleoli, distinct nuclear membrane.

III.15q   Imprint preparation of a Reed-Sternberg cell.

III.15r,s   Methyl-green-pyronin preparation displaying the plasma cells, the pyroninophilic nucleoli of the mononuclear Hodgkin cells and their slight cytoplasmic pyroninophilia.

CHAPTER IV

The normal architecture of the node is distorted or replaced to varying degrees by accumulation and/or proliferation of cells within the sinuses

ANALYTICAL
SUMMARY

1. **Sinus lymphocytosis:**

   Reactive; Hodgkin's disease; chronic lymphocytic leukaemia

2. **Sinus histiocytosis:**

   Sinus catarrh; reaction to neoplasm; steatorrhoea; dermatopathic lymphadenopathy; immunodeficiencies

3. **Foamy histiocytes in the sinuses:**

   Inborn lysosomal diseases; cystinosis; Wolman's disease; histiocytosis X; sinus histiocytosis with massive lymphadenopathy

4. **Foamy histiocytes in the sinuses with extracellular vacuolation:**

   Lymphangiography; lipogranulomatosis; lymphangiectasia; pneumatosis; Whipple's disease

5. **Sinus histiocytosis with phagocytosis:**

   Histiocytic medullary reticulosis (Malignant histiocytosis); haemophagocytic syndromes; familial haemophagocytic reticulosis with immunodeficiency

6. **Metastatic neoplastic cells in the sinuses:**

   Carcinoma

7. **Nodal angiomatosis:**

   Vascular transformation of the sinuses; Kaposi's sarcoma

IN A PREVIOUS CHAPTER dealing with follicular proliferation, there was a discussion (p. 72–3) of some conditions in which significant cellular proliferation also occurs in the sinuses. Here consideration will be given to lymphadenopathies in which the proliferation is predominantly in the sinuses, while there is negligible reactivity in the follicles or paracortical regions of the node. Nevertheless, as many of these conditions are particular forms of general reactive hyperplasia, the demarcation between moderate and negligible follicular proliferations is not sharp. In essence this chapter is concerned with those conditions in which the low power view of the lymph node reveals a racemose pattern of dilated, usually palely staining, sinuses, separated by narrow projections of darker staining lymphoid tissue, in which follicles may or may not be present. The conditions will be considered in relation to the cellular content of the sinuses.

1. Sinus Lymphocytosis

In reactive lymph nodes one may on occasions find distinct sinuses or channels, lined by flattened endothelium with a tenuous reticulin framework, containing packed lymphocytes of varying sizes, ranging from small lymphocytes to transformed type cells (immunoblasts). Occasional neutrophils or eosinophils may also be present, but histiocytes are not commonly present and plasma cells are almost never seen. These channels are most prominent in the paracortical area where they are easily distinguished from the post-capillary venules, which have *Sinus* prominent endothelium and a distinct formed wall. The obvious medullary sinuses *lymphocytosis* may also contain numerous lymphocytes and are probably in continuity with these paracortical lymph channels.

Fig. IV.1   The existence of this 'sinus lymphocytosis' is usually most pronounced in prolonged florid hyperplasia, but may also be seen in lymph nodes during the *Hodgkin's disease* initial stages of involvement by a lymphoma – such as *Hodgkin's disease*. In *Chronic* *chronic lymphocytic leukaemia*, during the early stages, the appearance of these *lymphocytic* *leukaemia* channels may be of some diagnostic value for they contain a relatively monomorphic population of small lymphocytes rather than the mixed population of small lymphocytes and transformed lymphocytes seen in reactive hyperplasia.

2. Sinus Histiocytosis

Sinus catarrh   Marshall (1956) suggested that a pure *sinus histiocytosis*, in the absence of significant follicular or paracortical hyperplasia, is distinctly uncommon, but may *Fig. IV.2* occur in haemolytic anaemias and leukaemias. Marshall made the analogy with animal studies where a pure proliferation of phagocytic cells may be seen following intense vital staining and may be associated with some giant cell formations. Similar reactions in man (so-called *sinus catarrh*) may be those of mediastinal lymph nodes containing much carbon, where the sinuses are often dilated and prominent, being packed with large pink histiocytes containing numerous carbon particles. The extremes of this reaction occur in anthracosis, where the histological picture may however be complicated by degrees of fibrosis due to siliceous elements also present. Likewise, the histiocytosis of haemosiderosis may be a hyperplastic response of the phagocytic system to the presence of particulate haemosiderin.

Reaction to   Sinus histiocytosis, sometimes with follicular or paracortical hyperplasia, also *neoplasm* occurs quite commonly in lymph nodes draining adjacent foci of malignant disease (even in the absence of preceding lymphangiograms). This florid sinus histiocytosis may be seen as a reaction to carcinoma or to Hodgkin's disease, and is undoubtedly related to the occurrence of definite histiocytic granulomata which constitute the sarcoid reaction already described in association with these conditions (p. 89).

It has long been suggested that in carcinoma of the breast, the degree of sinus histiocytosis in the axillary lymph nodes provides evidence as to prognosis, but

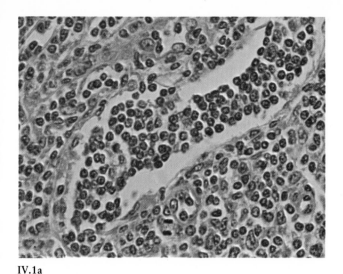

IV.1a

IV.1b

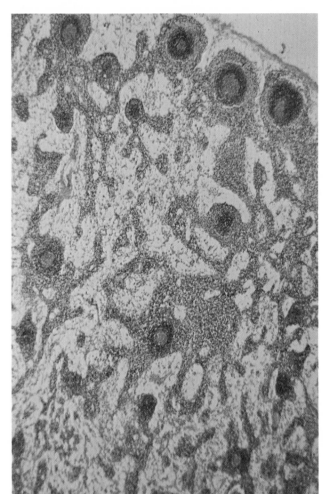

IV.2a

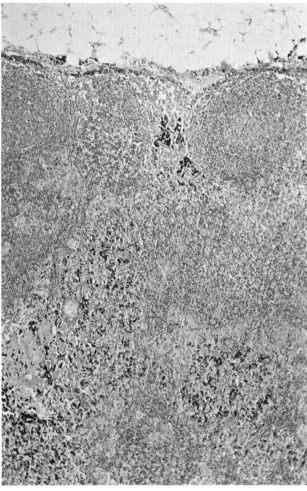

IV.2b

IV.1a-b   Sinus Lymphocytosis and Histiocytosis

IV.1a   Chronic Lymphocytic leukaemia. The sinus is filled with uniform small lymphocytes and the paracortical tissue is also infiltrated by leukaemic cells.

IV.1b   Sinus lymphocytosis in Hodgkin's Disease; in contrast to the lymphocytosis associated with chronic lymphocytic leukaemia, here it can be seen that there is a mixed cellular population in the sinus. A mononuclear Hodgkin cell can be seen in the lower left corner and though it would not be possible to make a diagnosis, the perisinusoidal cellular tissue is polymorphic.

IV.2a-b   Sinus Histiocytosis

IV.2a   This mesenteric node shows the typical pattern of a sinus histiocytosis, in this case in the early stages of steatorrhoea lymphadenopathy. The larger abnormal histiocytes can just be discerned in the dilated sinuses, but the diagnosis could not be suspected from a low power view such as this.

IV.2b   Sinus histiocytosis in a mediastinal lymph node in which many of the histiocytes are laden with carbon pigment.

129

as yet no satisfying analysis of this hypothesis has been presented (Friedell et al, 1974).

Early stages of steatorrhoea and dermatopathic lymphadenopathy

Fig. IV.2a

In the early stages of *steatorrhoea* and of *dermatopathic lymphadenopathy* paracortical proliferation may be negligible and the striking feature is the sinus change. In *steatorrhoea lymphadenopathy* the sinuses are dilated, but are not filled with cells and it is usually possible to recognise the occasional abnormal histiocyte with a large pachychromatic nucleus, a cellular change that extends into the paracortical tissue as the characteristic feature of the condition (p. 73).

The early phase of *dermatopathic lymphadenopathy* cannot be distinguished from sinus catarrh, but a stage will be reached when there is an admixture of eosinophils and histiocytes many of which contain melanin and lipoid and it is legitimate to interpret the lesion as dermatopathic lymphadenopathy (p. 72).

Histiocytosis in immunodeficiencies

Omenn (1965) and Barth et al (1972) have described a family in which a number of children during the first month of life developed an erythematous rash, generalised lymphadenopathy and hepatosplenomegaly with eosinophilia, hypogammaglobulinaemia and rapidly succumbed to infections. The lymph nodes showed marked lymphoid hypoplasia with eosinophilia and extreme sinus histiocytosis in which the cells had large hyperchromatic nuclei but scant cytoplasm and no phagocytosis. It is clear that this condition is distinct from familial haemophagocytic reticulosis (p. 140), chronic granulomatous disease with lipochrome pigmented histiocytes (p. 84), or the mucocutaneous lymph node syndrome (Tanaka, 1976), but is related to the combined immunodeficiencies.

3. Foamy Histiocytes in the Sinuses

There are a range of conditions in which the dilated sinuses are filled with histiocytes with an abundant eosinophilic cytoplasm which may be granular or finely vacuolated. This is the characteristic appearance in heterophagic sinus histiocytosis, of which one example is the change occurring when *lipoid materials* are carried along the lymphatics to the lymph node. A similar reaction occurs in association with either exogenous lipoid materials, such as liquid paraffin or cod liver oil, or endogenous lipoids released as a result of local tissue break down, tumour necrosis, or obstruction to excretion, as in lipoid retention pneumonia or mammary duct occlusion. Sinus histiocytosis of this type was mentioned in the section dealing with lipoid granulomata (p. 94), but it should be appreciated that histiocytes, of similar morphological appearance in paraffin embedded sections,

Inborn lysosomal diseases

Gaucher's disease

Fig. IV.3

Wolman's disease

may occur in a whole range of metabolic storage disorders. In the *inborn lysosomal diseases* (e.g. Gaucher's disease) the morphological changes are usually more marked in the histiocytes in the paracortical tissue than in those of the lymph sinuses, but on occasions, as in *cystinosis*, the histiocytosis is limited to sinus histiocytes and their homologues; however it is only possible to display the doubly refractile cystine crystals in alcohol fixed material. Similarly in Wolman's disease (acid esterase deficiency) the lipoid histiocytosis is limited to the sinuses

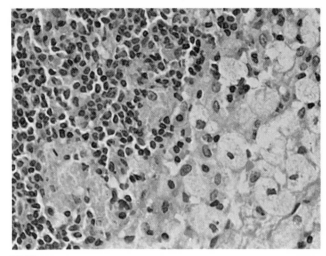

IV.3b

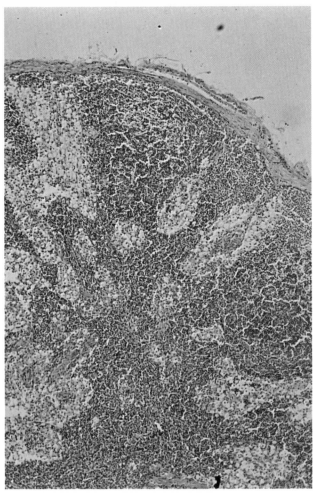

IV.3a

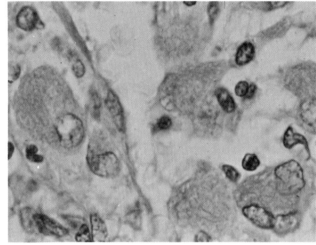

IV.3c

IV.3a-c   Gaucher's Disease

IV.3a   Sinuses are dilated with foamy macrophages.

IV.3b   The appearances are in no way specific and the siderosis that is usually apparent in the littoral cells in Gaucher's cells is not apparent in this case.

IV.3c   In this section stained with PAS-tartrazine, the characteristic structures are apparent in the cytoplasm of the Gaucher cells both in and outside the sinuses.

(Leclerc et al, 1970). Rarely in kappa light chain myelomatosis there is widespread deposition of red shaped crystalline immunoglobulin throughout the cells of the reticulo-endothelial system, with the result that the plasma cell element is quite inconspicuous and the crystal storage histiocytosis may simulate cystinosis but is *Histiocytosis X* not dissolved in aquaeous solutions (Terashima et al, 1978). In *histiocytosis X* the cellular proliferation may exceptionally be restricted to the sinuses, but here there is invariably an admixture of eosinophils with the lipoid containing histiocytes, which tend to coalesce into masses which may undergo karyolysis, while electron microscopy will reveal the Langerhans granules (Reid et al, 1977).

Silicone lymphadenopathy Symmers (1968) has described the *lymphadenopathy associated with granulomatous prosthetogenic mastitis* consequent on the injection of silicone fluids to enhance the bust dimensions. There was marked vacuolation of the sinus histiocytes, which contained finely particulate doubly refractile particles first noted by Sternberg et al (1964); polyvinylopyrrolidone (povidone) may induce similar changes.

Another condition with a marked sinus reaction, which can be confused with histiocytosis X was described by Robb-Smith (1947) as 'giant cell sinus reticulosis *Sinus histiocytosis with massive lymphadenopathy* in children' and has been termed *'sinus histiocytosis with massive lymphadenopathy ('SHML')'* by Rosai and Dorfman (1969, 1972). It would appear to be *Fig. IV.4* a benign condition manifested by massive bilateral cervical lymphadenopathy, though other nodes may also be involved and has most commonly been described in black children; there is mild anaemia, neutrophil leucocytosis and hyperglobulinaemia. In the majority of cases the lymphadenopathy gradually recedes and it has been suggested that it may be an unusual reaction to klebsiella infection (Lainport and Lennert, 1976).

Histologically there is a marked dilatation of the sinuses with corresponding reduction of cortex and paracortex and attenuation of the medullary cords which contain large collections of plasma cells. The tortuous dilated sinuses are packed with large histiocytes having abundant eosinophilic cytoplasm, usually with a granular or foamy appearance, or with marked vacuolation. The nuclei are vesicular in type, round and regular and possess prominent nucleoli which usually have an eosinophilic staining reaction. Histochemically there is a minimal amount of neutral fat and scanty diastase labile PAS positive granules in the histiocytes. The most characteristic feature is the constant finding of well preserved lymphocytes and occasionally plasma cells or erythrocytes within the distended cytoplasm of the histiocytes.

Distinction from histiocytic medullary reticulosis This appearance of relatively large histiocytes containing intact lymphocytes or plasma cells has sometimes been misinterpreted as evidence of a histiocytic medullary reticulosis (malignant hystiocytosis). The diagnostic distinction largely depends upon the extreme regularity of the nuclei in sinus histiocytosis with massive lymphadenopathy as opposed to the atypical nuclei and cellular pleomorphism found in histiocytic medullary reticulosis. However, in both conditions histiocytes may overrun the sinuses and infiltrate paracortex and cortex giving

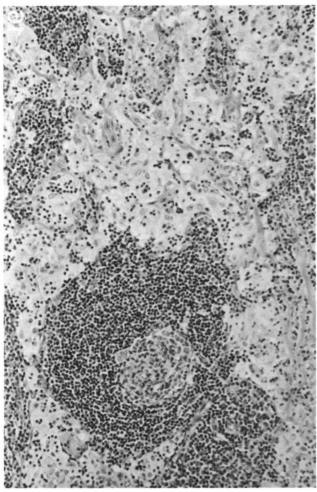

IV.4a

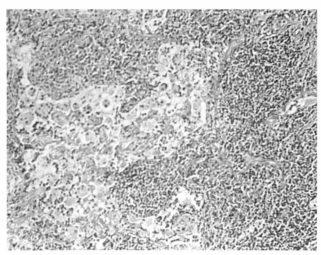

IV.4b

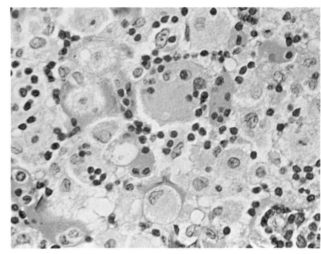

IV.4c

IV.4a-c   Sinus Histiocytosis with Massive Lymphadenopathy

> **IV.4a**   This is the typical low power view. Good preservation of the follicles and paracortex and great dilatation of the sinuses with lymphocytes in the histiocytes.

> **IV.4b**   This shows very clearly the sinus dilatation.

> **IV.4c**   The mature histiocytes with an eosinophil cytoplasm containing lymphocytes and plasma cells are liable to be mistaken for multinucleate macrophages.

benign sinus histiocytosis with massive lymphadenopathy a distinctly aggressive appearance which, however, belies its behaviour. Sometimes multinucleated histiocytes are present, but these show a uniform nuclear structure resembling the mononuclear cells, and there is no true destruction of the lymph node or invasion of capsule or pericapsular tissue. Necrosis is much less common than in histiocytic medullary reticulosis.

4. Foamy Histiocytosis of the Sinuses with Extracellular Vacuolation

In the previous section the striking appearance was the great dilatation of the sinuses filled with large uniform acidophil histiocytes, but there is another group of sinus histiocytoses, in which the most notable feature in paraffin sections is the presence in the sinuses of numerous extracellular vacuoles of varying size. This is often associated with paracortical fibrosis so that the sinus outlines are *Lymphadenopathy* not so readily seen. An excellent example of this change is the *lymph node* *following* *lymphangiography* *reaction to lymphangiography*, an investigation now much used in the staging of the lymphomas and in visualising the pelvic and para-aortic lymph nodes in cases *Fig. IV.5* of suspected metastatic carcinoma. Selected lymph nodes, judged to be abnormal on lymphangiography are often removed subsequently and presented to the pathologist for interpretation and recognition of involvement by secondary neoplasm (e.g. from uterus or testis) or malignant lymphoma (e.g. in staging laparotomy for Hodgkin's disease).

In these circumstances the presence of lymphangiograph dye (an oil based iodine containing compound – Ethiodol or Lipiodol being two commonly used forms) produces quite characteristic and occasionally radical changes in nodal morphology which may cause confusion, and may obscure small deposits of metastatic carcinoma or focal infiltration by Hodgkin's disease. The changes in response to lymphangiographic dye or oil are well recognised and were described by Harrison (1966) and Ravel (1966). Ravel reviewed groups of nodes from 67 cases in which lymphangiography had been performed prior to radical hysterectomy for uterine carcinoma. There was considerable variation in the response in different patients and even between adjacent lymph nodes from a single patient. The most characteristic feature was the presence of the oil itself within the node in the form of globules (seen as clear spaces in the sections, as the oil had dissolved during tissue processing) varying from a few microns to hundreds of microns in size, situated within the sinus system, or distributed within the paracortex, or even within the lymphoid follicles of the cortex. The oil globules were surrounded by a rim of compressed pink histiocytes with flattened nuclei, and associated larger foamy histiocytes. There was almost invariably a marked sinus histiocytosis, whether or not actual oil droplets were present. The follicles were less prominent than usual (unless reacting for other reasons) and occasionally were largely obscured by the developing granulomatous response, with epithelioid type histiocytes and foreign body giant cells. Distinct foreign body granulomata

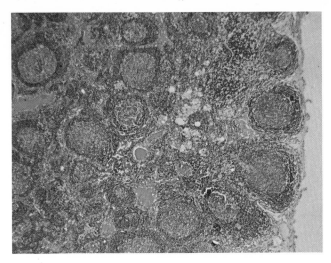

IV.5a

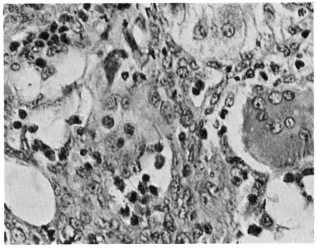

IV.5b

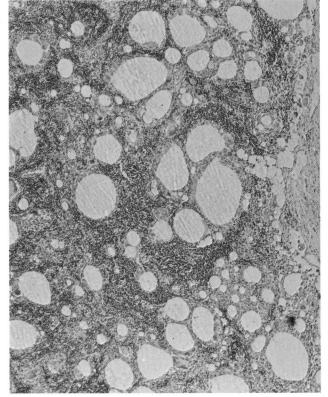

IV.5c

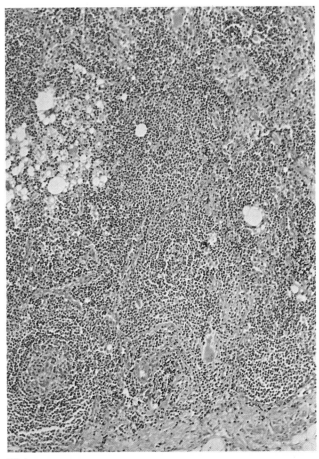

IV.6a

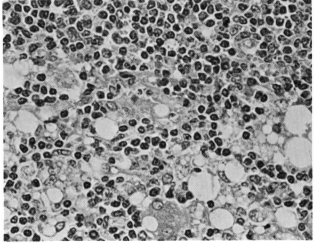

IV.6b

IV.5a-c   Lymph Node Reaction to Lymphangiography

IV.5a   In the early stages the vacuolation in the macrophages and fat droplets in the sinuses are the most striking features.

IV.5b   This reveals the details of the early reaction to the lipoid – acidophil multinucleate giant cells, transformed lymphocytes some binucleate (top right), having a superficial resemblance to Reed-Sternberg cells, and eosinophils; it is understandable that this can be mistaken for Hodgkin's disease.

IV.5c   In the later stages the fatty vacuoles are much larger and there is a marked fibrous reaction around the vacuoles and in the paracortical tissue.

IV.6a-b   Liquid Paraffin Lymphadenitis

IV.6a   In contrast to lipiodol, the droplets tend to be smaller and many of the macrophages have a foamy cytoplasm, furthermore there is much less tendency to a fibrous reaction.

IV.6b   Details of cellular reaction which is very different from the reaction to lipiodol (Fig. IV.5b).

were present as early as four days after lymphangiography, and sometimes persisted for months, though there was gradual regression, as fibrosis finally developed within the node. An initial acute inflammatory response, sometimes associated with eosinophils, subsided after a week or so, and plasma cells subsequently became prominent. The presence of eosinophils in the first week is of importance in the assessment of nodes removed at staging laparotomy for Hodgkin's disease, as the presence of focal collections of eosinophils is often regarded as a valuable pointer to early involvement by Hodgkin's disease.

Histological changes resembling those following lymphangiography may be chance findings in lymph nodes removed at laparotomy (Spain, 1957; Kelsall and *Lipogranulomatosis* Blackwell, 1969). In some cases this lipogranulomatosis may be consequent on *Fig. IV.6* *liquid paraffin ingestion* but this does not account for all cases; ceroid bodies may be present and, as they are acid-fast, could be confused with tubercle bacilli. *Lymphangiectasia* *Lymphangiectasia* may be confused with the lymphangiographic change though *Fig. IV.7* *pneumatosis intestinalis* has greater similarities, as there are clear spaces (containing gas) in the sinuses which are surrounded by histiocytes and there may be a granulomatous reaction.

The other condition in which fatty extracellular vacuoles may be seen in *Whipple's disease* relation to the sinuses is *Whipple's disease* and this possibility should always be *Fig. IV.8* considered in abdominal lymph nodes in which unexpected fat vacuoles are present; staining with PAS will usually resolve the problem, and if material has been set aside for electron microscopy, a specific diagnosis can be achieved.

The lymph node changes in Whipple's disease are very variable in degree within any one node, and also in the extent of nodal involvement. Mesenteric lymph nodes are most commonly involved but more than half of the patients carefully studied by Entzinger and Helwig (1963) also showed changes in cervical or axillary nodes.

In the early stages the basic lymph node architecture persists and there may be mild degrees of follicular hyperplasia. Scattered within the sinuses and paracortex are occasional large foamy histiocytes, together with a few clear spaces, which mark the site occupied by lipoid material prior to processing. The presence of these lipids can be demonstrated in frozen sections, using a range of fat stains. In prolonged disease the number of foamy cells increases remarkably within medullary, cortical and marginal sinuses, and spills over into the substance of the node. In addition, some epithelioid type cells may be present, but giant cells are sparse. In these circumstances lipoid spaces may be numerous and chiefly occupy the medullary sinus area. These lipoid spaces are commonly bounded by flattened eosinophilic histiocytes or giant cells. The pale histiocytes in marginal sinuses are quite characteristic and contrast clearly with the underlying cortical lymphocytes. In later stages fibrosis may be extensive and only small clusters of cells may remain in an otherwise totally scarred lymph node. Many of the foamy histiocytes contain small rod-like inclusions, which are not readily seen in haematoxylin-eosin preparations, but are strongly PAS positive and diastase resistant, and have a characteristic electronmicroscopic appearance. These are believed to correspond to the aetiological agent of Whipple's disease and the demonstration of such PAS positive granules is valuable in distinguishing this condition from the other lipoid granulomata.

It has been suggested that it is possible to diagnose Whipple's disease on the basis of PAS positive inclusions in histiocytes in an axillary or cervical lymph node, but this is not absolutely true as isolated PAS positive histiocytes may occur as chance findings.

5. Sinus Histiocytosis with Phagocytosis

While describing the appearance of 'sinus histiocytosis with massive lymphadeno-pathy' there was mention of possible confusion with the highly lethal condition of *histiocytic medullary reticulosis*, or *malignant histiocytosis* which is charac- *Histiocytic medullary reticulosis* terised by a proliferation of atypical and actively phagocytic histiocytes in the sinus spreading into the paracortex (Bodley Scott and Robb-Smith, 1939; Warnke *Fig. IV.9* et al, 1975; Rilke et al, 1978; Lapert et al, 1978). In the initial involvement of the node, this histiocytic proliferation is limited to the sinuses and the notable feature is the cytological atypia of the histiocytes in which there are large hyper-chromatic and pleomorphic nuclei with prominent nucleoli, and a faintly baso-philic cytoplasm. Multinucleate forms somewhat resembling megakaryocytes are not uncommon, and the less abnormal histiocytes show marked erythrophago-cytosis with negligible haemosiderosis; ingestion of leucocytes is uncommon. As the process advances, the proliferation of abnormal histiocytes – termed prohis-tiocytes by Scott and Robb-Smith (1939) – spreads out into the paracortical tissue so that the nodal architecture is obliterated, and the process may eventually extend into the periadenoid tissue. It is not unusual to find numerous erythrocytes in the sinuses and paracortical tissue so that on occasions the appearances suggest an infarcted node. This may cause difficulty in diagnosis as there is usually active erythrophagocytosis in the normal reactive histiocytes of an infarcted node. However, such histiocytes show no evidence of cellular atypia, and this is also true in agranulocytic nodes which may also show erythrophagocytic histiocytes. It should be appreciated that Byrne and Rappaport (1973) used 'malignant histiocytosis' as a collective term to embrace a whole range of conditions involving abnormal histiocytes, including sarcomata, whereas 'histiocytic medullary reticulosis' was the name proposed for a clinico-pathological entity with a char-acteristic natural history and histopathology and this usage has been adopted by most writers; however there have been references (Chandra et al, 1978) to 'transient histiocytic medullary reticulosis' in conditions, probably reactions to infections, in which there was cytophagocytosis but lacking the cellular abnor-malities of the lethal condition. Risdall et al (1979) have given an admirable account of a 'viral haemophagocytic syndrome' which they emphasize is a benign proliferative condition quite distinctive from histiocytic medullary reticulosis.

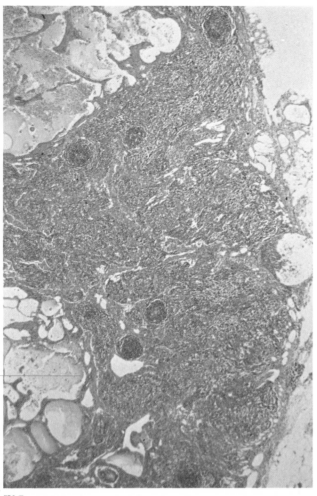

IV.7

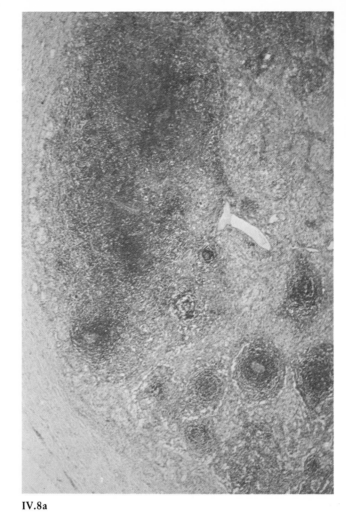

IV.8a

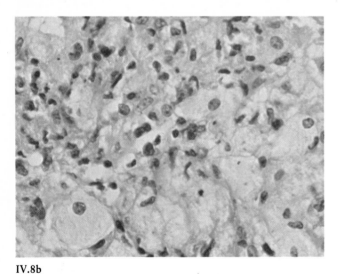

IV.8b

IV.8c

IV.7   Lymphangiectasia

It has been suggested that this may be confused with the lymph-angiographic change but in reality the appearances are very different.

IV.8a-c   Whipple's Disease

IV.8a   The extensive zone of foamy histiocytes in the sinuses and paracortex with commencing fibrosis is characteristic and zones of lipoid vacuolation can be seen in the medulla.

IV.8b   In ordinary stained preparations the histiocytes have a very fine granularity somewhat resembling epithelioid cells and may be interspersed with vacuolated cells from which lipoid has been extracted.

IV.8c   Section stained with PAS-tartrazine revealing the rod-like inclusions.

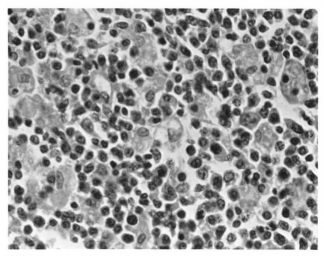

IV.9b

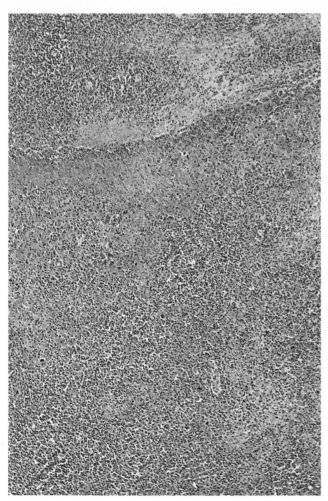

IV.9a

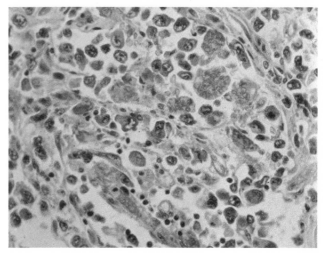

IV.9c

IV.9a-d   Histiocytosis with Phagocytosis

IV.9a-c   Histiocytic Medullary Reticulosis

IV.9a   The involvement has become very extensive. It is difficult to define the distended sinuses as there has been widespread proliferation in the paracortex and this has spread into the extra-capsular tissue; there are foci of necrosis and the larger prohistiocytes can be recognized.

IV.9b   A distended sinus filled with a range of histiocytic forms and multinucleate macrophages containing red cells. The nuclear atypia of the malignant histiocytes can often only be appreciated by examining many cells in different areas.

IV.9c   High power view from another case in which there are numerous macrophages with marked phagocytoses together with large numbers of abnormal, non-phagocytic prohistiocytes.

IV.9d   Familial Haemophagocytic Reticulosis

It can be seen that there is an extensive replacement of the node by macrophages showing erythrophagocytosis, but they are all mature cells and no abnormal forms are present. The plasma-cytoid lymphocytes are apparent on the left-hand side of the field.

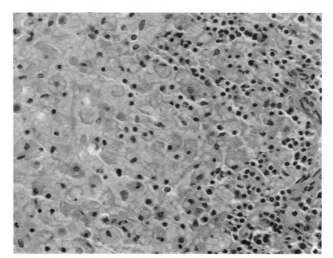

IV.9d

It is of paramount importance to appreciate the difference as these reactive haemophagocytic conditions often, but not invariably, arise in patients under immunosuppression and heroic exhibition of immunosuppressive and cytotoxic therapy can have disastrous effects. Reactive histiocytes are very labile and often present bizarre, giant or multinucleate forms which the unwary may interpret as indications of malignancy, but the abnormal histiocytes in histiocytic medullary reticulosis have, as has already been mentioned striking nuclear changes and such cells are not usually phagocytic. Menelsohn et al (1980) have correlated the lysozyme activity of the abnormal histiocytes with the degree of differentiation. It is unfortunate that Isaacson et al (1978, 1979) have adopted 'malignant histiocytosis' as the term to describe the lymphoproliferative intestinal condition associated with steatorrhoea lymphadenopathy (p. 73). It is of course correct that there may be a progression in this disorder to a histiocytic sarcoma (p. 177). There has also been confusion between histiocytic medullary reticulosis and a grave familial disorder of childhood variously known as *'familial haemophago-*

Familial haemophagocytic reticulosis with immunodeficiency

Fig. IV.9d

cytic reticulosis' (Bell et al, 1968) or *'familial lymphohistiocytosis'** (Donohue et al, 1972), associated with immunodeficiency; the lymph nodes lack germinal centres, the paracortical area is enlarged and rich in plasmacytoid lymphocytes, while the sinuses are full of relatively normal histiocytes showing active erythrophagocytosis and nucleophagocytosis. A particular variant, named the X-linked lympho-proliferative syndrome (formerly Duncan's disease) showed a defective response to Epstein-Barr virus and a high incidence of immunoblastic sarcoma (Purtilo et al, 1978; Pattengale et al, 1979).

6. Metastatic Neoplastic Cells in the Sinuses

Mention has already been made of the florid sinus histiocytosis which may occur in lymph nodes draining carcinomata, and of the early involvement of peripheral sinuses by metastatic carcinoma cells. Such carcinoma cells occurring in small numbers may be difficult to distinguish morphologically from histiocytes, but when present in large numbers the diagnosis is usually more obvious. However, some metastatic adenocarcinomata show an extensive eosinophilic cytoplasm and surprising uniformity of nuclear morphology with only occasional atypical and obviously malignant forms being present. Widespread involvement of the sinuses by carcinoma or melanoma cells may thus resemble a sinus histiocytosis and the superficial resemblance of malignant melanoma cells to histiocytes has already been considered.

Carcinoma

Fig. IV.10

There are several especial difficulties in the recognition of metastatic cells in the lymph sinuses. A small mammary carcinoma in the axillary tail may only manifest itself by enlarged axillary lymph nodes, in which the anaplastic carcinoma cells with an acidophil cytoplasm may be remarkably uniform and their

* Chelloul (1973) used 'adult histiolymphocytosis' as a synonym for 'hairy cell leukaemia'.

bland appearance may cause them to be mistaken for histiocytes; however, the nuclear membrane of carcinoma cells is usually sharper than that of a histiocyte while the nucleoli are larger and hyperchromatism is present.

Another difficulty can arise in the recognition in a cervical lymph node, of a poorly differentiated nasopharyngeal squamous cell carcinoma, the so-called *lympho-epithelioma*, which may be associated with quite marked lymphotropism; the carcinoma cells, which often have considerable morphological resemblance to transformed lymphocytes (immunoblasts) tend to spread from the sinuses into the paracortical tissue, and so the condition may be mistaken for a reactive lymphadenopathy; this has been considered in chapter III (p. 109). A further diagnostic hazard which is not widely appreciated is that this type of nasopharyngeal carcinoma may occur in children and adolescents and as the primary growth is often small and symptomless the only manifestation may be the cervical lymphadenopathy.

Lympho-epithelioma

Fig. III.11

Fig. V.13c

Diffuse sinus infiltration by malignant melanoma cells with their acidophil cytoplasm may be mistaken for sinus histiocytosis with massive lymphadenopathy or malignant histiocytosis, but the absence of cytophagocytosis and the presence of large nuclei with prominent nucleoli should render one hesitant of diagnosing a histiocytosis. In equivocal cases a positive histochemical reaction for melanin is of great value, but it should be recognized that the pseudo-histiocytic type of melanoma cell is most often seen in amelanotic melanomas, and that it is necessary to show that the pigment is not only argyrophilic, but is also bleached by oxidising agents, before it can be accepted as melanin; nor can we accept an intracytoplasmic PAS reaction as indicative of a mucous secreting adenocarcinoma, for histiocytes often reveal PAS positive materials.

Melanoma

7. Nodal Angiomatosis

There are a group of conditions with superficial morphological similarities which are characterised by fibrosis of the sinuses associated with vascularisation. 'Vascular transformation of the sinuses' (Haferkamp et al, 1971; Fayemi and Toker, 1975) is usually to be found in congested lymph nodes in relation to extra-nodal venous thrombosis, consequent on surgery, or dense fibrosis. The general feature is an enlarged node with loose fibrosis of the cortical sinuses, in which there are also prominent endothelial lined spaces. There is no follicular or paracortical reaction. At a later stage, the cortical and medullary sinuses undergo hyalinisation. Thick-walled arterioles and venules develop in these areas and the fibrosis may extend into the paracortex, occasionally associated with dilatation of the cortical sinuses.

Vascular transformation of the sinuses

Fig. IV.11

The early phase of nodal angiomatosis may be difficult to distinguish from early lymph node involvement in *Kaposi's angiosarcoma* (Lubin and Rywlin, 1971; Templeton, 1972; O'Connell, 1977) where there is also an angiomatous change in the cortical sinuses, but in Kaposi's sarcoma this is associated with a

Kaposi's sarcoma

141

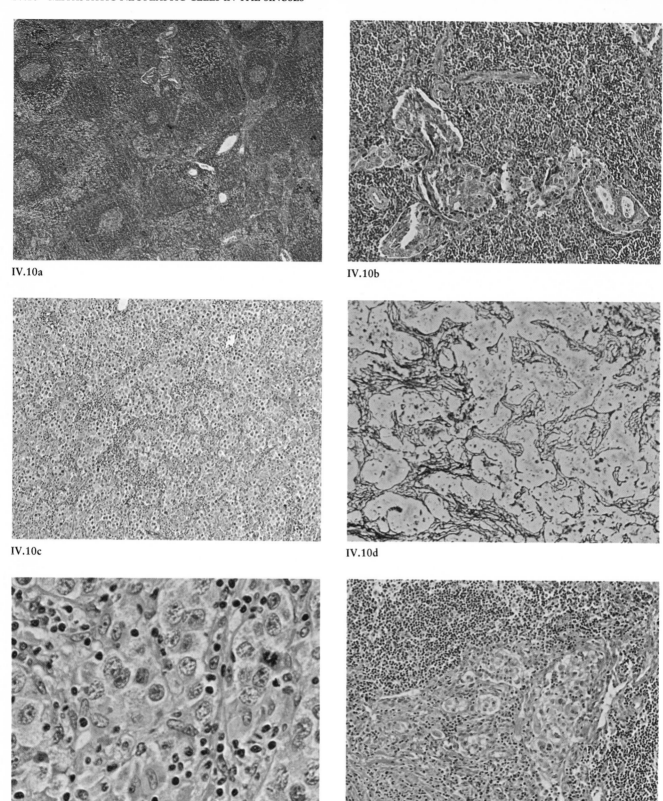

IV.10a

IV.10b

IV.10c

IV.10d

IV.10e

IV.10f

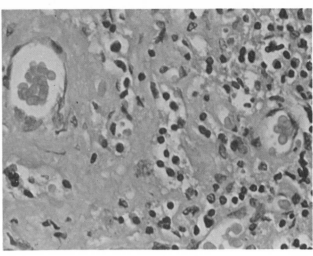

IV.11b

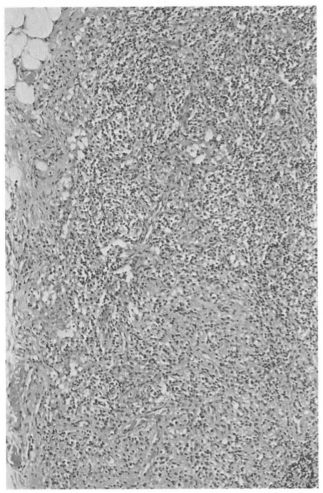

IV.11a

IV.11a-b   Vascular Transformation of the Sinuses

IV.11a   The capsule is thickened and vascularized and the fibro-vascular tissue is spreading from the sinuses into the paracortex.

IV.11b   This shows the hyalinization of the capsule in which small vessels are lying.

◀**IV.10a-f   Metastatic Neoplastic Cells in the Sinuses**

IV.10a   This illustrates how inconspicuous a small deposit of adenocarcinoma can be as the node as a whole appears normal.

IV.10b   The focus, once identified, is obvious.

IV.10c   The appearance suggests a diffuse paracortical proliferation with the possibility of a primary lymphadenopathy.

IV.10d   The reticulin impregnation shows that the neoplastic cells are restricted to the proliferated sinuses.

IV.10e   The high power confirms that the sinus is infiltrated by a poorly differentiated carcinoma.

IV.10f   Another example of invasion of the sinus by carcinoma; with initial confinement of carcinoma cells within the sinuses.

proliferation of spindle-shaped cells, rather than the loose fibrosis of vascular transformation. As the angiosarcoma progresses, the cellular proliferation, in which there are vascular slits containing red cells, becomes more prominent, gradually spreading to replace the whole node. Haemosiderin-containing histiocytes are widely scattered between the spindle cells, which, though they may show nuclear variability, do not display much mitotic activity.

In this chapter an attempt has been made to describe the lymph node changes in which a sinus proliferation was predominant. However it was emphasized initially and was apparent in the discussion, that the demarcation is not absolute, as it is common to have changes in the follicles and paracortex in association with sinus proliferation. Nevertheless, there is the group of conditions considered here, in which the sinus proliferation is such a striking feature that it becomes the pivot on which the diagnosis is based.

CHAPTER V

Follicles and sinuses are inconspicuous or absent and the normal architecture of the node has been replaced by a diffuse cellular process or by fibrosis

ANALYTICAL
SUMMARY
(continued)

d) Lymphocytes, immunoblasts, large folded cells: *Mycosis fungoides*

e) Extramedullary haemopoiesis: *Myelosclerosis*

f) Lymphocytes, immunoblasts, plasma cells, fibrosis: *lymphadenopathy of Sjögren's syndrome*

4. **Diffuse involvement, reduced cellularity, fibrosis or infarction**

a) Diffuse fibrosis: *Fibrosis in chronic reactive lymphadenitis; Hodgkin's disease lymphocyte depleted; sclerosing malignant lymphoma*

b) Massive infarction: *Hodgkin's disease lymphocyte depleted; metastatic tumours; infective lymphadenitis; polyarteritis nodosa*

IN THE EARLIER CHAPTERS, the initial diagnostic determinant was the prominence of follicles or follicular-like structures, or of sinuses. Finally consideration must be given to a large group of lymphadenopathies, in which these architectural features are ill-defined and the whole substance of the node is occupied by a diffuse monomorphic or polymorphic process, or by fibrosis.

Whether this diffuse cellular proliferation originates in paracortex or cortex is often a matter of conjecture for any given lymph node biopsy. However, the observation of early infiltration with a zonal pattern may be of diagnostic value in chronic lymphocytic leukaemia, hairy cell leukaemia, and Sézary's syndrome, while in Hodgkin's disease focal paracortical involvement may be observed in the initial stages. Clearly in any diffuse process, residual lymph node structures may remain but in most cases the pattern of involvement is not of diagnostic value and the diagnosis must be made on the basis of the nature of the cellular infiltrate itself. On this basis, the diffuse cellular proliferations will be considered according to the type or types of cells present, for the precise diagnosis is dependent upon cytological features, with some assistance from special staining methods and from evidence of architectural disruption or new fibre formation as seen in reticulin preparations.

1. Absent follicles though the general cellular pattern is normal or there is reduced cellularity in the cortex or paracortex

Conditions resulting in a diffuse reduction of cellularity throughout the node, with absence of follicular structures, are uncommon and will seldom be found in biopsy material. When present, however, they are invariably associated with *Immunodeficiencies* some degree of immunodeficiency and, as was mentioned earlier, the identification of the particular type is dependent not so much on the biopsy appearances as on an adequate clinical and family history, together with haematological and immunoglobulin studies (Good, 1973).

In the most severe forms of primary combined immune deficiency (reticular dysgenesis, Swiss agammaglobulinaemia, thymic alymphoplasia, etc.) death occurs before the second year, and the lymph nodes are extremely small, revealing a loose framework of fibrocytes and histiocytes, and occasional lymphocytes, but

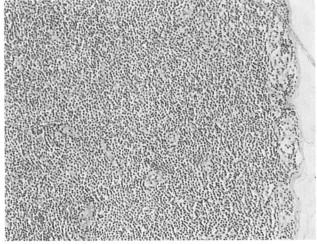

V.1a

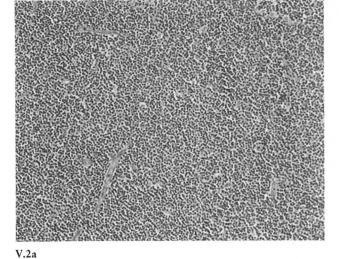

V.2a

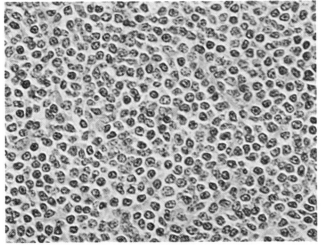

V.1b

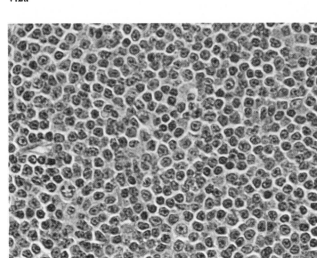

V.2b

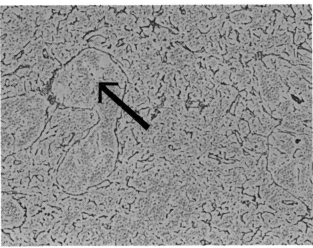

V.1c

V.1a-c   Chronic Lymphocytic Leukaemia (CLL)

V.1a   Monotonous small lymphocytic replacement of whole node, in which follicles cannot be recognized, and the cortical sinuses persist.

V.1b   The vast majority of the cells are mature type small lymphocytes. A small proportion of the cells are of the large prolymphocyte type (i.e. an early phase of the transformation process). These constitute the so-called proliferative foci often seen in this condition. There is no evidence of mitotic activity or cellular atypia. (See p. 109.)

V.1c   A reticulin impregnation revealing that the infiltration involves cortex and paracortex but the sinuses are dilated and filled with lymphocytes. The arrow indicates a focal proliferation centre (transformed lymphocytes).

V.2a-b   Diffuse Small Lymphocytic Lymphoma (well-differentiated)

The appearances are indistinguishable from those seen in chronic lymphocytic leukaemia. In the high power view there may be a slightly higher proportion of larger cells and an occasional transformed type cell, but these differences are not significant. However, it is important to note the absence of mitoses, atypical cells or small cleaved cells.

no plasma cells; indeed it may be necessary to display the sinus pattern by a reticulin impregnation to achieve a confident recognition that the material is a lymph node.

In the Bruton type of sex-linked agammaglobulinaemia, the lymph nodes are usually of normal size, lacking follicles, though the sinuses may be apparent; there is a reasonable lymphoid cellularity, sometimes with immunoblasts in the paracortex, but no plasma cells.

In the Wiskott-Aldrich syndrome and acquired idiopathic hypogammaglobulinaemia, the lymph nodes may be increased in size, but as already mentioned (p. 53), the histological appearances are variable. Some cases show persistence of follicles, which may be enlarged. In others there is follicular loss with lymphoid hypoplasia together with proliferation of immature histiocytes. It is in this group of immune deficiencies that there is an increased risk of developing lymphoreticular neoplasms which may complicate the histological findings. There is increasing evidence that many of these neoplasms, formerly classified as reticulum cell sarcomas or histiocytic lymphomas (Hansen and Good, 1974) are varieties of immunoblastic sarcoma, most probably of B-cell type (Hertel et al, 1977; Taylor, Russell, Davis, Lukes, 1978).

Iatrogenic lymphadenopathy It should not be forgotten that reduced cellularity in a lymph node, somewhat resembling the changes in immunodeficiency, may be of iatrogenic origin. Radiotherapy, high dose steroid therapy and quadruple chemotherapy may all induce radical cellular depletion of varying degree in lymph nodes.

In addition cellular proliferation, manifested by the presence of many transformed lymphocytes, in the post-therapeutic regenerative phase, may occasionally mimic a neoplastic condition.

2. Diffuse cellular proliferation, predominantly of one cell type

2a. *Small Lymphocytes*

Chronic lymphocytic leukaemia (CLL)
Fig. V.1
Small lymphocytic lymphoma

2a(i) *The predominant cell is the small lymphocyte* or so-called well differentiated small lymphocyte. The term 'well differentiated' seems inappropriate and will tend to be avoided here in view of the ability of the small lymphocyte to undergo lymphocyte transformation.

The monotonous monomorphic appearance of a lymph node replaced by lymphocytes ('CLL cells') in *chronic lymphocytic leukaemia** has been discussed (pp. 108, 128). It was emphasized that in many cases a few residual sinuses or inconspicuous follicles persist. Such residual structures are often best seen in reticulin preparations and may be displayed in cases which, upon examination of haematoxylin-eosin preparations, are believed to be entirely diffuse in type.

*Synonyms: Chronic lymphocytic leukaemia B-cell type (Kiel); Diffuse lymphocytic lymphosarcoma (WHO); Diffuse well differentiated lymphocytic lymphoma (Rappaport); B-cell small lymphocytic lymphoma (Lukes and Collins); Lymphocytic well differentiated diffuse lymphoma (NLI); Small lymphocytic diffuse lymphoma (Dorfman). The bracketed designations are explained in Appendix I.

It should be recognized that this histological appearance may also be found in patients presenting with a single enlarged lymph node, a localised mass of nodes, or with generalized lymphadenopathy without overt leukaemia. If there is only a localized lymphoid mass, the lymphocyte count is often not raised (on occasions there may even be a lymphopenia), nor is there evidence of increase of lymphocytes in the bone marrow; on the other hand where there is a generalized lymphadenopathy it is more usual to find a persistent lymphocytosis, though it may be less than 10,000 per cu.mm. It has been customary in recent years to suggest that a histological distinction can be drawn between the lymph nodes in chronic lymphocytic leukaemia and the diffuse lymphocytic 'well differentiated' lymphoma or lymphosarcoma, rather than adopting the older collective term of 'lymphoid leukosis' for both conditions.

Fig. V.2

Pangalis et al (1977) take the more reasonable view that 'the well differentiated lymphocytic type is histologically and cytologically similar but clinicopathologically different from chronic lymphatic leukaemia'. Furthermore they emphasized, and this has also been our experience, that there is little tendency for patients, whose lymph nodes show the changes of well differentiated lymphocytic lymphoma to develop chronic lymphocytic leukaemia, if the initial lymphocyte count is normal. In both forms of clinical presentation, the lymph nodes are widely infiltrated by sheets of lymphocytes of uniform size having a compact condensed nucleus and a thin rim of cytoplasm showing variable basophilia. Mitoses are scarcely ever observed. It is not unusual to find a spread of lymphocytes beyond the capsule, with foci in the periadenoid fat, but the connective tissue structure of the node is not destroyed. Thus these two forms of small lymphocytic neoplasia are best regarded as part of a single spectrum of disease, though we remain in ignorance of the factors which govern whether or not the lymphocytes circulate or are retained in the tissues. In the majority of these cases the lymphocytes can be shown to the B-cells.

Lennert (1975) stressed the occurrence of focal or pseudo-follicular proliferation centres of 'lymphoblasts' (i.e. large cells with more open nuclei and prominent nucleoli that may be regarded as partially transformed lymphocytes) in chronic lymphocytic leukaemia and inferred that this was restricted to the B-cell type. It is true that this appearance is a good indication of this form of lymphocytic proliferation, but it is only found in a proportion of typical cases of chronic lymphocytic leukaemia.

Fig. V.16c

Occasionally rectangular unstained cytoplasmic inclusions may be found in chronic lymphocytic leukaemia. By immunofluorescence these may be shown to contain IgM, while electron microscopy reveals a crystalline structure. In these cases there is usually no increase of monoclonal immunoglobulins in the serum, and plasmacytoid lymphocytes of the Waldenström type are absent (Hurez et al, 1972; Feremans et al, 1978).

Fig. V.4

There has been considerable confusion as to whether or not chronic lymphocytic leukaemia of T-cell type exists. The critical studies of Brouet et al (1975)

T-cell chronic lymphocytic leukaemia

make it clear that it does occur, albeit rarely. Smears or frozen sections of lymphocytes in these cases give a localized positive acid phosphatase reaction, while in paraffin section the cytoplasm is curiously pellucid with a sharp cytoplasmic margin and the nuclear outline is often irregular. Lennert (1978) has stressed the prominence of post-capillary venules and absence of proliferation centres. The neoplastic cells form spontaneous E-rosettes with sheep red blood cells and react with various anti-T-cell sera. So-called 'parallel tubular arrays' are visible at electron microscopy which are thought to correspond to the cytoplasmic azurophil granules observed by light microscopy. Clinically skin involvement is common and there is no doubt that confusion with Sézary's syndrome has occurred; splenomegaly is frequent, though lymphadenopathy is much less marked. There is preliminary evidence that T-cell chronic lymphocytic leukaemia may tend to involve younger patients than B-cell chronic lymphocytic leukaemia. In several recent reports it appeared that approximately 5% of cases of chronic lymphocytic leukaemia are of T-cell type (Toben and Smith, 1977; Marks et al, 1978).

Plasma cells do not form an intrinsic part of small lymphocytic lymphoma, though a few may be found at the periphery of involved lymph nodes. If plasmacytoid cells are present in significant numbers, a diagnosis of lympho-plasmacytoid lymphoma, with possible clinical evidence of Waldenström's disease, should be considered. Morphological and functional studies (Lennert, 1978; Taylor, 1979) have shown that the characters of the lymphoid cells in the small lymphocytic lymphoma and the lympho-plasmacytoid lymphoma form a continuous interrelated spectrum of B-cell dysplasia, although nosologically, distinct clinical syndromes, which are a reflection of the predominant cell types, can be identified. It has been emphasized that it is the monotonous uniformity of sheets of small lymphocytes that is so characteristic of small lymphocytic lymphoma and thus areas of fibrosis or necrosis, or clumps of granulocytes or histiocytes, must immediately raise doubts as to the diagnosis.

In contrast to Lennert's pseudo-follicular proliferation centres in lymphocytic leukaemia, Lukes and Collins described the occurrence of scattered larger cells more closely resembling transformed lymphocytes, occurring singly or in small foci. The presence of these cells can be regarded as a manifestation of lymphocyte transformation, indicative of sites of proliferation of the neoplastic cells. This appearance, particularly in young adults in whom chronic lymphocytic leukaemia is uncommon, demands a critical examination of the node, bearing in mind the possibility that the scattered large cells may be mononuclear Hodgkin cells, and that the diagnosis is in reality lymphocyte predominant Hodgkin's disease.

Differentiation from lymphocytic predominant Hodgkin's disease

Fig. III.13

The typical features of the pure *lymphocytic predominant Hodgkin's disease*, occurring in diffuse form, are analogous to those of the nodular variety already described (chapter III, p. 112). Indeed, in the diffuse variety, there may be a suggestion of nodule formation, although clearly defined nodules are absent. Usually a few scattered histiocytes are present and these should not be confused with mononuclear Hodgkin cells; sometimes the histiocytes may be more numerous, merging into the lymphocyte/histiocyte and epithelioid varieties of lymphocytic predominant Hodgkin's disease to be described subsequently. Occasionally Reed-Sternberg type cells are quite prominent and in such cases the diagnosis is straightforward, but more often the recognition of the special variant of the Hodgkin cell points to the diagnosis. It should be appreciated that in this variety of Hodgkin's disease, eosinophils occur rarely and there is little fibrosis.

There is usually little difficulty in distinguishing the small 'well-differentiated' lymphocytic lymphoma from the small cleaved (or centrocytic) forms of follicular lymphoma. Pseudo-follicular proliferation centres are distinct from the neoplastic follicles of follicular lymphoma, for in the latter at least a proportion of the cells comprising the follicle have cleaved or folded nuclei. These cleaved cells are never found in the small lymphocytic lymphoma. Nevertheless, the follicular pattern may be inconspicuous, and some cases are clearly diffuse. In poorly fixed preparations the cleaved cells may not be easily identified, so causing problems in diagnosis. These difficulties can often be resolved by examining a reticulin impregnation which may reveal a previously unnoticed follicular pattern. *Differentiation of small lymphocytic lymphoma from follicular lymphoma*

Problems of nomenclature and classification will be dealt with in detail in the appendix. Suffice it to say that it is undesirable to include the term 'lymphosarcoma' in the description of the small lymphocytic lymphoma. Lymphosarcoma is an ambiguous term which can embrace a range of morphological conditions, yet it always has the inference of a malignant invasive neoplasm, whereas small ('well-differentiated') lymphocytic lymphoma or chronic lymphocytic leukaemia is rightly classed by Lennert as a 'low grade malignant lymphoma' (he also eschews the term lymphosarcoma). A high grade malignant lymphoma which is commonly confused with the well-differentiated lymphocytic lymphoma is the tumour often known as a *lymphoblastic malignant lymphoma* with or without leukaemia (p. 161). The nuclei are round, not convoluted, and have a finer chromatin structure than the small lymphocyte, while nucleoli are not usually prominent. It is the marked mitotic activity and the extensive destructive invasion of the surrounding tissue which distinguishes this lymphocytic neoplasm from the small lymphocytic lymphoma. There is good evidence that on occasions chronic lymphocytic leukaemia may terminate in a 'blast' crisis (Richter, 1928) in which the poorly differentiated cells retain the immunoglobulin characters of the original B-lymphocytic clone (Brouet et al, 1976; Armitage et al, 1978). This then resembles a B-cell immunoblastic sarcoma. *Differentiation from lymphoblastic malignant lymphoma* *Figs. V.9,10* *Fig. V.14c*

2a(ii) *The predominant cell with its condensed nuclear chromatin resembles a small or medium-sized lymphocyte, but mitotic activity is marked and many of the cells have definite cleaved or folded nuclei. The cytoplasm is scanty with a variable degree of basophilia. There may be periadenoid infiltration with stromal destruction*

This epitomises the essential characters of the *diffuse small cleaved cell malig-*

Diffuse small cleaved cell malignant lymphoma

nant lymphoma*, an uncommon tumour of small cleaved cells; these cells were characterized in chapter III (p. 104) when dealing with follicular lymphadeno-pathies, as the diffuse and follicular forms of this lymphoma are very similar cytologically: a critical examination makes it apparent that it is made up of a range of lymphocyte forms, closely resembling the varieties normally found in the reactive centre of a follicle. In addition to the small cells with their darkly staining cleaved or folded nuclei, there will be a small number of larger cells with abundant usually pyroninophilic cytoplasm and an oval nucleus with fine chromatin and a nucleolus related to the nuclear membrane, corresponding to the centroblast or non-cleaved follicular centre cell.

Fig. V.7

It was on this morphological evidence that Lukes and Collins (1975) and Lennert and his colleagues (1975) put forward the view that these tumours were derived from follicle centre cells (germinoblast and germinocytes of Lennert, later called centroblasts and centrocytes) but proliferating diffusely rather than main-taining a nodular pattern; sometimes ill-defined aggregates of cells may be found suggesting a residual follicular pattern. This may be more obvious in a preparation stained for reticulin, which is usually scanty, though masses of hyaline are oc-casionally present. Another feature in support of the follicular centre cell origin is that a monoclonal (monotypic) immunoglobulin can be demonstrated in the cytoplasm of a small proportion of the cells, while surface immunoglobulins and cell surface receptors for complement can usually be detected, as in the corre-sponding follicular tumours. However it is the diffuse replacement of this node by the small cleaved cells that is so characteristic of this tumour and partial nodal involvement or persistence of reactive follicles must immediately raise doubts as to the diagnosis. In contrast to the follicular form, there appears to be little tendency for the diffuse tumour to transform into large cell or sarcomatous phase, though marrow involvement may occur and abnormal cells can be found in the peripheral blood in about 10% of cases on morphological evidence; but immu-nological techniques reveal a much larger proportion of abnormal cells. Evans et al (1978) have suggested that an aid to the recognition of this tumour is a mitotic count, in which these tumours may show over 30 mitoses in twenty high power fields; this corresponds to the figures given by Lennert et al (1978), but Lukes and Taylor expect few mitoses in this tumour.

Distinction between small cleaved cell and centrocytic malignant lymphoma

It should be appreciated that while the terms small cleaved cell and centrocyte are synonymous, this is not true for the definition of the corresponding neoplasms. In the Lennert classification the presence of even a few centroblasts requires the tumour to be classed as a diffuse centrocytic-centroblastic lymphoma; whereas a small proportion of non-cleaved cells within the predominant small cleaved cell

*Synonyms: Diffuse follicular centre cell lymphoma (Lukes), Centrocytic lymphoma (Kiel); Diffuse lympho-sarcoma, prolymphocytic (WHO); Diffuse lymphoma, lymphocytic intermediately differentiated (NLI); Diffuse lymphoma, atypical small lymphoid (Dorfman); Diffuse poorly differentiated lymphocytic lymphoma (Rappaport). The bracketed designations are explained in Appendix I.

population does not affect assignment to the small cleaved follicular centre cell lymphoma of Lukes and Collins. It is uncertain what influence the presence or absence of centroblasts (non-cleaved cells) has on the clinical characters of this tumour, but it certainly has a worse prognosis than follicular lymphoma.

In the past malignant lymphomas comprised of small cleaved follicular centre cells (centrocytes) have been classed, on the basis of their variable cell morphology, as moderate to poorly differentiated lymphocytic malignant lymphoma, or have been included in the lymphosarcoma or lymphoblastic lymphoma group; this inferred a worse prognosis than the tumour deserves and it would be better to class it in an intermediate category.

2b. *The Predominant cell is lymphoid in appearance but intermediate in size*

The lymphadenopathies in which there is a diffuse involvement with 'large' or 'medium' lymphocytes can be subdivided into several different types, segregation which is justified both on histological and clinical features. Firstly there are conditions in which there are abnormal lymphoid cells in the blood stream, but lymphadenopathy is not a presenting feature and a lymph node biopsy would seldom be required to arrive at the diagnosis. There are two principle disorders which fall into this category – Sézary's syndrome and Hairy cell leukaemia.

2b(i) *The predominant cell is lymphoid in character, larger than the small lymphocyte, with a complex folded (cerebriform) nucleus*

Sézary's syndrome is a dermatological disorder, usually occurring in the fifth and sixth decades, characterized by erythrodermia, alopecia and palmar keratodermia. In Sézary's syndrome it is unlikely that a lymph node biopsy would provide the diagnosis, but it may be helpful in determining prognosis. The peripheral blood shows variable leucocytosis and a proportion of the lymphocytes possess a complexly folded (cerebriform) nucleus and a swirled chromatin pattern. The cytoplasm frequently contains PAS positive vacuoles arranged in a 'necklace' around the nucleus. Electron microscopy reveals the striking cerebriform nucleus. Surface marker studies show that these cells have features of T-lymphocytes, while Lawrence et al (1978) classed them as 'helper type' T-cells. Skin biopsies commonly show a characteristic appearance quite distinct from that seen in classical mycosis fungoides; there is a focal or bandlike monomorphic lymphoid infiltrate in the superficial dermis and the majority of the infiltrating cells reveal a cerebriform nucleus on electron microscopy. It is unusual to see elongation of the rete pegs or an intra-epidermic infiltrate. In the later stage of the disease when invasive nodules may develop, the histology resmbles that of a lymphoblastic malignant lymphoma of the convoluted cell type (p. 162).

There is a moderate generalized lymphadenopathy, the nodes being discreet and mobile, in the early stages. Histology may initially show a dermatopathic lymphadenopathy (p. 72) but later there is a diffuse paracortical replacement of

Sézary's syndrome

Fig. V.5

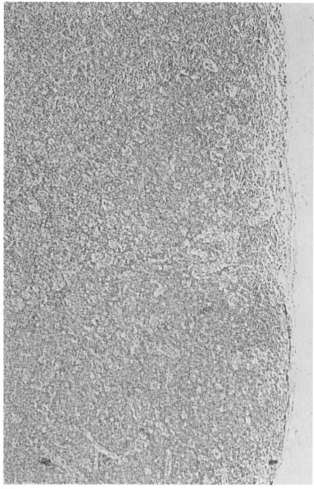

V.3a

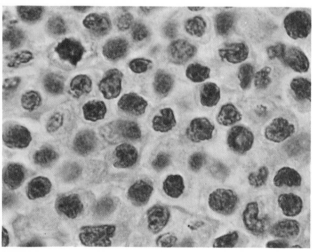

V.3b

V.3c

V.3a-c   Sézary's Syndrome

V.3a   In the low power all that can be recognized is a loss of landmarks consequent on a diffuse monomorphic replacement by lymphoid cells. There has been no infiltration outside the capsule nor any stromal destruction.

V.3b,c   The high power displays the complex folded nuclei with a broad rim of acidophil cytoplasm; mitotic division is quite common. A small proportion of the cells are larger, with a dense nuclear membrane and a prominent nucleolus; these less mature cells correspond to the pale areas seen in the low power.

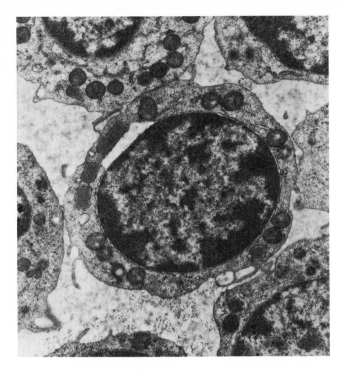

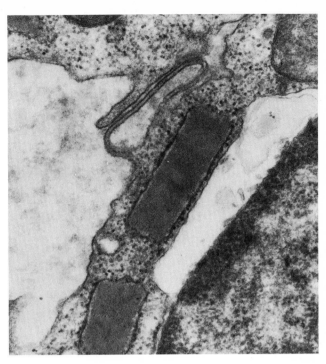

V.4a-b   Chronic Lymphocytic Leukaemia with IgM Inclusions

V.4a The rectangular cytoplasmic inclusions are easily seen. (×8,000)

V.4b High power revealing the laminated structure of the inclusions. (×42,000)

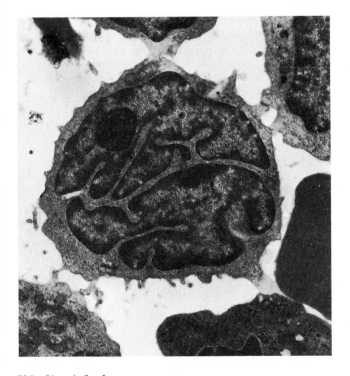

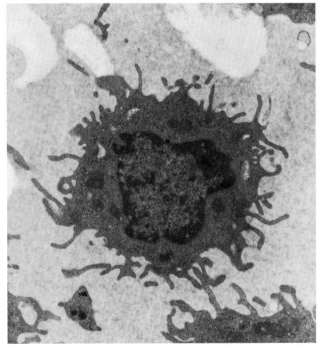

V.5   Sézary's Syndrome

The complex folding of the nucleus is well shown. There is considerable condensation of the chromatin and a small nucleolus is apparent.(×10,000)

V.6   Hairy Cell Leukaemia

The morphological characters are lymphoid; the numerous villi or hairs are obvious. (×9,500)

the node by the Sézary cells, without stromal destruction. The infiltrating cells are larger than small lymphocytes and more variable in size and nuclear outline. The most striking feature is the cerebriform or convoluted nuclear morphology.

Fig. V.3 There may be an occasional cell with a large indented nucleus which could be classed as a giant cell; the fact that occasional cells show mitotic division should not, per se, be interpreted as indicative of a sarcomatous change. When the sarcomatous change has taken place in the dermis, the nodes also become extensively infiltrated, so that the nodal pattern is destroyed and the malignant process, resembling a lymphoblastic lymphoma, spreads into the periadenoidal tissue (Winkelmann et al, 1974). It is generally agreed that Sézary's syndrome and mycosis fungoides form part of a spectrum of hyperplastic and neoplastic conditions of the T-lymphocyte series that may also include T-cell chronic lymphocytic lymphoma and T-zone lymphoma (Lutzner et al, 1975). However the clinical features and tissue changes in Sézary's syndrome are very different from those in mycosis fungoides, of which the nodal characters will be discussed in a later section (p. 213).

2b(ii) *The predominant cell is lymphoid in character, larger than the small lymphocyte, with more extensive cytoplasm and a 'hairy' margin*

Hairy cell leukaemia **Hairy cell leukaemia** (leukaemic reticulo-endotheliosis) is a form of chronic leukaemia predominantly affecting adult males and associated with pancytopenia,

Fig. V.6 haemorrhagic manifestations, and marked splenomegaly. Lymphadenopathy is often not significant. Diagnosis is usually achieved by sternal puncture, though there may be a dry tap (Katayama and Finkel, 1974), or by the recognition of the abnormal mononuclear cells in films of peripheral blood. The histological features in the spleen may also be diagnostic (Burke et al, 1974, 1976).

In films of peripheral blood the mononuclear 'hairy cells' measure 10–18 μm in diameter, with a pale cytoplasm which may contain azurophilic granules. The nucleus is often situated eccentrically and may show one or more indentations, often having a 'monocytoid' appearance. The nuclear membrane is distinct, the chromatin dispersed and the nucleolus sometimes prominent. The diagnostic feature, however, is the presence of numerous fine cytoplasmic projections which are seen with difficulty in Romanowsky preparations, but are well displayed by phase contrast microscopy, and better still by electron microscopy, in particular using the scanning electron microscope (Roath and Newell, 1975; Möbius et al, 1975). A specific feature which can be demonstrated in smears or frozen sections is a strong tartrate resistant acid phosphatase reaction in the cytoplasm (Katayama and Yang, 1977, Appendix II).

The diffuse interfollicular involvement of the lymph node by the leukaemic cells has been clearly described by Catovsky et al (1974) and Burke et al (1974), though Lennert et al (1974) suggested that the initial lesions was confined to the B-zone (cortex). However, it is the histology of tissue from splenectomy that is best known. There is widening and expansion of splenic cords by a dense infiltrate of the pale mononuclear cells with a darkly staining round or indented nucleus surrounded by an extensive clearly defined pale eosinophilic cytoplasm, and there is usually some reticulin increase in the stroma (Burke et al, 1976).

There has been dispute as to the origin of the hairy cell, the evidence from morphology, histochemistry and function studies being conflicting with individual features in support of the B-lymphocyte, monocyte or histiocyte. One current view, put forward by Burns et al (1977), is that the 'hairy' cell should be regarded as a dysplastic haemic cell. Catovsky (1977), in an excellent review of current evidence, favours a lymphocytic origin.

2b(iii) *The predominant cell resembles a medium-sized lymphocyte, but mitotic activity is marked, while the large nucleus has peripheral chromatin and one or more prominent nucleoli*

This malignant *lymphoma*, which must perforce be designated *'lymphoblastic'*, *The problem of* is composed of medium-sized lymphocytes which do not have the compact dense *malignant* *lymphoma* chromatin of the small lymphocyte, but instead show an enlarged nucleus with reduced chromatin clumping and often one or two distinct nucleoli; the nucleus is centrally situated and is not extensively folded as in the cleaved follicle centre cell. The cytoplasm is increased in amount and shows variable basophilia, but the cells do not appear plasmacytoid in form, and there is no suggestion of a 'hof'. It should also be remembered that, as a malignant cell, this cell form may show atypical features such as nuclear hyperchromatism, coarsely blocked chromatin, distinct nuclear membrane, and the occurrence of abnormal mitoses. These are the cells that have been called 'lymphoblasts' and are believed to represent an intermediate stage of lymphocyte transformation. However, it must be admitted that the usage of the term 'lymphoblasts' varies widely in different centres, including sometimes the neoplastic cell characteristic of acute lymphoblastic leukaemia, the neoplastic cell of childhood mediastinal T-cell lymphoma whether or not obviously convoluted; and also, in former times, intermediate-sized 'blastic' lymphocytes that we now recognize to be stages of lymphocyte transformation occurring diffusely within the paracortex or within the follicular centres (in the latter situation they are designated small non-cleaved cells or centroblasts). These problems of usage cannot be resolved by our exhortations, but only by widespread subliminal indoctrination. Since that seems far off, we will proceed cautiously to review some *'lymphoblastic lymphomas'** but in every instance will attempt to explain our usage of the term. Mathé (1977) in a thoughtful review of the classification of lymphoid tumours wrote 'As long as we call "lymphoblastic"

---

* Synonyms: Lymphoblastic lymphoma (Kiel); Diffuse lymphoblastic, non-convoluted, lymphoma (Rappaport); Diffuse lymphoblastic lymphosarcoma (WHO); Small non-cleaved follicular centre cell B-cell lymphoma (Lukes and Collins); Lymphocytic poorly differentiated non-Burkitt lymphoma (NLI); Lymphoblastic non-convoluted lymphoma (Dorfman). The bracketed designations are explained in Appendix I.

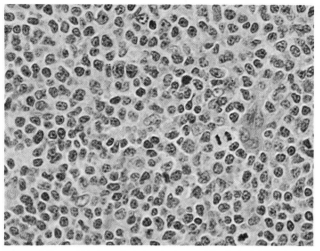

V.7a

V.8a

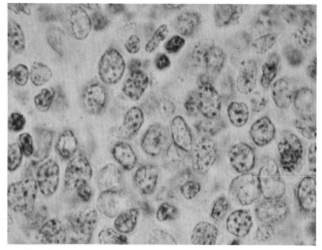

V.7b

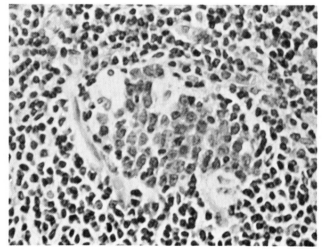

V.8b

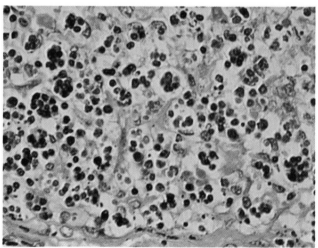

V.8c

V.7a-b   Small Cleaved Cell Malignant Lymphoma

V.7a   Diffuse replacement by small cleaved and a very few small non-cleaved cell types; small cleaved cells predominate.

V.7b   Immunoperoxidase preparation showing brown staining of immunoglobulin in a minority of the non-cleaved cells. Cleaved cells can be seen at the bottom right and bottom left, but generally do not contain detectable cytoplasmic immunoglobulin, though they bear surface immunoglobulin when examined in cell suspensions.

V.8a-c   Acute Lymphoblastic Leukaemia

V.8a   Low power showing a diffuse infiltration although the vascular and stromal landmarks have been preserved.

V.8b   High power view showing a lymph sinus packed with leukaemic lymphoblasts which is surrounded by the normal paracortical tissue of the node.

V.8c   Early stage of lymph node involvement showing phagocytosis of the leukaemic lymphoblasts.

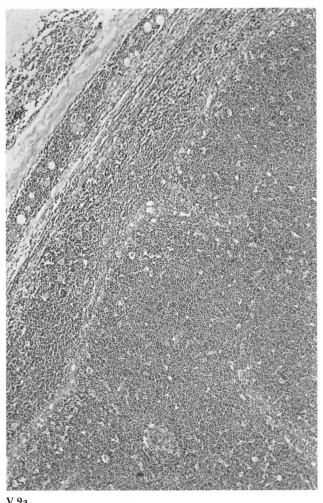

V.9a

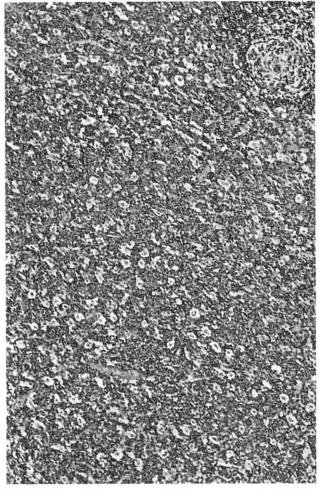

V.10a

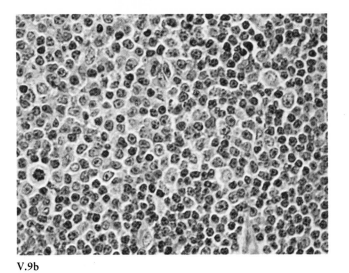

V.9b

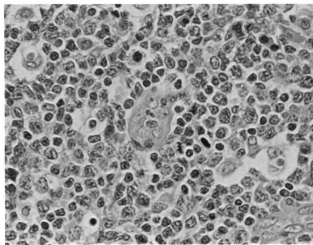

V.10b

V.9a-b   Lymphoblastic Malignant Lymphoma

V.9a   Low power showing diffuse infiltration of the node by lymphoblasts and complete loss of architecture, together with periadenoid infiltration and stromal destruction.

V.9b   High power showing the variable character of lymphoblasts with obvious nucleoli, diminished chromatin and active mitoses. A few larger cells are also present.

V.10a-b   Lymphoblastic Malignant Lymphoma (small non-cleaved type)

V.10a   Low power showing a diffuse infiltration of the node by lymphoblasts with scattered reactive histiocytes resulting in a 'starry sky' appearance.

V.10b   High power showing the range in the morphology of the lymphoblastic infiltrate including a minority of cleaved cells (centrocytes).

the typical blasts of so-called acute lymphoid leukaemia, we cannot use another term for the cells morphologically and immunologically similar which characterise a form of lymphosarcoma'. While Jaffe and Berard (1978) provided an editorial entitled 'Lymphoblastic lymphoma: a term rekindled with new precision', with reference to an article by Rosen et al (1978) 'Convoluted lymphocytic lymphoma in adults', in which the term 'lymphoblastic' did not appear; Mann et al (1979) have analyzed very clearly a number of studies on 'lymphoblasts'. Lymphoblastic proliferation may manifest itself as a systemic disorder with leukaemia (acute lymphoblastic leukaemia), or as a localized tumour mass which may metastasize or become generalized throughout the lymphoid tissue.

Mathé and colleagues (1974, 1975) and Chessells et al (1977) have shown that it is possible, using haematological staining techniques, to distinguish several types of acute leukaemias (prolymphocytic, microlymphoblastic, macrolympho-blastic, prolymphoblastic, and immunoblastic), which appear to be significant in relation to therapeutic response. In leukaemia, the bone marrow is invariably involved from the very beginning, but lymph nodes in the early stages may merely show partial infiltration, with preservation of some follicles and paracortical tissue. It is only in the later stages that there is infiltration of the capsule and periadenoid tissue, and there is little evidence of the extensive stromal destruction that characterizes the primarily nodal forms, which only subsequently develop leukaemic manifestations.

Acute lymphoblastic leukaemia (ALL)

Fig. V.8

It is important to be aware that the follicular structures can be preserved in the early phases of nodal involvement by *acute lymphoblastic leukaemia (ALL)* for this may result in a failure to recognize that the node is abnormal. The para-cortical infiltration with lymphoblasts may be interpreted as a normal reactive change, an error that is particularly likely to be made in poorly fixed and stained material. In good preparations it should always be possible to see the sharp line of demarcation between the spreading sheet of pale staining lymphoblasts, in contrast to the more darkly stained densely packed small lymphocytes of the paracortex. Furthermore the cellular population of the paracortex is mixed, whereas a lymphoblastic invasion is essentially monomorphic with numerous mitotic cells, though there may be 'starry sky' macrophages scattered between the sheets of lymphoblasts. There is no infallible method for avoiding this diag-nostic error, save that one should never make a diagnosis of reactive hyperplasia or nonspecific lymphadenitis until the node has been examined very critically for early evidence of specific lesions, as was discussed in chapter II. One should always be alarmed if there are monomorphic areas, rich in mitotic cells, in the

Fig. V.8c

paracortex. In some cases of early acute lymphoblastic leukaemia, we have observed extensive phagocytosis of the leukaemic cells by mononuclear histiocytes resulting in a striking appearance. It has been claimed that the early pattern of invasion of the different forms of lymphoblasts are characteristic; for example that the T-cell form initially invades the paracortex preferentially, though we have never seen a convincing example of this.

Ten to twenty percent of cases of acute lymphoblastic leukaemia show T-cell morphological markers, while 5% or less mark as B-cells (Taylor et al, 1978). The remaining 80% or so, are designated non-B, non-T or null cell type. The majority of these 'null' cell cases show a high proportion of cells reacting with anti-ALL serum, directed against the so-called common ALL antigen (Greaves et al, 1975). The significance of these different immunological variants remains to be elucidated, though it does appear that null cell ALL (the common or typical childhood form) carries a much better prognosis than either the T-cell or B-cell variety. The T-cell form has affinities with the lymphoblastic or convoluted lymphocytic lymphoma and the B-cell form with Burkitt's or small non-cleaved follicular centre cell lymphoma, both of which are discussed subsequently.

The appearances in a leukaemic involved node must be contrasted with the destructive invasion of the solid or sarcomatous variety of the primary *malignant* *lymphoma composed of 'lymphoblastic' cells*. Cytologically the cells cannot be distinguished with certainty from those in acute lymphoblastic leukaemia, although the degree of nuclear hyperchromatism, pleomorphism, and the high mitotic rate would all favour a diagnosis of malignant lymphoma (sarcoma), while evidence of invasion and extensive stromal destruction would render this definite. However, examination of the peripheral blood and bone marrow is necessary to exclude a leukaemic process, for these conditions constitute a nosological spectrum ranging from the predominantly leukaemic to the solid aggressive neoplasm without any detectable leukaemic phase. Even in such cases, examination of peripheral blood buffy coat may reveal occasional malignant cells in the circulation, and the numbers may increase and justify a diagnosis of leukaemic lymphoblastic sarcoma. The interrelationship between malignant lymphoma and leukaemia is particularly obvious in childhood (Coccia et al, 1976; Williams et al, 1978) leading to the suggestion that all these neoplasms should be regarded as aleukaemic or leukaemic lymphoblastic sarcomas which can be segregated into various types of clinical and cytological features. The presence of some cleaved cells in cases which would otherwise be classed as lymphoblastic lymphoma, suggests a diagnosis of *diffuse follicle centre malignant lymphoma of* *small non-cleaved type*, the group to which Lukes and Collins have also assigned the Burkitt lymphoma. The resemblance to typical Burkitt's lymphoma may be heightened by the presence in some cases of numerous reactive 'starry sky' histiocytes and these may be associated with leukaemia. In contrast to the Burkitt tumour, the nuclei of leukaemic lymphoblasts are often considerably smaller than the nuclei of the histiocytes and much less uniform. The precise interrelationship of these various forms of leukaemia and malignant lymphoma is, however, far from clear. Nor is it known whether the distinctions are significant from the point of view of prognosis or response to treatment. However, it does appear that overt leukaemic manifestations are less common in those cases in which definite cleaved cells are present.

The relationship of these lymphoblastic conditions to the Sternberg sarcoma

Lymphoblastic malignant lymphoma

Fig. V.9

Small non-cleaved cell malignant lymphoma

Fig. V.10

161

(T-cell mediastinal or convoluted malignant lymphoma) is discussed in the next section.

2b(iv) *The predominant cell resembles a medium-sized lymphocyte, but a significant proportion of the cells show multiple complex folding or convolution of the nuclear membrane*

These cells have been termed 'convoluted cells' (Barcos and Lukes, 1975; Lukes and Collins, 1975). The complex folding is distinct from the single deep fold or cleft seen in follicle centre cells, and in addition the nuclear chromatin is finely dispersed (primitive) in convoluted cells.

Convoluted cell malignant lymphoma

Fig. V.11

The recognition of *Convoluted Cell Malignant Lymphoma** is important for they are frequently associated with a distinct clinical syndrome – the so-called Sternberg leuko-sarcoma (Sternberg, 1916). This syndrome is characterized by the occurrence in children and young adolescents (especially males) of a malignant lymphomatous mediastinal tumour, associated with early bone marrow involvement and a leukaemic blood picture. The prognosis is much worse than 'common' acute lymphoblastic leukaemia.

The tumour, or involved lymph node, is made up of uniformly packed small to medium sized lymphocytes with a high mitotic rate. The cytoplasm is scanty, and non-pyroninophilic, with an ill-defined cell border. It is the nucleus that is most striking, with an irregular multilobed outline giving a convoluted or cerebriform pattern; the nuclear chromatin is finely dispersed and though nucleoli may be present they are not prominent. It is apparent that this cell is very similar morphologically to the Sézary or Lutzner cell already discussed (p. 153), except that the chromatin is more finely dispersed ('primitive') in the convoluted cell. The nuclear configuration is more apparent in ultra-thin or electron microscopic preparations or in imprints. Using cell suspensions it is possible to demonstrate the 'T-cell' nature of this cell by the sheep red cell rosette method, and characteristic focal punctate staining is usually found in the acid-phosphatase reaction (Catovsky, 1975). Accordingly all the evidence would support the view that this convoluted lymphoma is a malignant lymphoma of T-cell origin.

In addition to local invasion with stromal destruction and more distant lymph node involvement, bone marrow invasion occurs early in the progress of the disease, resulting in a frankly leukaemic blood picture that may be indistinguishable from acute lymphoblastic leukaemia. Although the majority of case reports conform to Sternberg's clinical description, a significant number of cases have been reported with the characteristic histology but without a mediastinal mass. In most of these the tumour ultimately involved the cervical lymph nodes.

---

* Synonyms: Convoluted cell-type, lymphoblastic malignant lymphoma (Kiel); Convoluted lymphoblastic lymphoma (Rappaport); T-cell type convoluted lymphocytic lymphoma (Lukes and Collins); Diffuse lymphoblastic lymphosarcoma (WHO); Convoluted cell mediastinal lymphoma (NLI); Diffuse lymphoblastic convoluted lymphoma (Dorfman). The bracketed designations are explained in Appendix I.

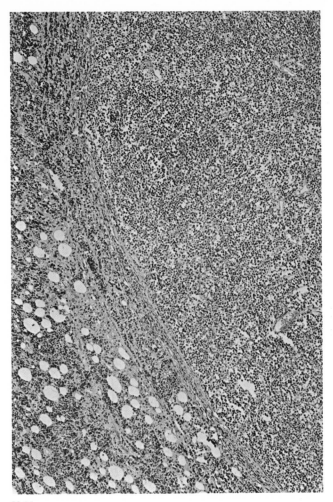

V.11a

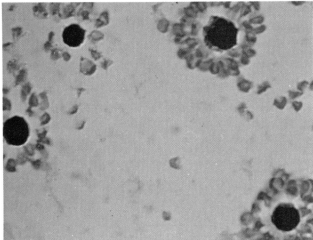

V.11b

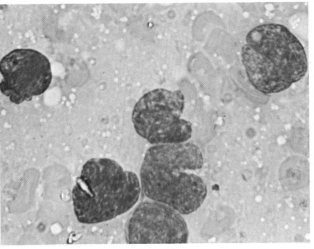

V.11c

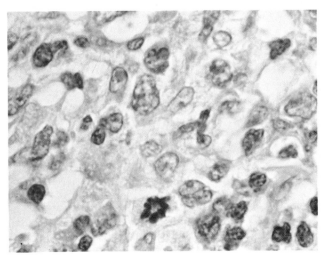

V.11d

V.11a-d   Convoluted Cell Malignant Lymphoma

V.11a   Diffuse destruction of the lymphnode with invasion of the capsule and periadenoid fat.

V.11b   Cytocentrifuge preparation showing formation of spontaneous 'E rosettes' (with non-sensitized sheep red cells) by the convoluted cells; nuclear details are not well seen in this specimen.

V.11c   Lymph node imprint showing multiple nuclear folds, having some resemblance to cleaved cells except for the 'primitive' finely dispersed chromatin. More complex folded 'clover leaf' or convoluted forms are present at the lower left and upper right.

V.11d   It is only possible to display the irregular nuclear morphology in ultra thin sections; some cells can be seen to contain small nucleoli.

In many cases, as Barcos and Lukes (1975) recognized, in addition to the convoluted nuclear cells, there is an admixture of non-convoluted cells conforming closely to the classical lymphoblast (p. 157). Nathwani, Kim and Rappaport (1976) have studied this finding in detail, reviewing a series of thirty cases of 'lymphoblastic malignant lymphoma.' They found that 16 were of the convoluted cell type and 14 non-convoluted, while just half of the cases with mediastinal involvement were of the convoluted cell type. However, they could find no clinical distinction between the cases with convoluted cells and those with non-convoluted cells, save that the latter had a slightly higher mean age. Rosen et al (1978) have also emphasized the occurrence of this tumour in adults. Thus, while the finding of convoluted 'lymphoblasts' is of value in the diagnosis of this distinctive form of leukaemic malignant lymphoma, the lack of identifiable convoluted cells does not exclude the possibility that one is dealing with this syndrome. For this reason some consider the term 'convoluted lymphocytic lymphoma,' proposed by Barcos and Lukes (1975), to be inappropriate. Nathwani and colleagues prefer instead to use 'lymphoblastic lymphoma' for this condition, recognizing that convoluted cells, when present, serve as valuable diagnostic aids.

2b(v) The predominant cell is obviously lymphoid, is of medium size and very uniform, resembling the 'lymphoblast', but is interspersed with large pale histiocytes, giving the tumour a 'starry sky' pattern.

Burkitt's lymphoma
Fig. V.12   This is a succinct description of the Burkitt's lymphoma* but it is neccessary to characterize the cytological features more precisely. The principal cell is of lymphoid type and has a relatively large central nucleus (12–15 μm in diameter), in which the dense clumped chromatin is irregularly distributed in a relatively clear parachromatin, resulting in a vesicular appearance in mercuric chloride fixed material. Two or more rounded nucleoli are often present, and may be prominent. The nuclear membrane is distinct and rarely shows any evidence of deep folding (clefts) or convolutions. These are important distinguishing features from the cleaved follicular cell lymphoma and the lymphoblastic (convoluted) Sternberg lymphoma, reviewed in the previous sections. Mitotic activity is high.

The cytoplasm of the neoplastic cells is strongly pyroninophilic in methyl green-pyronin preparations, and exists as a narrow, occasionally slightly eccentric, amphophilic rim (when stained by haematoxylin) around the nucleus. Examination with the high power often reveals cytoplasmic vacuoles, some of which, in frozen sections or imprint preparation, may be shown to contain lipids. Under the electron microscope, the striking features are the uniformity of the tumour

---

* Synonyms: Lymphoblastic lymphoma, Burkitt's type (Kiel); Burkitt's tumour (Rappaport); Small non-cleaved follicular centre cell diffuse lymphoma (Lukes and Collins); Diffuse lymphosarcoma, Burkitt's tumour (WHO); Lymphocytic poorly differentiated (lymphoblast) diffuse lymphoma, Burkitt's tumour (NLI); Burkitt's lymphoma (Dorfman). The bracketed designations are explained in Appendix I.

cells, the abundance of polyribosomes and large vacuoles, and the relative paucity of endoplasmic reticulum in the cytoplasm. In the nucleus, the chromatin is clumped at the nuclear membrane and around the nucleoli, but the interchromatin substance is relatively clear, giving an impression of emptiness.

The histiocytes are present in varying numbers, interspersed throughout the tumour. They characteristically possess a rounded or oval nucleus, with a fine nucleolus, and extensive clear cytoplasm, in which nuclear fragments are often present.

These appearances can be considered diagnostic of Burkitt's lymphoma, the particular features being the uniformity of the neoplastic lymphoid cells, the interspersed histiocytes, and the diffuse replacement of the lymph node architecture. Nodular forms of Burkitt's lymphoma have only recently been described *Fig. V.12* (Mann et al, 1976) and certainly are not characteristic of the condition, possibly occurring only in the early evolution of the process. One should not consider a diagnosis of Burkitt's lymphoma unless diffuse areas of tumour are present, for vigorously reacting follicles may show many of the features of Burkitt's lymphoma, with uniform medium sized lymphoid cells, a high mitotic rate, and 'starry sky' histiocytes.

Burkitt's lymphoma represents a distinct clinical and pathological entity which, though most common in Africa, is not restricted to that continent. The histological features in most cases are sufficiently characteristic for a confident diagnosis of Burkitt's lymphoma, particularly if additional information from touch preparation, frozen section and electron microscopy is available. However, in simple formalin fixed paraffin sections the differential diagnosis may be more difficult, embracing the different diffuse neoplasms of medium and large lymphoid cells already discussed in this section, as well as the large cell malignant lymphomas about to be considered.

On occasions all these tumours and other lymphoreticular disorders, such as acute myeloid leukaemia, may present as sheets of cells interspersed with reactive histiocytes containing nuclear debris and so may be confused with Burkitt's lymphoma. Indeed the presence of a tessellation of histiocytes is not specific to any particular tumour, but is probably a response to the presence of rapidly dividing cells and is comparable to the tingible body macrophages occurring in florid reactive centres or in acute thymic involution (Henry, 1967, 1968). It is the particular cytological characters of the malignant lymphoid cells of the Burkitt's tumour that is diagnostic rather than the pattern of the tumour. This has been well discussed in the excellently illustrated WHO monograph on this tumour (Berard et al, 1969).

2b(vi) *The predominant cell type replacing the lymph node may be mistaken for a lymphoid cell*

The hazards of confusing a *metastatic anaplastic carcinoma* with a primary

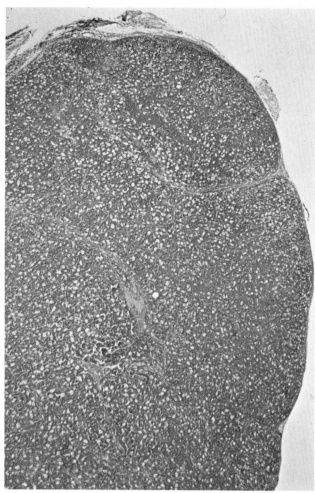

V.12a

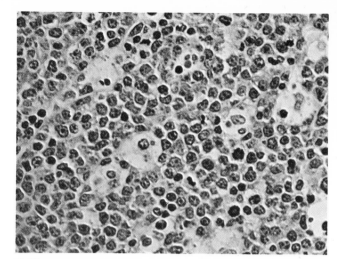

V.12b

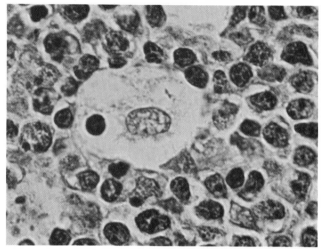

V.12c

V.12a-c   Burkitt's Lymphoma

V.12a   Typically starry sky appearance with a diffuse infiltrate throughout the node.

V.12b-c   Higher magnifications which emphasize the monomorphic character of the tumour. There is marked mitotic activity, while the chromatin is clumped and nucleoli are obvious. In Fig. 12b, the majority of the tumour cell nuclei are of the same size or larger than the histiocytic nuclei, but in Fig. 12c the histiocytic nucleus is unusually large and so many of the tumour cell nuclei appear smaller!

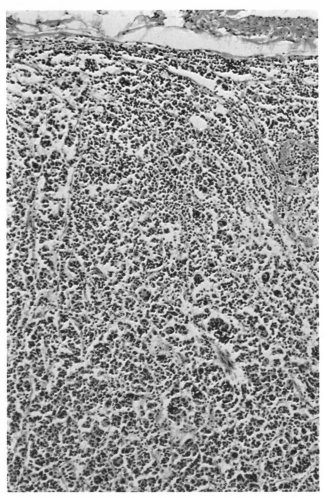

V.13a

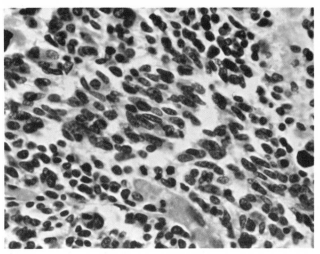

V.13b

V.13a-c   Metastases of Anaplastic Carcinoma

V.13a,b   Low and high magnification of a lymph node diffusely replaced by a secondary oat cell carcinoma from a bronchus. While confusion with a malignant lymphoma is not often a problem, difficulties may arise if there is distortion of the material, a crush artefact or only a very small fragment of material. Oat cells may occasionally closely resemble lymphoid cells as may be seen in the upper right hand corner of Fig. 13b.

V.13c   High power of metastasis of a nasopharyngeal carcinoma which can be mistaken for Hodgkin's disease, though the nuclear characters of a malignant epithelial cell are very different from those of a Hodgkin's cell.

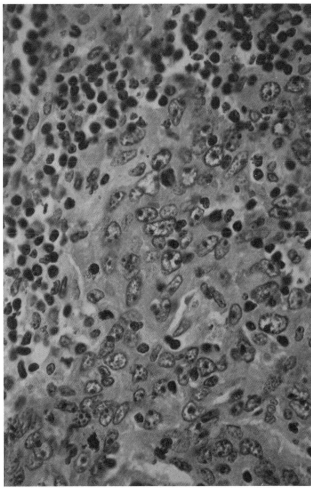

V.13c

Metastatic tumours lymphadenopathy, or vice versa, have been referred to (pp. 109, 141). It is worth emphasizing that secondary deposits of an oat cell carcinoma or a seminoma, in
Fig. V.13 which the rounded or ovoid cells may occur diffusely, or occasionally in a crude nodular pattern, can closely resemble a diffuse or nodular small or intermediate cell malignant lymphoma. Neuroblastomas can also cause difficulties as the nuclei of the neoplastic cells closely resemble those of lymphoblasts; pseudo-rosettes are often difficult to discern but a characteristic feature is that the tumour cells surround small amorphous acellular areas of homogeneous pale pink material. Special silver methods may on occasions display neurites projecting from the cells into these amorphous zones.

The problem of distinguishing secondary neoplasms from primary malignant lymphomas are, of course, compounded by poor quality preparations.

2c. *The predominant cell type is very large and has some resemblance to the transformed lymphocyte or immunoblast*

This group includes neoplasms of varying appearance which have previously been classified as reticulum cell sarcomas or malignant lymphomas of stem cell or histiocytic type. However, it is now believed that the majority of these tumours can be related to the morphological forms of lymphocyte, observed during the transformation process within the follicle centres and in the paracortical areas. Nevertheless, there is uncertainty amongst lymphoid systematists as to whether this group of tumours should receive a noncommital title such as 'large cell lymphoma' or should be designated 'immunoblastic sarcoma'. The specific term is gaining popularity and will be adopted here, in spite of the fact that there is a lack of unanimity, well emphasized by Dorfman (1977), as to what should be included under the term immunoblast, which is certainly not being used in the sense of its originator, Dameshek (1963).

It is convenient to segregate the large cell malignant lymphomas, simulating the transformed lymphocyte, into four groups:

(i) Immunoblastic sarcoma (B- or T-cell) lacking obvious plasmacytoid features

(ii) Immunoblastic sarcoma with plasmacytoid features

(iii) Plasma cell sarcoma

(iv) Pleomorphic immunoblastic sarcoma.

2c(i) *Immunoblastic sarcoma lacking obvious plasmacytoid features**

Immunoblastic sarcoma is a strikingly handsome tumour. The malignant cell population consists of large monomorphic cells resembling the fully transformed lymphocyte or immunoblast. There is usually some variation in size and shape and nuclear form, but the majority of cells are still clearly recognizable as immunoblasts. A variable number of widely scattered macrophages may be associated with the neoplastic cells. The tumour cells are characterized by a large vesicular nucleus (20 μm or more in diameter) with some peripheral clumped chromatin, a sharply defined nuclear membrane and usually a single central prominent nucleolus. The nuclear outline varies from round to oval, but there is usually little lobulation or folding. The cytoplasm is pale or lightly basophilic and may be quite extensive, in which case the nucleus is often eccentrically placed though other plasmacytoid features are not present. Mitotic activity is present but is not a prominent feature.

Immunoblastic sarcoma

Fig. V.14

In many instances, particularly where fixation appears to be inadequate, the cell boundaries are not defined, and the nuclei appear to lie in a continuous poorly defined synplasma (the syncytial reticulosarcoma group of Robb-Smith, 1938). Small numbers of multinucleate forms may be present and if they are more numerous the appearances merge with the pleomorphic immunoblastic sarcoma to be described shortly. Interspersed histiocytes may be present, but the cytological characters and the large size of the tumour cells precludes any reasonable confusion with Burkitt's sarcoma.

In some of our cases a small proportion of the neoplastic cells could be shown to contain cytoplasmic immunoglobulin in monoclonal pattern; these like others with more obvious plasmacytoid features are probably B-cell derived. Indeed Lennert (1975) would class 'large cell lymphomas' as centroblastic (p. 180) rather than immunoblastic if immunoglobulins were not detectable, though it seems that a diagnosis of centroblastic malignant lymphoma is only willingly made by Lennert if centrocytes are also present in the tumour. On the other hand, Lukes and Collins (1975), comparing the cells of *large non-cleaved follicular centre cell lymphoma* with those of immunoblastic sarcoma, maintain that the latter are larger and have a more abundant amphophilic cytoplasm, whereas a residual follicular pattern, occasional cleaved cells, absence of plasma cells and smaller but more numerous nucleoli, often apposed to the nuclear membrane, in the primitive cells, are features of the former type of malignant neoplasm. It remains to be seen whether these differences are correlated with the natural history of the tumours.

B-cell immunoblastic sarcoma

Large non-cleaved follicular centre cell lymphoma

Fig. V.15

Furthermore, immunological studies (Waldron et al, 1977; Lukes et al, 1978;

*Synonyms: Immunoblastic malignant lymphoma B- or T-cell series (Kiel); Diffuse immunoblastic lympho-sarcoma (WHO); Diffuse immunoblastic sarcoma (B- or T-cell), some large non-cleaved follicular centre cell lymphomas (Lukes and Collins); Poorly differentiated diffuse lymphoma with plasmacytoid features, histiocytic diffuse and undifferentiated diffuse (Rappaport); Undifferentiated large cell lymphoma (NLI); Large lymphoid lymphoma without plasmacytoid differentiation (Dorfman). The bracketed designations are explained in Appendix I.

V.14a

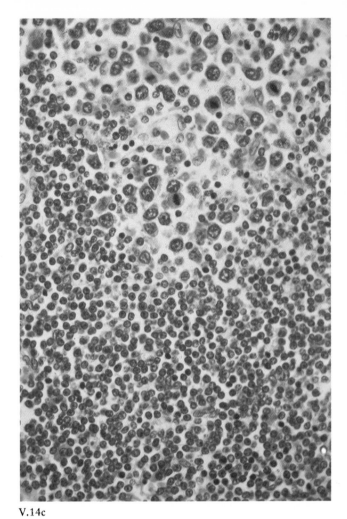

V.14c

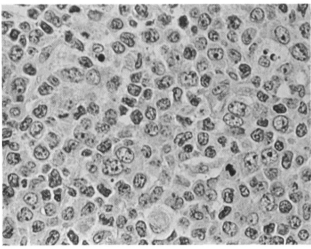

V.14b

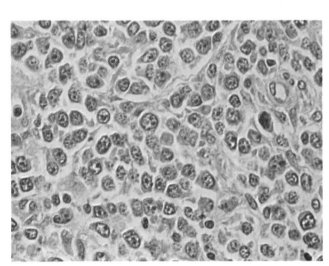

V.15

V.14a–c Immunoblastic Sarcoma

V.14a Diffuse replacement of lymph node by relatively monomorphic large cells.

V.14b Higher magnification showing close resemblance of some of the cells to transformed lymphocytes (immunoblasts) with thick nuclear membranes and often a prominent central nucleolus.

V.14c Richter's syndrome (Immunoblastic sarcoma in chronic lymphocytic leukaemia). There is a striking contrast between the sheets of small lymphocytes and the foci of malignant immuno-

blasts, but immunoperoxidase preparations show both cell types having the same monoclonal immunoglobulin.

V.15 Large non-cleaved Follicular Centre Cell Lymphoma for comparison with an Immunoblastic Sarcoma (see page 180)

The neoplastic cells show fine distinctions from the fully transformed lymphocyte. They are slightly smaller, the cytoplasm is less extensive and nucleoli are often multiple and situated at the nuclear membrane rather than centrally. Obvious cleaved cells are not present in this example, but usually are found in small numbers.

V.16a

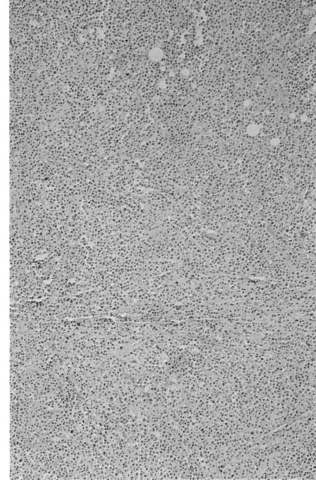

V.17a

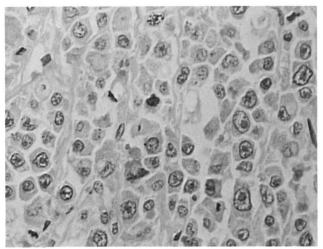

V.16b

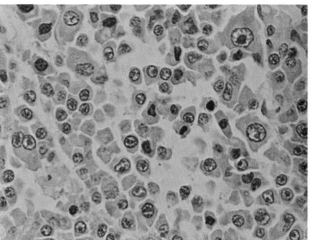

V.17b

V.16a-b   Plasmacytoid Immunoblastic Sarcoma

V.16a   Diffuse replacement of the node by large monomorphic cells.

V.16b   At higher magnification, the cells resemble the transformed lymphocyte but in addition there are early plasmacytoid features. The nuclear membrane is distinct, the cytoplasm extensive, while the nucleus is often eccentrically placed with a prominent central nucleolus.

V.17a-b   Plasma Cell Sarcoma

V.17a   There has been complete replacement of the node and the perinodal tissue, by neoplastic cells. Consequent on the stromal destruction no line of demarcation is apparent though this could still be displayed by a reticulin impregnation; in the haematoxylin-eosin preparation, it is only possible to identify the periadenoid tissue by the surviving fat spaces.

V.17b   The tumour cells resemble the immunoblastic sarcoma shown in Fig. 16a, but plasmacytoid forms (plasmablasts) are more obvious and there are numerous giant and bi-nucleate forms. Many of the smaller cells have the pyknotic nuclei of the more mature plasma cell.

T-cell immunoblastic sarcoma

Taylor, 1978) have provided evidence that a proportion of the immunoglobulin negative tumours of this group would appear to be T-cell derived. There is preliminary evidence (Taylor, 1978) that subtle morphologic features may serve to distinguish at least some cases of T-immunoblastic sarcoma from those cases of B-immunoblastic sarcoma that lack plasmacytoid features (the latter probably represent instances in which the neoplastic B-cells have lost the capacity for plasma cell differentiation; most cases of immunoblastic sarcoma of B-cell type do show some plasmacytoid features). The T-immunoblastic sarcoma has more extensive eosinophilic cytoplasm, more dispersed nuclear chromatin, smaller nucleoli and often some degree of complex nuclear folding (convolutions), particularly in the smaller cells. However, it must be confessed that at the present time the practical significance of these morphological distinctions amongst the immunoblastic sarcomata is uncertain, though some preliminary evidence, based on personal experience, suggests that T-cell immunoblastic sarcoma has a more favorable prognosis than B-cell immunoblastic sarcoma.

2c(ii) *Immunoblastic sarcoma with plasmacytoid features*

Plasmacytoid immunoblastic sarcoma

Fig. V.16

When the diffuse malignant proliferation consists of cells resembling transformed lymphocytes of fairly uniform type with a rounded nucleus, distinct nuclear membrane, and a prominent central nucleolus, mixed with smaller numbers of plasmacytoid cells, the appearances correspond to the immunoblastic sarcoma described by Lukes and Tindle (1975). These initial cases were manifestations of a sarcomatous transformation of immunoblastic lymphadenopathy, as also was the case described by Fisher et al (1976). Tumours of similar morphology have developed following abnormal immune states such as Sjögren's syndrome, and this tumour is typical of post-transplant malignant lymphoma (Matas et al, 1976). We feel that these *plasmacytoid immunoblastic sarcomas** are related morphologically, and by cell origin, both to the large cell immunoblastic sarcoma of B-cell type, lacking obvious plasmacytoid features, already described, and to those neoplasms consisting of obvious malignant plasma cells (the plasma cell sarcoma group), next to be considered. All three tumours arise from cells of the B-lymphocyte series and form part of a continuous spectrum of disease, but are distinguished here for the purposes of defining the diagnostic features. It is not yet clear whether there are significant prognostic differences, for all appear to be highly malignant aggressive tumours.

2c(iii) *The cellular proliferation is pleomorphic; and the morphology though bizarre, has a simulacrum to the plasma cell*

Plasma cell sarcoma

The *plasma cell variants of pleomorphic immunoblastic sarcoma (plasma cell sarcoma)* may present as sarcomatous transformation in myeloma (Holt and

---

* Synonyms: cf. p. 169 but qualified 'with plasmacytoid features'.

Robb-Smith, 1973; Taylor and Mason, 1974) or α-chain disease (Pangalis and *Fig. V.17* Rappaport, 1977; Galian et al, 1977; Brouet et al, 1977; Roth and Riecken, 1978) or as primary malignant tumours (Taylor, 1974, 1978), particularly in the gastro-intestinal tract (Henry and Farrer-Brown, 1977). In myeloma and α-chain disease, the tumours are clearly derived from the same progenitor clone as the neoplastic plasma cell population, and the malignant cells generally contain the same immunoglobulin as the original neoplastic plasma cells (Taylor and Mason, 1974; Pangalis and Rappaport, 1977).

There is a more cellular pleomorphism than in the other forms of immuno-blastic sarcoma described above, and the cells are larger, with a more prominent nuclear membrane and very conspicuous nucleoli. In addition, atypical plasma-cytoid cells are present, including multinucleate forms in which a juxta-nuclear 'hof' may still be visible. When such multinucleate cells are numerous the cyto-logical features obviously blend with the remainder of the pleomorphic immuno-blastic sarcoma group that lack plasmacytoid features and are described below. Occasionally plasma cell sarcomas, particularly those presenting de novo, consist of more uniform cells of plasmacytoid type with perhaps an equal proportion of neoplastic cells resembling the transformed lymphocyte. Such neoplasms have clear similarities to the immunoblastic sarcomas, but a high proportion of cells may contain immunoglobulin with a monoclonal staining pattern, and in some cases we have demonstrated the presence of a distinct serum paraprotein; ac-cordingly there appears to be a close functional relationship with the classical plasma cell neoplasms (including multiple myeloma).

2c(iv) *The cells are large with some resemblance to the transformed lymphocyte (immunoblast) but there is great variation in cell size and in addition to giant mononuclear cells, there are multinucleate and other bizarre nuclear forms*

The remainder of the *pleomorphic immunoblastic sarcoma group, lacking* *Pleomorphic immunoblastic sarcoma* *plasmacytoid features*, is a difficult group to categorise for it includes tumours which have been designated 'polymorphic reticulosarcoma', 'polymorphic reticu-lum cell sarcoma', 'Hodgkin's sarcoma' and 'pleomorphic immunoblastic *Fig. V.18* sarcoma'. These titles reflect the supposed morphogenesis of poorly differentiated neoplasma believed to be either of lymphoid or histiocytic derivation.

To make a confident diagnosis of *pleomorphic immunoblastic sarcoma*, it is necessary that the smaller and less bizarre cells in the tumour have the morpho-logical characteristics of malignant immunoblasts as described in the foregoing sections. In addition it should be possible to trace transitional cell forms between the malignant immunoblasts and the bizarre multinucleate forms. In contrast to the plasma cell sarcoma, giant binuclear forms are not common, whereas complex multinucleate giant cells, with a superficial resemblance to the megakaryocyte are often present, and bizarre mitotic forms are usually to be seen. As these tumours are 'poorly differentiated', both histochemistry and electron microscopy can often

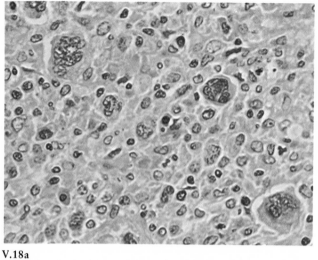

V.18a

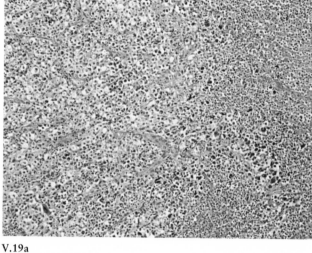

V.19a

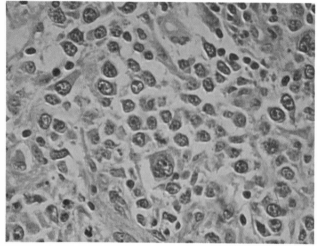

V.18b

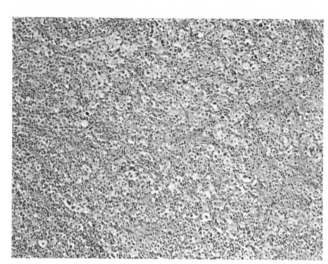

V.19b

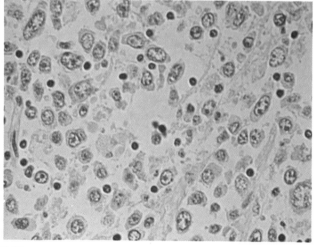

V.18c

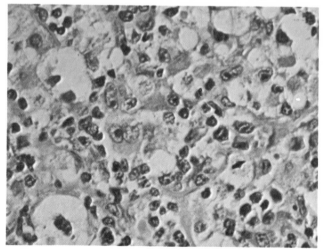

V.19c

V.18a-c Pleomorphic Immunoblastic Sarcoma

These are three examples of pleomorphic immunoblastic sarcomas. They all display a great variability in cell size but the smaller cells have the features of a malignant immunoblast and in spite of the great range of cell size, the cytological impression is of a homogeneous cell population.

V.19a-c Hodgkin's Disease Nodular Sclerosis, Diffuse Cellular Areas

V.19a-b Different aspects of diffuse cellular areas with minimal fibrosis from a case of nodular sclerosing Hodgkin's disease, which in other areas was quite typical as was displayed in Fig. III.15k.

Residual foci of small lymphocytes are to be seen in the top left hand corner of Fig. V.19a.

V.19c Higher magnification showing the somewhat bizarre appearance of the packed lacunar cells.

V.20a

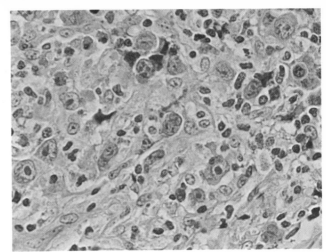

V.20b

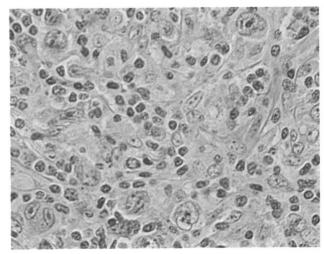

V.20c

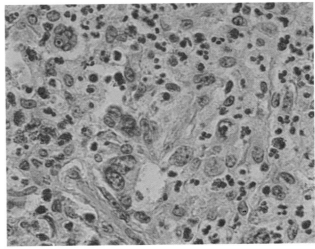

V.20d

V.20a-d   Hodgkin's Disease, Lymphocyte Depleted

V.20a   Diffuse replacement of the node by a cellular proliferation with minimal fibrosis.

V.20b   High magnification showing numerous mononuclear Reed-Sternberg variants which have very prominent nucleoli; there are also scattered lymphocytes and eosinophils.

V.20c   Another field from the same section showing appearances entirely consistent with mixed cellularity type Hodgkin's Disease; a small Reed-Sternberg cell is present at bottom left.

V.20d   This is another example in which there is a striking variability in the giant cells, very few of which are typical Reed-Sternberg cells, though the general morphology of the lesion is typical of lymphocyte depleted Hodgkin's Disease.

only provide equivocal information and a reticulin impregnation seldom gives any positive guidance, though fine strands may separate the tumour cells. On occasions a silver impregnation may reveal that a putative pleomorphic immunoblastic sarcoma is in reality a poorly differentiated metastatic carcinoma.

Distinction from Hodgkin's disease

It is clear that there is confusion and disagreement as to whether one can distinguish betwen pleomorphic (polymorphic) tumours of lymphoid or histiocytic type. As has already been mentioned this type of tumour has, in some

Fig. V.19

classifications, simply been called 'large cell lymphoma' thus evading the issue. Although the term 'Hodgkin's sarcoma' is rightly out of favour, there is sometimes diagnostic confusion between these pleomorphic sarcomas and Hodgkin's disease, particularly in the cellular type of nodular sclerosis and the lymphocytic depleted forms, the latter corresponding to the reticular form of the original Lukes and Butler (1966) classification.

The difficulty in distinguishing the cellular form of nodular sclerosis from the mixed cellular type of Hodgkin's disease has already been discussed (p. 116). On occasions lacunar type Reed-Sternberg cells may occur in closely packed groups, or may even extend throughout the node, so that the sheets of lacunar type cells, with multilobed nuclei and water clear cytoplasm, present a somewhat unusual appearance. This constitutes a particular problem if there is little evidence of a nodular pattern, and if the normal admixture of lymphocytes, plasma cells, fibrocytes and eosinophils is inconspicuous. Nevertheless in contrast to pleomorphic immunoblastic sarcoma, the lacunar cells and Reed-Sternberg cells seldom show much evidence of mitotic activity, and it is usually possible to recognize foci of typical nodular sclerosing Hodgkin's disease surrounded either by fibrosis or more normal lymphoid tissue.

Fig. V.20

The lymphocytic depleted or reticular form of Hodgkin's disease can present greater difficulties as the numerous bizarre Reed-Sternberg cells may simulate the giant cells of pleomorphic immunoblastic sarcoma. However, in Hodgkin's disease the characteristic admixture of normal fibrocytes, lymphocytes, plasma cells and eosinophils is usually still present and a small number of classical binucleate Reed-Sternberg cells may also be found. Furthermore sections taken at several levels will usually display the typical appearances of the diffuse variety of lymphocyte depleted Hodgkin's disease or of forms intermediate with mixed cellular Hodgkin's disease, thus betraying the true diagnosis.

2d. *The predominant cell is large and pleomorphic but does not resemble the transformed lymphocyte (immunoblast)*

In the previous section, consideration was given to malignant neoplasms which had some resemblance to the transformed lymphocyte, and were believed to be related to that cell, although such neoplasms had previously been classed as reticulum cell sarcoma or histiocytic lymphoma.

It is now necessary to consider a group of malignant neoplasms of undoubted morphological similarity, except that some observers believe that they are lacking the features which would justify regarding them as related to the transformed lymphocyte (immunoblast).

2d(i) *The cells are large and pleomorphic; the nucleus is somewhat angular and is rich in basichromatin with a prominent nucleolus; the cytoplasm is abundant, somewhat eosinophilic and opaque or foamy with a tendency to vacuolation*

These are the features that are regarded by many histologists as indicative of a *histiocytic sarcoma*,* but the acceptance or rejection of this concept is still under debate. The recognition that the transformed lymphocyte corresponded in appearance to many of the cells previously designated as reticulum cells induced the idea that all the large cell tumours known as reticulum cell sarcomas were tumours of malignant transformed lymphocytes and that true histiocytic malignant tumours were very rare, if they existed at all (Gérard-Marchant et al, 1974; Lukes and Collins, 1975; Lennert et al, 1975). However, Henry (1975) described the ultrastructural features of malignant histiocytes, while Taylor (1976) identified similar cases by immunocytochemical methods demonstrating the presence of cellular lysozyme (muramidase), and this has been endorsed by Motoi et al (1978), and Wright and his colleagues (Isaacson and Wright, 1978; Isaacson, Wright, Judd and Mepham, 1978), using histochemical methods. Lennert (1978), in the light of the work of Müller–Hermelink et al (1974), and Motoi et al (1978), has now accepted the existence of histiocytic sarcomas. These observations confirmed the morphological features of the malignant histiocytic neoplasm that Whitehead (1968) and Robb-Smith (1964, 1975) believed to be the sarcomatous phase of the progressive histiocytic hyperplasia associated with idiopathic steatorrhoea. In addition to the appearances summarized above, in the better differentiated tumours, the nucleus is often reniform or slightly folded, while multinucleate forms are not uncommon. Some authors have stressed the importance of phagocytosis as a diagnostic feature, and valuable though this is, it should be remembered that phagocytosis may not occur in poorly differentiated histiocytes, while malignant cells of non-histiocytic origin may show cytoplasmic inclusions and may reveal phagocytosis in tissue culture. Many, but not all histiocytic sarcomas have a closely set reticulin framework, conforming with the characters of the dictyocytic reticulo-sarcomata of Robb-Smith's (1938) classification.

Histochemistry can display nonspecific esterase activity in fresh specimens (Yam et al, 1971) while the immunoperoxidase technique may reveal lysozyme (muramidase), α^1-antitrypsin (Isaacson et al, 1979, 1980) and a range of immunoglobulins, presumably representing phagocytosis of immune complexes.

Histiocytic sarcoma
Figs. V.21,22

---

* Synonyms: Diffuse histiocytic malignant lymphoma (Rappaport, Dorfman); Histiocytic cell lymphoma (NLI); Histiocytic malignant lymphoma (Lukes and Collins); Reticulo-sarcoma (WHO; Lennert et al, 1978); Other malignant lymphoma (Kiel). The bracketed designations are explained in Appendix I.

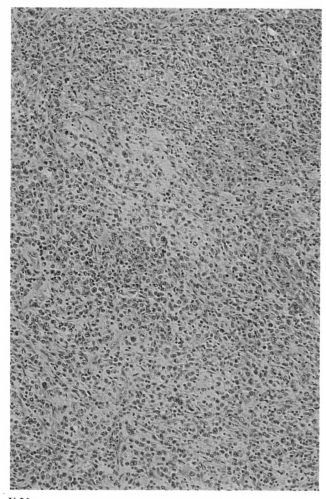

V.21a

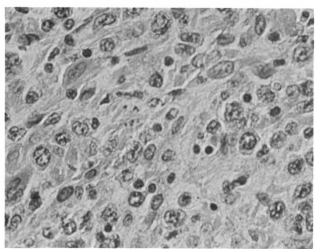

V.21b

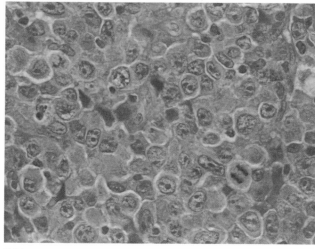

V.21c

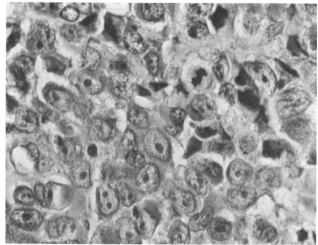

V.21d

V.21a-d Histiocytic Sarcoma

V.21a Diffuse replacement of nodal architecture by large pale cells.

V.21b High magnification showing the presence of large polymorphic cells having a superficial resemblance to sarcomatous immunoblasts, but the majority of the nuclei are oval with irregular outlines, often reniform or slightly folded, while the basichromatin is coarse, nucleoli are obvious and multinucleate forms are frequent. Furthermore the cytoplasm is abundant, opaque and foamy and in many instances (e.g. top and bottom left) is markedly eosinophilic.

(The diagnosis of histiocytic sarcoma in this instance was confirmed by histochemistry and ultra-structural studies.)

V.21c Another tumour in which the morphological features of a histiocytic sarcoma are well displayed. The cytoplasm is acidophil and somewhat opaque with a polygonal cellular outline. The nuclei are large and there is a dense nuclear membrane with few strands of basichromatin and a prominent nucleolus. There is little variability in cell character and mitotic activity is marked.

V.21d Immunoperoxidase preparation stained for muramidase shows the positive reaction in the cytoplasm of the malignant histiocytes.

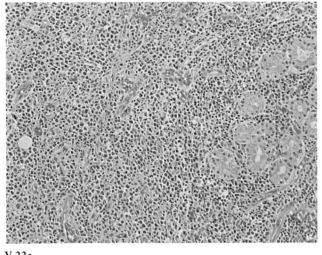

V.22a

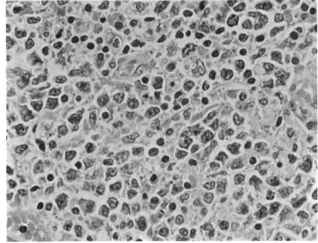

V.22b

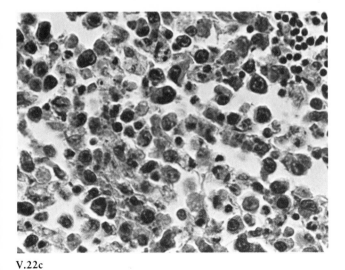

V.22c

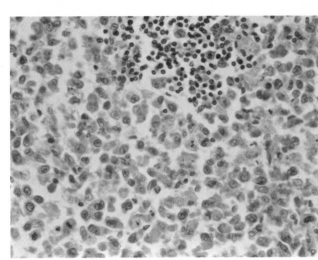

V.22d

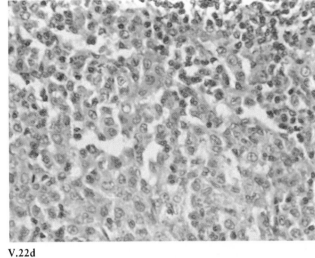

V.22e

V.22a-e   Histiocytic Sarcoma arising in Steatorrhoea Lymphadenopathy

V.22a   There is diffuse infiltration and destruction of all layers of the gut wall.

V.22b   High power showing the polygonal outline of the nuclei, rich in basi-chromatin and a prominent nucleolus while the cytoplasm is markedly eosinophilic; a few lymphocytes and plasma cells are scattered between the malignant cells.

V.22c,d,e   Other examples of sarcoma arising in steatorrhoea lymphadenopathy in which a range of immature and atypical histiocytes are displayed, but both the nuclear and cytoplasmic characters are consistent and characteristic.

Ultrastructural studies may display scattered lysosomes, short stacks of rough endoplasmic reticulum, evidence of phagocytosis ('phagosomes') and interdigitating cell borders (Henry et al, 1978).

2d(ii) *The cells are large and a variable proportion possess an irregular shaped nucleus having a distinct deep region of folding (cleaved cells). There is a delicate nuclear membrane and the chromatin shows slight peripheral clumping together with two or three small and relatively inconspicuous nucleoli. The cytoplasm is clear or faintly basophilic*

Large cleaved and non-cleaved malignant lymphoma or centroblastic sarcoma

This is the appearance of a tumour named by Lukes and Collins (1975) diffuse follicle centre cell lymphoma of the large cleaved and large non-cleaved cell types (centrocytic, centroblastic) but it is more realistic to call it a *large cleaved or non-cleaved malignant lymphoma* or *centroblastic sarcoma*.* These diffuse tumours are related to the diffuse small cleaved cell malignant lymphomas already described (p. 152) and to the follicular lymphomas themselves. Indeed an identical morphology is seen in the large cell follicle centre cell lymphoma (formerly termed 'nodular reticulum cell sarcoma' or 'nodular histiocytic lymphoma') developing in a pre-existing lymphoma with an obvious follicular pattern. Usually in these cases a transition can be seen from the follicular to the diffuse phase. However,

Fig. III.7

as was mentioned in chapter III (p. 108), a malignant diffuse lymphoma of this type can arise primarily as a localized nodular mass, whereas when it occurs in association with a pre-existing follicular lymphoma it is usually multicentric. Bizarre cells and mitotic activity are usual and become more marked as the proportion of large non-cleaved cells (centroblasts) rises. There is often an admixture of macrophages but a starry sky appearance is distinctly uncommon. This is one of the tumours which was formerly classed with reticulum cell sarcoma or malignant lymphoma, histiocytic or mixed, diffuse (Rappaport, 1966). In 1975 De Vita et al reported that chemotherapy was curative in 30% − 40% of patients with diffuse histiocytic lymphoma with advanced disease, and this observation has been confirmed from other centres, but it was for some unclear as to what was meant by 'diffuse histiocytic lymphoma'. However, Strauchen et al (1978) have analyzed a series of 66 cases diagnosed under this title, and shown that about a third of the cases were more accurately classed as large-cleaved and non-cleaved malignant lymphoma, and these were the patients who responded so well to chemotherapy, particularly the cleaved cell type; there was a smaller proportion of mixed follicle cell tumours with a moderate response, while the 'blastic' and pleomorphic pyroninophilic types − corresponding to the poorly differentiated immunoblastic sarcomas − had a very poor prognosis. Li and Harrison (1978) in a review of 90 'large cell lymphomas' came to analogous conclusions, finding

---

* Synonyms: Centroblastic malignant lymphoma (Kiel); Histiocytic malignant lymphoma (Rappaport); Large cleaved or large non-cleaved diffuse follicule centre cell lymphoma (Lukes and Collins); Reticulosarcoma, unclassified malignant lymphoma (WHO); Undifferentiated large cell lymphoma (NLI); Undifferentiated diffuse lymphoma (Dorfman). The bracketed designations are explained in Appendix I.

that 57% were of B-cell follicular origin, 23% were immunoblastic, 14% were of T-cell origin and only 5% were histiocytic. Van den Tweel et al (1979) showed that a group of composite lymphomas on critical analysis merely reflected a mixture of transformed cells in various stages.

All the tumours in this group consist of an admixture of large cleaved and non-cleaved cells, with a variable proportion of smaller cells, but by definition the large cells predominate. Recognizing that these tumours consist of a mixture of large cleaved and large non-cleaved cells, the criteria adopted by Lukes and Collins (1975) to determine whether a tumour should be classed as either large cleaved or large non-cleaved are somewhat arbitrary. It is not simply a matter of *Large non-cleaved malignant lymphoma* which cell type predominates. Rather, the designation of large non-cleaved is reserved for the more aggressive tumours in this group, and a tumour of this *Fig. V.15* type should be classed as large non-cleaved if 25% or more of the cells are of the large non-cleaved type. Thus more than half the cells of a tumour may be of the cleaved cell type (large or small) yet the overall classification would still be large non-cleaved, implying an unfavourable prognosis. This is consistent with current views of lymphocyte transformation and proliferation, for the large non-cleaved cell represents a late stage in the transformation process and as such may be regarded as a measure of the proliferation rate of the tumour cells. There are often strands of reticulin dividing large blocks of tumour cells, thus corresponding to the dictyosyncytial reticulo-sarcoma of Robb-Smith (1938).

Large cleaved cell malignant lymphoma, in which large cleaved cells predom- *Large cleaved malignant lymphoma* inate, though they may be mixed with a small proportion of small cleaved cells or non-cleaved cells, is believed to carry a much better prognosis than the large non-cleaved variety, though the evidence of clinical trials to support this conten- *Fig. V.23* tion is only just becoming available.

It is necessary to distinguish the immunoblastic sarcoma (p. 169) from these tumours of large follicle centre cells (large cleaved and large non-cleaved cells) since they may also contain a proportion of cells that closely resemble immuno-blasts. This is not surprising if it is recognized that the follicle cells and B-cell immunoblasts represent a continuous spectrum of cell types. Large cleaved cell lymphomas are usually distinguishable by the prominent nuclear cleavage planes and inconspicuous nucleoli. Differentiation of large non-cleaved tumours from immunoblastic sarcoma is more difficult, and depends on recognition of some-what subtle features; smaller nucleus, smaller nucleoli often apposed to the nuclear membrane, pale cytoplasm, an admixture of cleaved cells, a residual follicular pattern typify the large non-cleaved tumour.

2d(iii) *The predominant cell is large with a round nucleus, but there are also cells of a similar size with a reniform or folded nucleus, and smaller cells with a dense bi- or tri-lobed nucleus may also be present*

The appearance, in a haematoxylin-eosin preparation, of a uniform pale pink

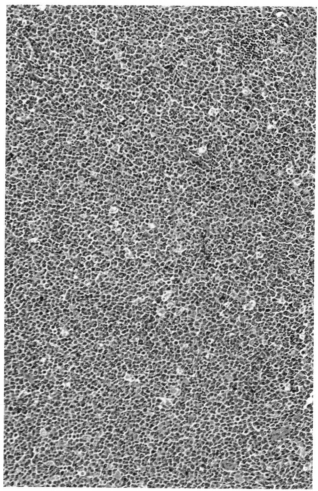

V.23a

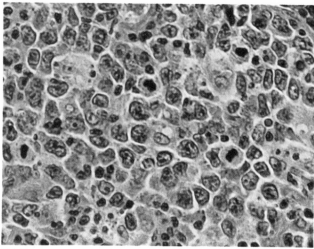

V.23b

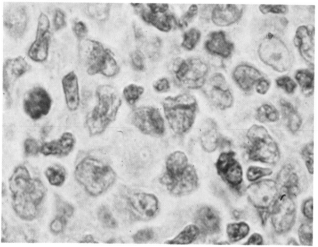

V.23c

V.23a-c Large Cleaved Malignant Lymphoma or Centroblastic Sarcoma

V.23a Diffuse replacement of nodal architecture. The clear areas are scattered macrophages.

V.23b High power showing an admixture of cleaved and non-cleaved cell types. There are numerous cells in mitoses and several macrophages are apparent; in general the prognosis worsens with a rising proportion of non-cleaved cells. In the Lukes-Collins classification the designation 'non-cleaved' is given to tumours in which 25% or more of the cells are of the non-cleaved type (compare with Fig. V.15).

V.23c This shows very clearly the nuclear detail of the cleaved cells and the pale and tenuous cytoplasm. Immunoperoxidase stain shows a single positive plasmacytoid cell. Generally the follicle centre cells show little staining though in a minority of cases, a distinct monoclonal pattern is observed. (However as in the case shown in Fig. V.7b, monoclonal surface immunoglobulins could be demonstrated in cell suspensions.)

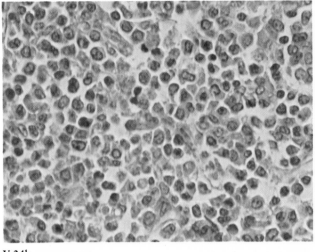

V.24b

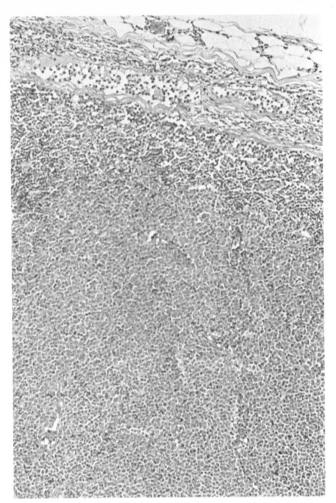

V.24a

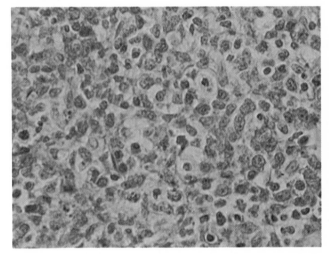

V.24c

V.24a-c   Myeloid Metaplasia

V.24a   Diffuse infiltration of node with initial sparing of the subcapsular cortex.

V.24b   Higher magnification showing cytoplasmic eosinophilia and variable nuclear morphology. Eosinophil myelocytes, a valuable diagnostic indicator are present but are not well displayed in this section.

V.24c   Chloroacetate esterase reaction showing positive red staining in the more mature cells.

Myeloid transformation

Fig. V.24

paracortical replacement of a node, with focal remnants of basophilic lymphoid tissue, should suggest the possibility of *myeloid metaplasia* of the node. The suspicion can become almost a certainty when the high power examination reveals that the larger cells have a round or reniform nucleus with a curious blurred eosinophilic cytoplasm. The identification of myelocytes (particularly eosinophilic promyelocytes) and cells with a bi- or tri-lobed nucleus and a truly granular cytoplasm is dependant on the degree of differentiation of the neoplastic granulocyte population. Confirmation is achieved by the use of a Romanowsky stain and a positive reaction with naphthol-AS-D chloracetate esterase. In addition many of the cells react positively for muramidase (lysozyme) by immunoperoxidase methods. Electron microscopy may reveal cytoplasmic granules that cannot be resolved with the light microscope. It is true that in chloromatous

Granulocytic sarcoma

tumours (myeloid or granulocytic sarcoma) there is invasion of the periadenoid tissue with stromal destruction, but ordinarily in the early stages of myeloid metaplasia, whether associated with myeloid leukaemia or indeed other myeloproliferative conditions, the basic lymph node structure is preserved and islands of lymphocytes survive. There are reports of cases of chronic myeloid leukaemia, following chemotherapy, undergoing crises in which there is lymphadenopathy and the histology in addition to the myeloid metaplasia reveal sheets of undifferentiated 'blast' cells (Beard et al, 1976; Janossy et al, 1976).

There is a dispute as to whether monocytic and myelomonocytic leukaemias are distinct entities or variants of acute myeloid leukaemia. There are certainly morphological and cytochemical differences between the types of cell, but as far as a lymph node is concerned, if the cells are limited to the 'blast' cell phase distinction is very difficult and is dependent upon fine cytochemical distinctions.

2d(iv) *The cells are large with a round or reniform nucleus, but the cytoplasm is ill-defined in haematoxylin-eosin preparations and it appears as though the nuclei are lying in a loose eosinophilic synplasma*

Mast-cell disease

Fig. V.25

It is this curious appearance of the background that warrants consideration of *mast-cell disease*, though a proliferation of histiocytes may have similar appearances. Where individual cells can be defined, the cytoplasmic margin is somewhat angular and there may be, due to a preparation artefact, a clear zone around the cell. Once the possibility of mast-cell disease has been seriously considered, the diagnosis is easily confirmed by using a metachromatic stain such as toluidine blue or azure A. In such preparations the cytoplasmic granules become apparent, and it can be seen that the majority of the cells are somewhat oval or angular and are lying in a fine collagenous stroma. Indeed these zones of fibrosis are features that suggest mast-cell infiltration in a node. Also helpful is the fact that before the node is diffusely involved, the cell collections are most prominent around small vessels or lymph sinuses. Mast cell granules cannot be defined in a haematoxylin-eosin preparation, but apart from metachromatic staining they

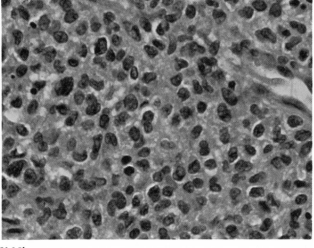

V.25b

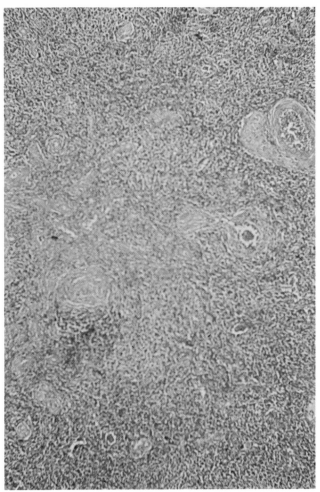

V.25a

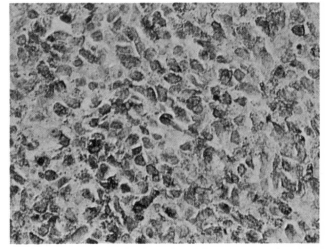

V.25c

V.25a-c   Mast Cell Disease

V.25a   General view of node showing a diffuse infiltration with widespread fine fibrosis as well as focal areas of collagen around blood vessels and hyalinization of the septa.

V.25b   Higher magnification showing the nuclear character of the mast cells in a haematoxylin eosin preparation and the false synplasmic appearance which may simulate histiocytes. Contrast this with the well defined cell outline of a myeloid infiltration (Fig. V.24b).

V.25c   Toluidine blue preparation showing the metachromatic cytoplasmic granules. This also defines the cell outline and makes clear that the synplasmic appearance in Fig. V.25b is a consequence of the stroma in which the mast cells are lying.

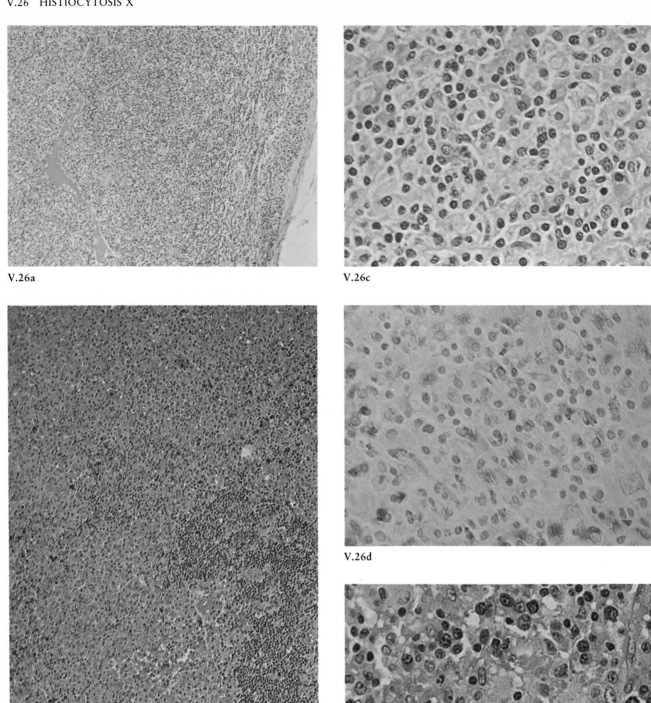

V.26a

V.26b

V.26c

V.26d

V.26e

V.26a-e   Histiocytosis X

V.26a   Diffuse monomorphic replacement of the node.

V.26b   Small islands of surviving lymphoid tissue contrast with the sheets of acidophil histiocytes.

V.26c   The diffuse histiocytic infiltration is obvious and it can be seen that the cells show no evidence of functional activity; the plasma cells and lymphocytes are not easily discerned.

V.26d   Immunoperoxidase stain for lysozyme (muramidase) showing a positive reaction in many of the histiocytes.

V.26e   Immunoperoxidase stain for immunoglobulins showing that there are many immunoglobulin containing plasma cells lying between the histiocytes; these were inconspicuous in the ordinary stained preparation (Fig. V.26c). The plasma cells are most numerous at the edge of the histiocytic infiltrate.

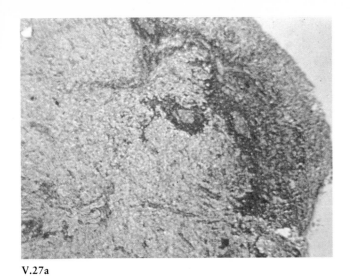

V.27a

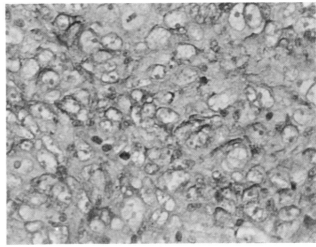

V.27c

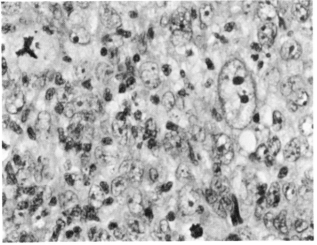

V.27b

V.27a-c   Metastases of a Non-lymphoid Tumour

V.27a   Metastatic carcinoma replacing the major portion of the node. Isolated islands of surviving lymphoid tissue are apparent and there is a sharp demarcation between the dark blue lymphoid areas and the pale pink sheets of neoplastic tissue.

V.27b   The high power displays the nuclear characters and the occasional giant nuclei, as well as the eosinophilic reticular cytoplasm; the presence of normal lymphoid cells scattered amongst the malignant cells may provide a clue, indicating that the tumour tissue is non-lymphoid.

V.27c   A section stained by PAS-tartrate tartrazine reveals the presence of intracytoplasmic mucin, confirming the diagnosis of adenocarcinoma.

can be displayed indifferently by trichrome methods; however, they are chloroacetate esterase positive and so a mast-cell proliferation might be mistaken for a myeloid infiltration (Lennert and Parwaresch, 1979).

As mast-cell disease is uncommon and the appearances in a haematoxylin-eosin preparation misleading, it is a diagnosis that rarely comes to mind when examining a lymph node, in the absence of any clinical information to guide one. Indeed the association of skin and bone lesions in a child or young adult might cause a misdiagnosis of Letterer-Siwe disease or some other manifestation of histiocytosis X, the mast cell infiltration being mistaken for histiocytes.

2d(v) *The cells are large with a round or oval nucleus rich in basichromatin; the cytoplasm is extensive, pale, eosinophilic, and somewhat vacuolated with a sharp cytoplasmic membrane, and a rather angular cell outline. There is little mitotic activity or cellular atypia*

Histiocytosis X This diffuse histiocytic proliferation is typical of certain forms of *histiocytosis X*. Immunocytochemistry often reveals the presence of cytoplasmic muramidase *Fig. V.26* while electron microscopy displays the pentalaminar X bodies ('Langerhans' granules). This histiocytic proliferation, without eosinophilia or necrosis, occurs in the subacute infantile Letterer-Siwe syndrome and in the chronic adult form of histiocytosis X, sometimes known as reticulum celled medullary reticulosis. This is essentially a paracortical proliferation, in which sinuses are inconspicuous and follicles are obscured, though on occasions there may be surviving islands of lymphoid tissue. The appearances in eosinophilic granuloma, which are very different have been described in chapter II (p. 77).

Monocytic leukaemia A somewhat similar appearance can be found in lymph nodes in chronic monocytic leukaemia, but the monocytes are discrete, smaller, and rounded in outline, with an oval nucleus and a relatively narrow cytoplasmic rim. However, histiocytic medullary reticulosis (malignant histiocytosis, see p. 137) is quite distinct as the mature histiocytes show marked cytophagocytosis and there is invariably an admixture of immature and atypical histiocytes.

The confusion that can arise between mast cell disease and histiocytosis X was mentioned in the previous section, but it should not be forgotten that metastases from a poorly differentiated spheroidal cell carcinoma – often seen in the axillary nodes draining a breast tumour – may be mistaken for a histiocytic proliferation.

2d(vi) *The cells are large but the cell outline may be ill-defined, with a faintly eosinophilic cytoplasm. The nucleus has a fine well-defined membrane and though nucleoli are striking, the basichromatin is scanty giving the nucleus an empty appearance. There may be surviving islands of lymphoid tissue*

Metastatic carcinoma The problem when presented with a node in which there is partial or complete replacement of the nodal tissue by sheets of large pale cells is whether this is a malignant lymphoma invading the node or a *secondary deposit of a poorly differentiated carcinoma.* The cellular features emphasized above – the pale faintly reticular cytoplasm with an 'empty' nucleus and prominent nucleoli would strongly favour a metastastic carcinoma, particularly if there is a sharp demarcation between surviving areas of normal lymphoid tissue and the neoplastic tissue. *Fig. V.27* Histochemical tests may help – demonstration of cytoplasmic mucin, melanin, or acid phosphatase supporting a carcinoma, while monotypic immunoglobulins would suggest a lymphoma. Unhappily in many cases such special methods are not helpful and so knowledge of cytomorphology must be the guiding principle. Malignant neoplasms of lympho-epithelial organs, such as the tonsils, may present particular difficulties. Reticulin impregnation can often help, as sheets of carcinoma cells will have no reticulin fibres between individual cells, whereas scattered fibres usually interlace the cells of a malignant lymphoma or the residual lymphoid tissue, and there is often a condensation of reticulin between the neoplastic and lymphoid tissues. The early nodular phase of lymph node infiltration by secondary deposit of carcinoma has already been discussed in chapter III (p. 109).

In the future immunocytochemical methods for identifying tumour cell products or tumour associated antigens may provide the pathologist with a means of positively identifying many of these tumours (Taylor et al, 1978).

2e. *The predominant cell is a plasma cell or is plasmacytoid in character*

In the first part of this chapter consideration was given to the interpretation of lymph node biopsies in which there was a diffuse involvement with cells resembling the lymphocyte in its various phases. Now it is convenient to consider the diagnosis of a node in which a plasma type cell is predominant. It is true that the plasma cell sarcoma has already been discussed (p. 172) in relation to immunoblastic sarcoma; however, in the group of conditions about to be reviewed, the initial impression is of a proliferation of plasma cells, rather than a proliferation of immunoblasts.

2e(i) *There is a diffuse replacement of the node by plasma cells, the majority being of mature type which are closely packed*

This is the appearance of a lymph node involved by a plasmacytoma, whether in *Plasmacytoma* classical myelomatosis or the extra-medullary type, and it is as monotonous and uniform as the nodes in 'well differentiated' lymphocytic lymphoma or chronic lymphocytic leukaemia. However, enlarged lymph nodes are seldom a presenting sign in multiple myeloma, and extramedullary myeloma is far from common (Wiltshaw, 1976), so the differential diagnosis to be seriously considered in a *Fig. V.28* solitary node replete with plasma cells must be a chronic reactive plasmacytic lymphadenitis. The striking uniform appearance, close packing and apparent maturity of neoplastic plasma cells in multiple myeloma has already been mentioned. Reactive plasma cells on the other hand often show a mixture of mature plasma cells and various differentiating forms intermediate between the plasma

189

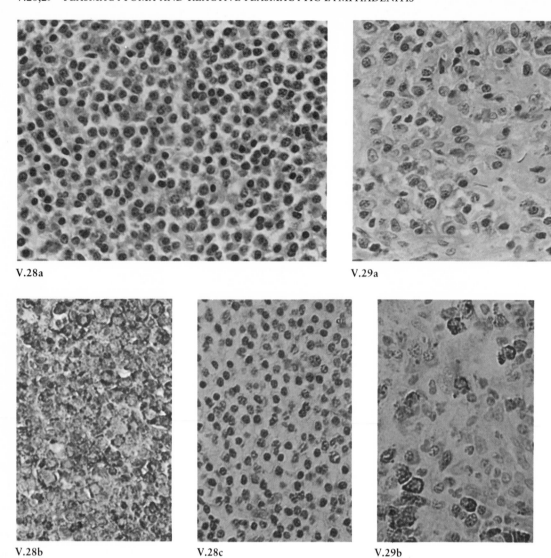

V.28a

V.29a

V.28b

V.28c

V.29b

V.28a-c Plasmacytoma (Multiple myeloma)

V.28a Diffuse infiltration of node by uniform 'mature' plasma cells.

V.28b-c The neoplastic nature of the infiltration is confirmed by a monoclonal staining pattern with immunoperoxidase on two adjacent sections. (**V.28b** Anti-λ light chain – positive; **V.28c** Anti-κ light chain – negative.)

V.29a-b Reactive Plasmacytic Lymphadenitis

V.29a In a reactive condition the morphology of the plasma cell population is quite variable with binucleate forms and cells in varying stages of maturation.

V.29b Stained by immunoperoxidase, a proportion of the plasma cells stained for κ-chain, and a proportion for λ-chain and positive and negative cells are to be seen side by side indicating their polyclonal nature.
This photo-micrograph shows a section stained with anti-κ chain antisera with positive cells. In a double stained preparation, the cells unstained by the anti-κ antisera would be positive for λ-chain.

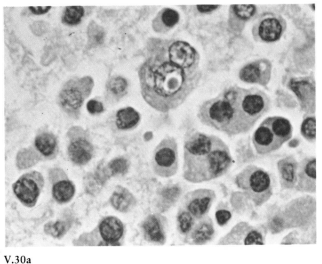

V.30a

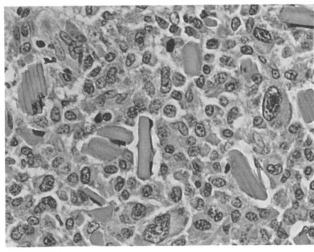

V.31a

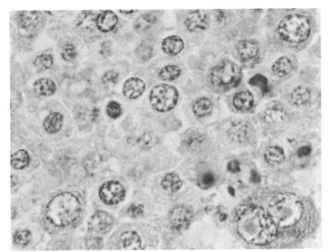

V.30b

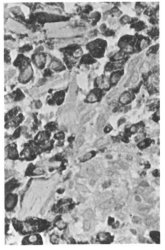

V.31b

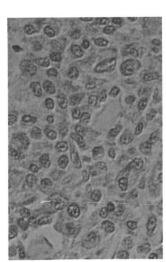

V.31c

V.30a-b   Poorly Differentiated Multiple Myeloma

V.30a   In this myeloma the majority of the cells are poorly differentiated although clearly of the plasma cell series, but included in the field is a binucleate cell with a superficial resemblance to a Reed-Sternberg cell.

V.30b   Immunoperoxidase technique shows a monoclonal staining pattern for immunoglobulin (in this case anti-κ chain) in all the immature plasma cells, including the 'pseudo-Reed Sternberg cell'.

V.31a-c   Plasmacytoid Immunoblastic Sarcoma

V.31a   This tumour presented as a nasopharyngeal mass in a forty-year-old man with no other evidence of disease. The section shows a tumour, which was infiltrating the surrounding structures and consists of immature plasma cells and immunoblasts with a proportion of giant nuclear forms and intra-cytoplasmic eosinophil paracrystalline masses.

V.31b,c   Immunoperoxidase preparation revealed a monoclonal staining pattern for γ-chain and a corresponding abnormality was subsequently demonstrated in the serum protein. **V.31b** Anti γ-chain positive. It should be noted that a proportion of the tumour cells and the inclusions fail to stain, though the thin rim of cytoplasm round an inclusion is positive. **V.31c** Anti-α-chain – negative.

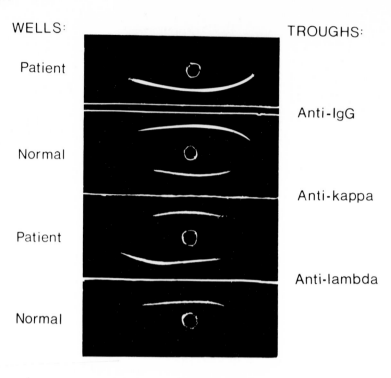

WELLS:

Patient

Normal

Patient

Normal

TROUGHS:

Anti-IgG

Anti-kappa

Anti-lambda

V.32 Immunoblastic Sarcoma

V.32a Immunoelectrophoresis of the patient's serum shows a prolongation of the band both with the anti-IgG and anti-lambda antisera confirming the secretion of lambda light chains.

Fig. V.29

Fig. V.30

Solitary plasmacytoma

Differentiation from reactive plasmacytosis

Fig. V. 29

cell and the transformed B-lymphocyte. Occasionally binucleate forms can be seen both in reactive and neoplastic conditions, but there is often more variation in the nuclear appearance (i.e. the full range of nuclear changes seen in the normal cell cycle) in a reactive plasma cell population than in a deposit of myeloma. The morphology of myeloma cells ranges from apparently normal plasma cells to obviously neoplastic cells with large atypical nuclei, thick nuclear membranes and very prominent nucleoli; in some cases these appearances approach those of the plasma cell sarcoma already discussed in this chapter (p. 173).

Solitary plasmacytoma can show a similar range of cell types, from mature plasma cells to 'dedifferentiated' forms analogous to the plasmacytoid type of immunoblastic sarcoma. In the solitary tumours crystalline or paracrystalline inclusions, as well as extra-cellular amyloid masses, are not uncommon. Nevertheless in a particular tumour, whether solitary or diffuse, there is commonly a uniformity of cell type, whether well or poorly differentiated, whereas in a reactive plasmacytic lymphadenitis it is usual for there to be a variety of cell types from transformed lymphocytes to plasma cells. Apart from the cytological differences, a chronic lymphadenitis will invariably retain the structural landmarks of a normal lymph node, which can be displayed by a reticulin impregnation, whereas in the neoplastic conditions these have ordinarily been obliterated. Also reactive plasmacytosis more commonly involves the medulla of the node, and less

V.32b

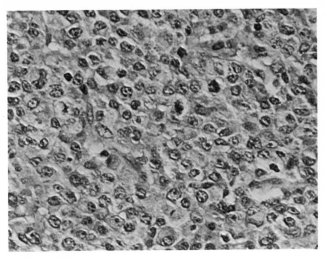

V.32c

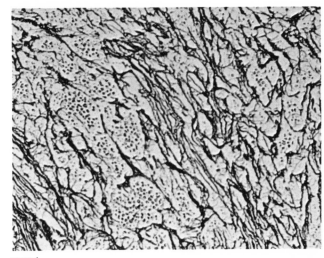

V.32d

V.32b-f   Immunoblastic Sarcoma

This case presented as a localized rib and soft tissue mass in a thirty-five year old man. Subsequent to the biopsy studies, the serum and urine were found to contain free λ-light chains (V.32a).

V.32b   Diffuse infiltration of soft tissues by a monomorphic tumour.

V.32c   High power shows that the majority of the cells resemble the transformed lymphocyte (immunoblasts) with a smattering of plasmocytoid forms. It could formerly have been classed as a lymphoblastic sarcoma or poorly differentiated reticulosarcoma.

V.32d   The reticulin impregnation shows the columns of tumour cells spreading along the reticulin sheaths of the muscle fibres. The interpretation of reticulin preparations necessitates familiarity with the normal connective tissue patterns of the various structures. In this example it might have been assumed, wrongly, that the reticulin was being induced by the tumour cells.

V.32e,f   Immunoperoxidase staining revealed that the neoplastic cells contained λ-light chains (brown granules) but were negative for κ-chains and all heavy chains.

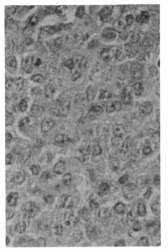

V.32e

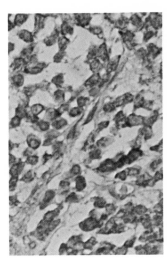

V.32f

often the cortex or paracortex. Furthermore in a plasmacytic lymphadenitis, the cells are commonly dispersed loosely in an oedematous or hyalinized stroma, in contrast to the closely packed myeloma cells, though this distinction does not always hold for the lymph nodes in α-chain disease. Differentiation between neoplastic and reactive plasma cells of mature types is facilitated by the demon-

Diagnostic value of immuno-globulin staining stration of intracellular immunoglobulin using immunoperoxidase methods (Taylor and Burns, 1974; Taylor and Mason, 1974; Taylor, 1977). Neoplastic plasma cells display a monotypic staining pattern for immunoglobulin compo-

Figs. V.28,29 nents, while reactive plasma cell populations appear polytypic (polyclonal).

Apart from differentiating reactive from neoplastic conditions, on occasions immunoglobulin staining may reveal the true identity of a malignant lymphoid tumour, which on cytological grounds might not have suggested a close relationship to the immunoglobulin forming tumours (immunocytomas). Examples of this are displayed by the cases illustrated in Figs. V. 31 and 32.

2e(ii) There is a diffuse replacement of the node by plasma type cells, loosely arranged, though the nuclear characters are lymphoid rather than plasmacytic

α-Chain disease This epitomises the features of lymph nodes in α-*chain disease*, but it is very doubtful if a confident diagnosis could be made without the help of clinical and

Fig. V.33 immunological information. On purely histological grounds the differential diagnosis would be myeloma and chronic plasmacytic lymphadenitis which have been discussed in the previous section. α-Chain disease (Mediterranean lymphoma – Seligmann, 1975; Galian et al, 1977; Brouet et al, 1977; Roth and Riecken, 1977) is essentially a gastro-intestinal disorder, though a few cases of respiratory involvement have recently been reported. Thus a mesenteric node and intestinal resection would ordinarily be the source of the material.

The morphological evolution of α-chain disease has similarities to that of steatorrhoea lymphadenopathy in that there is a range from a reactive proliferation to a progressive hyperplasia to a sarcoma. In α-chain disease these have been designated by Galian et al (1977) as stages A, B, and C.

In the reactive phase the normal architecture is maintained, but there is an increase of plasmacytic cells in the paracortical area. This proliferation becomes

Sarcomatous change more marked with the increasing obliteration of the follicles and sinuses till the phase of progressive hyperplasia is reached, when the nodal tissue is completely

Figs. V.33b,c replaced by a plasmacytic proliferation. There is no disagreement that a sarcomatous change develops in a proportion of cases with extensive infiltration in the gut wall and metastases. It is generally accepted that this represents an immunoblastic or plasma cell sarcoma (p. 173). However, recently Isaacson and Wright (1978) suggested that the sarcomatous tumour in α-chain disease is a true histiocytic sarcoma, analogous to that developing in steatorrhoea lymphadenopathy; this has not been confirmed by other workers.

In the progressive hyperplastic or 'B' stage of α-chain disease, the node is

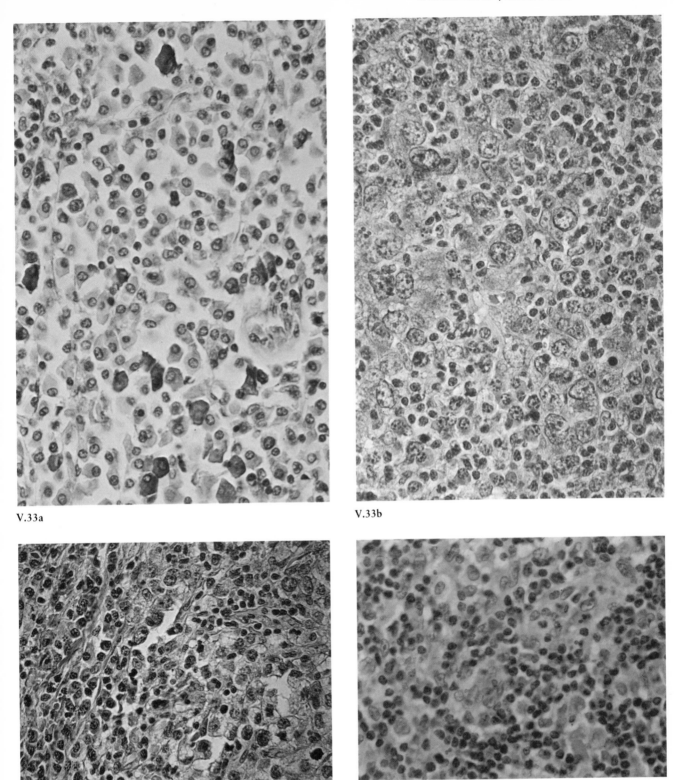

V.33a

V.33b

V.33c

V.33d

V.33a-c   α-Chain Disease

Diffuse infiltration of the node with plasmacytoid cells, the majority having lymphoid rather than plasmacytic type nuclei, but there are very few bizarre cells and very few cells resembling the transformed lymphocytes.

V.33a This is an immunoperoxidase preparation stained with anti-α chain specific antisera and it will be noted that only a small proportion of the cells have given a positive reaction.

V.33b,c α-chain disease with sarcomatous change. High power view showing plasmacytoid cells and malignant immunoblasts. V.33c is an immunoperoxidase preparation stained for anti-α and both the mature and malignant cells are positive.

V.33d   γ-Heavy Chain Disease

High power view showing the plasmacytoid cells interspersed with epithelioid cells; the eosinophils are not easily seen.

loosely infiltrated by plasma-like cells of which the majority have a bulky pale eosinophilic cytoplasm with an eccentrically placed nucleus; there are occasional binucleate forms, but giant forms and mitoses are uncommon. However, the majority of the nuclei have the character of the small lymphocyte rather than the plasma cell. This contrasts with Waldenström's disease in which the plasmacytoid type cell is admixed with typical plasma cells, small lymphocytes and immuno-blasts in varying proportions. Only a few immunoblasts are present in this phase of α-chain disease, and the observation of an increasing number of these cells should evoke suspicion that development of the sarcomatous phase is imminent.

In immunoperoxidase preparations, it will usually be found that only a small proportion of the cells stain with most orthodox anti-α chain specific antisera. It would appear that in α-chain disease, the cells secrete an imperfect α-chain fragment, lacking most of the variable amino-acid sequence portion of the α-heavy chain; furthermore the secreted fragment undergoes further enzymatic degradation in-vivo and hence may not be detectable as a defined spike in electrophoretic studies.

2e(iii) *There is a diffuse replacement of the node, in the main, with plasmacytoid lymphocytes, while typical plasma cells and lymphocytes are in the minority*

Lymphoplasmacytoid lymphoma

Waldenström's disease

It is the presence of the plasmacytoid lymphocytes admixed with small lympho-cytes that is so typical of lymphoplasmacytoid lymphoma or *Waldenström's disease**, as has been well described by Harrison (1972) and Staiger and Wester-hausen (1975). The nuclear characters are those of the small lymphocyte, but there is a clear rim of acidophil reticular cytoplasm, while the nucleus is usually central; only a minority have the eccentrically placed nucleus with the cytoplasmic 'hof' of the plasma cell. Many of the cells have large intranuclear inclusions

Fig. V.34 (Dutcher bodies) which are strongly PAS positive. Immunoperoxidase prepara-tions reveal that these inclusions contain large amounts of monotypic immuno-globulin. They are not specific for Waldenström's disease, for they have been described in other lymphoproliferative disorders and in some reactive conditions (Van den Tweel et al, 1977).

Although there is a general loss of the architectural features of the node, with a spread of the abnormal cells beyond the capsule into the periadenoid tissue, there is little stromal destruction, and almost no significant cellular atypia. Mi-toses are uncommon. The vessels in the node remain prominent and there is some orientation of the cells in relation to these vessels. The plasma in the vessels appears strongly eosinophilic and PAS positive, a consequence of the glycoprotein content of the large amount of released macroglobulin.

In some cases there is a higher proportion of transformed cells (immunoblasts)

* Synonyms: Lymphoplasmacytoid immunocytoma (Kiel); Waldenström's macroglobulinaemia (Rappa-port); Plasmacytoid lymphocytic malignant lymphoma (Lukes and Collins); Waldenström's primary ma-croglobulinaemia (WHO); Lymphocytic intermediately differentiated diffuse lymphoma with plasmacytoid differentiation (NLI); Small lymphocytic diffuse lymphoma with plasmacytoid differentiation (Dorfman). The bracketed designations are explained in Appendix l.

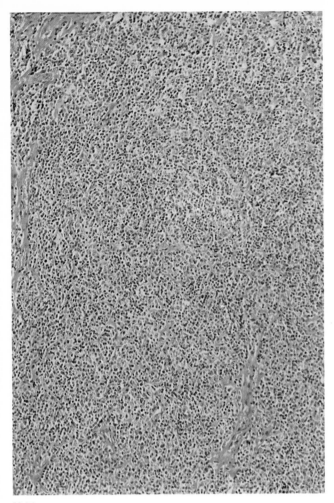

V.34a

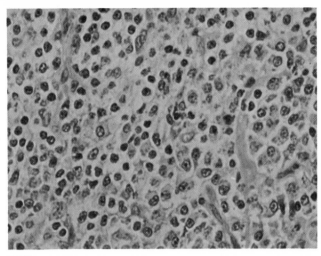

V.34b

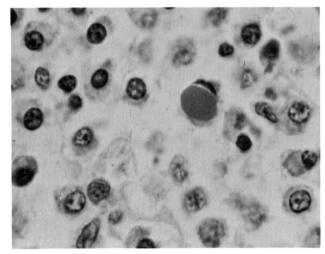

V.34c

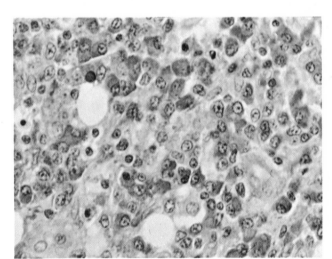

V.34d

V.34a-d   Lymphoplasmacytoid Lymphoma

V.34a   Diffuse infiltration of the node showing the uniform cellular replacement.

V.34b   Higher magnification showing the cellular characters ranging from lymphoid to plasmacytoid cells while the vessels are prominent. 'Supra-nuclear windows' reflecting the loss of intra-nuclear inclusions during processing can be seen in the upper right corner.

V.34c   This PAS-tartrazine preparation provides greater nuclear and cytoplasmic detail, while an intra-nuclear inclusion (Dutcher body) is strongly positive.

V.34d   Immunoperoxidase stain for μ-chain showing the presence of IgM in the plasmacytoid cells. A positive reacting intra-nuclear inclusion is apparent in the upper left corner.

and these tend to run a more aggressive coarse and may eventually undergo malignant transformation to an immunoblastic sarcoma.

Immunoperoxidase preparations stained for μ-chain reveal the presence of IgM in the plasmacytoid cells, but as Lennert (1975) and others have pointed out the occurrence of monoclonal macroglobulin is not restricted to Waldenström's disease. In addition, we have shown that other cases with identical morphology may contain monoclonal IgG or IgA, which may or may not be secreted into the serum in sufficient quantities for detection by immunoelectrophoresis.

γ-Heavy chain disease

The changes in the lymph nodes in γ-*heavy chain disease (Franklin's disease)* have not been very well described, but it would appear to have some morphological affinities to Waldenström's disease, save that there is a higher proportion of pleomorphic plasma cells, together with scattered foci of eosinophils and

Fig. V.33d

epithelioid cells (Frangione and Franklin, 1973; Bloch et al, 1973; Shirakura et al, 1976). Interestingly, early cases of this disease were misdiagnosed as Hodgkin's disease, consequent on the presence of atypical immunoblasts and eosinophils.

μ-Heavy chain disease

Recently a third form of *heavy chain disease of μ class* has been described (Franklin, 1975; Frangione et al, 1976) usually manifesting itself in patients with chronic lymphatic leukaemia, with minimal lymphadenopathy but marked hepatomegaly and splenomegaly. There may be excretion of a type of Bence-Jones protein in the urine. In the tissues in addition to small lymphocytes there were plasma cells with vacuoles in the vicinity of the Golgi apparatus, and in one case the cytoplasm contained μ-heavy chains and κ-light chains (Zucker-Franklin and Franklin, 1971).

3. Diffuse cellular proliferation, with increased cellularity, and admixture of two or more distinct cell types

In the previous sections, consideration was given to conditions associated with diffuse infiltration of the node by one particular neoplastic cell type, although there was sometimes a range of cells in various stages of development (e.g. lymphocytes, B-immunoblasts, plasma cells – all being B-lymphocyte derived), with varying degrees of differentiation and atypia, which might include giant or multinucleate cells. Also in certain conditions – of which Burkitt's tumour is a typical example – neoplastic cells were associated with large numbers of macrophages. It now remains to consider conditions in which the diffuse infiltration is characteristically polymorphic, consisting of an admixture of cells of the lymphoid and histiocytic series, together with myeloid and fibroblastic elements in some instances.

Hodgkin's disease is the classical example of this type of proliferation, but there are a number of other conditions, some of which are reactive and others neoplastic, which must be distinguished from Hodgkin's disease. In English speaking countries, the collective term 'granuloma' used to be applied to these polymorphic cellular proliferations, but nowadays in the main, this term is restricted to reactive conditions (Dhom, 1980). There is, however, still confusion as to the morphological features by which a diffuse reactive 'granulomatous' condition can be distinguished from its lymphoproliferative or neoplastic counterpart. In an attempt to overcome this, the unfortunate term 'pseudo-lymphoma' has been applied to some of these reactive conditions, thus perpetuating the conceptual chaos that was achieved nearly a century ago when Cohnheim wrote of pseudo-leukaemia.

There is no denying that it is difficult to provide precise structural and cytological criteria by which these distinctions can be made, as the determining factors are the overall pattern, the intimate relationship of the various cell types, the preservation of islands of normal but reactive lymphoid tissue, and the vascular response. In the lymphoproliferative conditions (including Hodgkin's disease) and malignant lymphomas, it is not only the cellular atypia, but also the destruction of the normal background in the involved area and the alteration in fibrous pattern, that influence the final decision. Several conditions falling into this differential diagnosis will be considered in turn.

3a. *There is a polymorphic infiltration consisting of lymphocytes (many being transformed), plasma cells, histiocytes and granulocytes lying in a somewhat oedematous stroma with areas of necrosis and prominent vessels, some showing fibrinoid change*

The various types of reactive lymphadenopathy in which there is both follicular (B-cell) and paracortical (T-cell) proliferation were discussed in chapter III. However, in some *reactive conditions* the follicular response (B-cell component) is minimal or is masked by an overwhelming and predominant paracortical T-cell response, in which large transformed lymphocytes (immunoblasts) predominate. This type of antigenically stimulated lymph node presents the appearances summarized above, and is very liable to be confused with a lymphoma of low or even high grade malignancy.

Reactive lymphadenitis

There are, however, a number of features which can guide one in recognizing these exuberant reactive conditions. As has already been emphasized, in a lymphomatous condition the majority of the cells, while atypical, are of one series, whereas in a reactive condition there will be an admixture of all types of lymphoid and histiocytic cells, and though there may be immunoblasts and immature histiocytes, there is no real cellular atypia. Mitotic activity is no guide as this may be marked both in reactive and lymphomatous conditions. Of the neoplastic lympho-proliferative conditions the only one likely to cause serious difficulty is Hodgkin's disease. Identification of angio-immunoblastic lymphadenopathy and Sjögren's lymphadenopathy is dependent on the diagnostic criteria accepted for these conditions and will be discussed later.

In Hodgkin's disease there is a mixed cellular infiltrate and the character of many of the lymphoid, histiocytic and myeloid cells is within the range found in reactive conditions. However, for a diagnosis of Hodgkin's disease, it is necessary

Differentiation from Hodgkin's disease

to identify typical cells of the Reed-Sternberg type. It should be remembered that though cells somewhat resembling Reed-Sternberg cells have been described in reactive conditions (Strum et al, 1970; Tindle et al, 1972), the general morphological background in which they occur does not really simulate Hodgkin's disease. Furthermore it is unusual to find diffuse involvement of the whole node in early Hodgkin's disease, whereas this is the rule in reactive lymphadenopathies.

Apart from the cytological distinctions, there are architectural features which are a far better guide in distinguishing reactive from neoplastic lymphadenopathies. In the first place there is no stromal destruction in reactive lymphadenopathies, unless there have been zones of necrosis with lysis of reticulin, while in mixed cellular and nodular sclerosing Hodgkin's disease an irregular increase of reticulin and collagen is invariable. Indeed it is these foci of acute necrosis, with

Hypersensitivity lymphadenopathy cellular debris, that are very characteristic of *hypersensitivity lymphadenopathy due to drugs* such a phenytoin (diphenyl hydantoin, dilantin, etc). In addition, in drug induced lymphadenopathy it is usual to find fibrinoid change in small vessels, often with thromboses, and the fibrinoid change may involve the perinodal tissue;

Fig. V. 35 it is seldom extensive, but the vascular necrotic change is a valuable diagnostic indicator. The particular cytological features of this type of lymphadenopathy, in addition to the immunoblastic proliferation, are the clumps of histiocytes that sometimes form Touton giant cells and the foci of eosinophils. Scattered or isolated eosinophils occur in a wide range of lymph node disorders, but local aggregates are uncommon, and are seldom seen except in conditions associated with hypersensitivity or in eosinophilic granuloma (Saltzstein and Ackerman, 1959; Krasznai and Szegedi, 1969).

Granulomatous lymphadenitis *Nonspecific granulomatous lymphadenitis* probably represents a variant of hypersensitivity lymphadenitis. There may be small giant cell granulomata scat-

Fig. V.36 tered amongst the sheets of immunoblasts, plasma cells and histiocytes and prominent post-capillary venules, features that tend to merge both clinically and morphologically with the angio-immunoblastic lymphadenopathy group. The diffuse type of reactive lymphadenopathy with inconspicuous follicular involvement may also occur, albeit uncommonly, in viral lymphadenitis (e.g. infectious mononucleosis). In all the diffuse reactive lymphadenopathies, in contrast to the neoplastic disorders, there is usually an increase of interstitial fluid, often giving an impression of oedema, with engorgement of vessels and lymph sinuses. This may even be apparent in the periadenoid tissue.

3b. *There is a polymorphic infiltration consisting of small and large lymphocytes, immunoblasts, numerous plasma cells and variable number of histiocytes lying in a markedly vascularized oedematous stroma*

This is an epitome of the lymph node changes in the clinico-pathological syn-
Angio-immunoblastic lymphadenopathy drome which Lukes and Tindle (1973, 1975) termed *immunoblastic lymphadenopathy*. The basic features, with some variations, have been endorsed by other

workers; Rappaport's (1974, 1975) angio-immunoblastic lymphadenopathy is apparently becoming the preferred designation, though Lennert (Radaszkiewicz and Lennert, 1975) has used the unfortunate term 'lymphogranulomatosis X' for what appears to be a closely related or identical condition.

It would seem from Lennert (1972) that the earliest discussions concerning this condition occurred at the U.S.-Japanese Seminar on malignant diseases of the haematopoietic system held at Nagaya in 1971, when Lukes classed it as an 'immunoblastic lesion', Katayama as 'Hodgkinoid or specific granulomatosis', and Dorfman, following Hutchinsonian precepts, spoke of Puckett's disease; these discussions were not published in the Gann monograph (Akazaki et al, 1973).

Lukes and his colleagues believed that it was more likely to be a hyperimmune reactive disorder than a neoplastic lymphoproliferative condition. They initially (cited by Dorfman and Warnke, 1974) described three histological forms: type I being related to hypersensitivity lymphadenopathy; type II was immunoblastic lymphadenopathy just described and type III corresponded to Lennert's lympho-epithelioid lymphoma (Lennert, 1975). Subsequently Lukes abandoned these subdivisions.

The condition occurs most commonly in the fifth and sixth decades, with fever, weight loss, rashes, generalized lymphadenopathy and hepato-splenomegaly. Polyclonal hyperglobulinaemia and cutaneous anergy are often found. In a proportion of cases there is a haemolytic anaemia. The course is stormy and unpredictable, many of the patients succumbing to intercurrent infections, perhaps precipitated by cytotoxic chemotherapy. The striking histological feature in the *Fig. V.37* lymph node is the generalised prominence of post-capillary venules, with marked endothelial proliferation and thickening of the basement membrane. Interspersed throughout the node are large numbers of transformed lymphocytes, some of which show plasmacytoid features and a polyclonal pattern of immunoglobulin staining; occasionally a small proportion of the immunoblasts may be multi-nucleate. In addition there are variable numbers of mature plasma cells and lymphocytes. There is usually an admixture of histiocytes; these may be prominent, with epithelioid and giant cell forms, occurring diffusely or in clusters. Eosinophils are noticeable in about a third of the cases. In addition to the cytological features there is a background of amorphous eosinophilic PAS positive material between the cells giving an overall hypocellular appearance; the PAS positive material may be extensive, in association with perivascular fibrosis. In a proportion of the cases residual follicles can be recognized, though by the strictest definition of Lukes and Tindle follicles are not present. The most detailed cytological study, including electron microscopy, has been made by Neimann et al (1978), who were able to confirm the light microscopical appearance. In addition they showed that the amorphous stromal material consists of debris from dead and dying cells. Wright et al (1976) confirmed by marker studies that this is predominantly a B-cell proliferation, associated with a deficit in the T-cell

V.35a

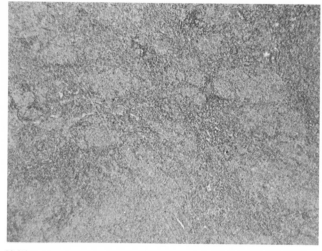

V.36a

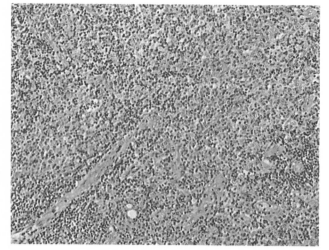

V.35b

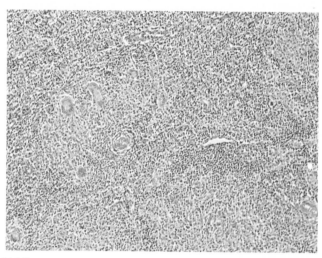

V.36b

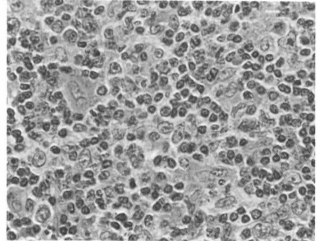

V.35c

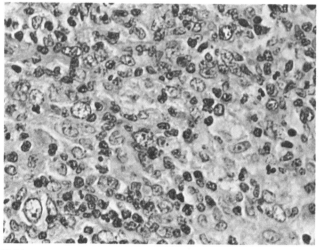

V.36c

V.35a-c Hypersensitivity Lymphadenopathy

V.35a Diffuse loss of normal architecture.

V.35b This infiltrate is somewhat irregular with small islands of surviving lymphoid tissue. It is usual to find foci of necrosis though these are not displayed here.

V.35c At high magnifications, the polymorphic infiltrate is clearly seen consisting of lymphocytes, plasma cells, reactive histiocytes, eosinophils and transformed lymphocytes. There is little cellular atypia and the binucleate histiocytes have only the most superficial resemblance to the Reed-Sternberg cell.

V.36a-c Non-specific Granulomatous Lymphadenitis

V.36a Diffuse and patchy infiltration of the node by sheets and clusters of large pale cells. The architecture of the node is obscured but a reticulin impregnation would display the structural landmarks.

V.36b Residual islands of lymphocytes remain, while there are foci of histiocytes and histiocytic giant cells associated with transformed lymphocytes.

V.36c At high magnification the infiltrate can be seen to consist of lymphocytes, plasma cells, histiocytes and immunoblasts, but once again there is very little cellular atypia.

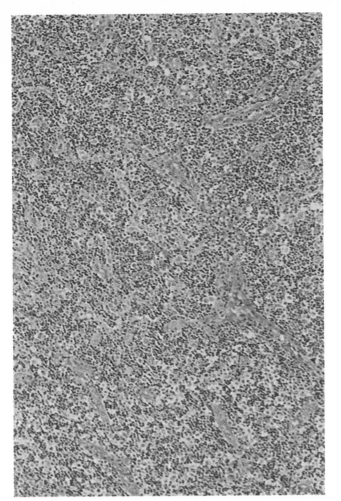

V.37a

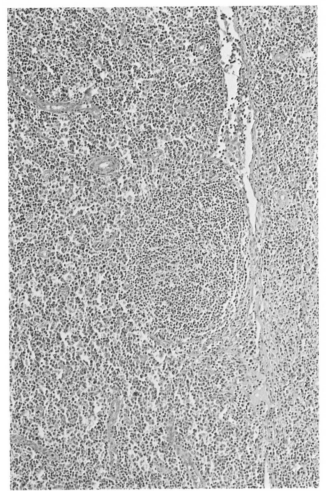

V.37b

V.37a-c Angio-Immunoblastic Lymphadenopathy

V.37a The normal architecture is obscured by a polymorphic cellular infiltrate interspersed by prominently interlacing small vessels with marked endothelial thickening.

V.37b Similar low power view save that there is a surviving follicle.

V.37c This shows the hyperplastic post-capillary venules surrounded by immunoblasts, lymphocytes, immature plasma cells, histiocytes and eosinophils but there is little cellular atypia. The amorphous eosinophil matrix is apparent, giving an overall hypocellular appearance.

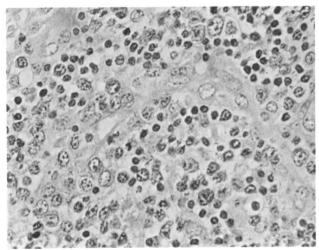

V.37c

system. In a later study Jones et al (1978) suggested that a type with a preponderance of B-cells and plasma cells had a good prognosis, while cases with a T-cell preponderance and a B-cell deficiency which were associated with a proliferation of B-immunoblasts and a paucity of plasma cells had a poor prognosis; Schnardt et al (1979) has come to similar conclusions.

Lukes and Tindle, in their original account (1975), mentioned that three of the cases had evolved to an immunoblastic sarcoma. Nathwani, Kim and Rappaport (1978) have set out the cytological features by which they recognize 'malignant lymphomatous change' in angio-immunoblastic lymphadenopathy. There appears to be a correlation between prognosis and cellular atypia. In brief the occurrence of 'multiple clusters or islands of compactly arranged large lymphoid cells (immunoblasts) constituted the initial histologic evidence of immunoblastic lymphoma'. Three variants of immunoblastic lymphoma were observed by Nathwani and colleagues: the first lacking plasmacytoid features, the second consisting of immunoblasts with some plasmacytoid differentiation, the third showing extreme plasmacytic differentiation resembling 'plasma cell sarcoma'. However their criteria for immunoblastic lymphoma differed from those adopted here for immunoblastic sarcoma. Lennert et al (1979) in an excellent discussion on pre-lymphomas also question the criteria adopted by Nathwani et al for recognizing a sarcomatory evolution which they claimed occurred in 50% of cases of angio-immunoblastic lymphadenopathy. Lennert et al analysed a series of 172 cases and concluded that using strict criteria only 6% underwent sarcomatous change, but with equivocal evidence this could increase to 13%: this corresponds closely to our experience.

It should be emphasized that we fully endorse the histological features recognized by Nathwani et al (1978) for identifying the poorly differentiated form of angio-immunoblastic lymphadenopathy and its prognostic importance. In particular the finding of focal collections of immunoblasts, that lack evidence of normal plasmacytoid maturation, and so appear monomorphous, is of sinister import.

All of this does little to simplify the diagnosis of this condition. Frizzera et al (1974) wrote that no single histological feature is pathognomic of angio-immunoblastic lymphadenopathy, but the diagnosis is a cumulative one. In the differential diagnosis, reactive hyperplasia and Hodgkin's disease present the greatest difficulty. As has already been said, the distinction between the non-specific granulomatous lymphadenitis and angio-immunoblastic lymphadenopathy is dependent on the criteria adopted, and it would seem that Rappaport and his colleagues have broader criteria than Lukes and Tindle, who demand total involvement of the node by a process that is wholly diffuse. On the other hand provided the biopsy material is of good quality there should not be difficulties in distinguishing Hodgkin's disease from angio-immunoblastic lymphadenopathy, always assuming that one's diagnostic criteria of Hodgkin's disease are precise.

Nevertheless in the past this form of lymphadenopathy was designated 'Hodgkinoid granulomatosis', 'lymphogranulomatous X' and perhaps included under Lennert and Mestdagh's 'epithelioid cell lymphogranulomatosis' (p. 92), and it is clear that there was confusion. This is understandable as all the cell types found in angio-immunoblastic lymphadenopathy – lymphocytes, plasmacytes, immunoblasts, histiocytes, eosinophils – are to be found in Hodgkin's disease, but the basic difference is the vascular pattern and the lack of Reed-Sternberg cells in angio-immunoblastic lymphadenopathy. Hyperplastic post-capillary venules can be found in a whole range of reactive lymphadenopathies, but their presence in a lymph node should make one very unwilling to make a diagnosis of Hodgkin's disease. Conversely some degree of general or local fibrosis is characteristic of Hodgkin's disease, whereas in angio-immunoblastic lymphadenopathy the reticulin is solely related to the vascular element. From a cytological point of view it is the cellular distribution and the absence of fibroblasts or 'Hodgkin cells,' whether mononuclear, Reed-Sternberg or lacunar, that should make one hesitate to consider a diagnosis of Hodgkin's disease in a lymph node with a diffuse polymorphic cellular replacement. Finally it should not be forgotten that angio-immunoblastic lymphadenopathy is a clinico-pathological syndrome and there are a number of clinical features which help distinguish it from Hodgkin's disease, e.g., the higher age group, the generalized lymphadenopathy and polyclonal hypergammaglobulinaemia.

3c. *There is a polymorphic infiltration consisting of lymphocytes, of which only a small minority are transformed, giant cells of Reed-Sternberg and mononuclear Hodgkin type, plasma cells, histiocytes, eosinophils and fibrocytes*

This summarizes the essential cytological features of *Hodgkin's disease of the mixed cellularity type*. A diagnosis of Hodgkin's disease depends not only on the cell types present but also on the architectural pattern. Most commonly the whole node is replaced by the polymorphic infiltration and, though there may be thickening of the capsule and fibrosis of the periadenoid fat, it is unusual for the infiltrate to extend into the periadenoid area. Where there is incomplete involvement of a node the infiltrate is restricted to focal areas in the cortical and paracortical zones, with preservation of follicles, but subsequently the fibrocellular infiltrate extends like a curtain across the node. A rather characteristic lesion is the hyalinisation of the trabeculae with a laminated arrangement of collagen around the trabecular vessels.

Hodgkin's disease mixed cellularity

Fig. V.38

Figs. III.15g,h

Fig. V.38c

Turning to the cellular details, there is, in the mixed cellular form of Hodgkin's disease, no overall patterning of the infiltrate. In contrast to the other conditions associated with a diffuse polymorphic cellular infiltrate, in this form of Hodgkin's disease an interlacing network of fibroblasts is always prominent; this is clearly seen by use of a reticulin impregnation, and it is between this fibrous network that the mixed cell infiltrate lies. The other feature that is of diagnostic importance is that apart from the 'Hodgkin' giant cells, the remaining cells are essentially normal in appearance. The effect, therefore, is of a fibroblastic network in which

V.38a

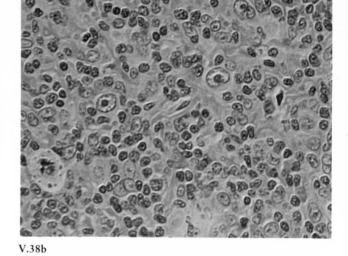

V.38b

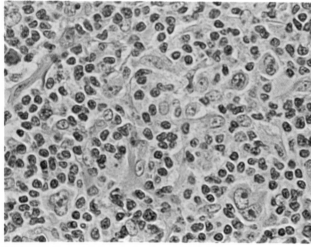

V.38c

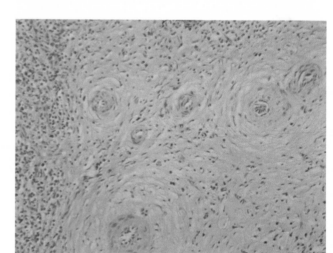

V.38d

V.38a-d   Hodgkin's Disease Mixed Cellularity

V.38a   The normal architecture is completely obscured by a mottled pattern due to the mixed cellularity. Coarse fibrosis is not seen but there are areas of necrosis.

V.38b   High power shows the mixed cell population lying between the interlacing fibroblasts. There are several mononuclear Hodgkin cells and occasional multinucleate histiocytes.

V.38c   Another field in which a classical Reed-Sternberg cell is apparent. This again emphasizes the morphological normality of the cells in Hodgkin's disease except for the giant cells, and mononuclear Hodgkin cells.

V.38d   This shows an area of hyalinization of a trabecle with the characteristic laminated arrangement of the collagen around the trabecular vessels. The Hodgkin tissue is apparent at the edge of the photo-micrograph.

V.39a

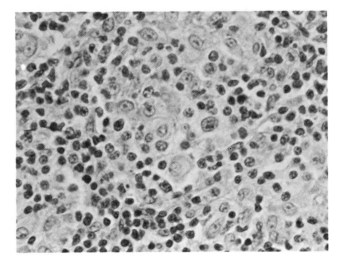

V.39b

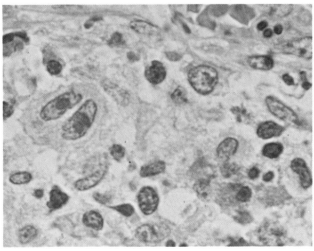

V.39c

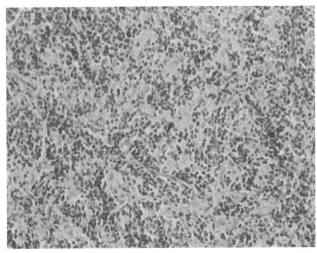

V.39d

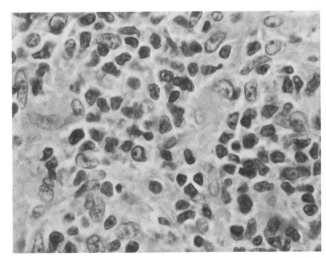

V.39e

V.39a-e   Lymphocytic and Histiocytic preponderant Hodgkin's Disease and Lympho-epithelioid (Peedell-Lennert) Lymphoma

Lymphocytic and Histiocytic preponderant Hodgkin's Disease

V.39a   The node has been replaced by lymphoid cells and scattered clumps of epithelioid histiocytes which tend to coalesce into large foci in contrast to the patterned distribution of the congeries in the lympho-epithelioid (Peedell-Lennert) lymphoma.

V.39b   The high power shows an admixture of epithelioid histiocytes and mononuclear Hodgkin cells; the majority of the lymphocytes are small mature forms.

V.39c   This field happens to include a Reed-Sternberg cell and some eosinophils which are uncommon in the lymphocyte preponderant Hodgkin's disease.

Lympho-epithelioid (Peedell-Lennert) Lymphoma

V.39d   Low power showing the diffuse distribution of epithelioid cells in the lymphoid stroma.

V.39e   High power showing the irregular nuclear outline of the T-type lymphocytes surrounding the epithelioid groups.

are lying normal lymphocytes, plasma cells and eosinophils, together with a few histiocytes and transformed lymphocytes. Scattered in this matrix are the striking giant cells that characterise the condition. Blood vessels are inconspicuous apart from those in the trabeculae which have already been mentioned. It is not uncommon to find small zones of focal necrosis. Rarely necrosis may be massive.

It is convenient here to recapitulate the essential features of the various forms of Hodgkin giant cell.

The Reed-Sternberg Cell

The overall dimensions of the cell exceed 15–20 μm. The appearance of the cytoplasm may vary with fixation; in well fixed material it is usually sharply defined and is weakly basophilic or amphophilic. Marked cytoplasmic eosinophilia is only seen in association with other evidence of cell degeneration such as nuclear pyknosis, and is associated with the 'necrobiotic' change which Cross (1969) considered to be characteristic of Hodgkin's disease. Some of the larger Reed-Sternberg cells may show cytoplasmic collapse in formalin fixed tissues, but this is rarely observed with Zenker fixation.

Figs. III.15p,q
Fig. V.38c

The nucleus is large in proportion to the cytoplasm and is multi-lobular; commonly the cell contains two or more nuclei. In the classical 'mirror image' Reed-Sternberg cell, two closely similar nuclei are opposed one to another in the same cell. The nucleus possesses some characteristic features. The nuclear membrane is distinct and relatively thick. The nuclear chromatin is dispersed, with small clumps occurring in relation to the nuclear membrane, giving the nucleus an overall clear vesicular appearance. In the centre of the nucleus there is usually a single large acidophil nucleolus (approximately one quarter the size of a red cell). These nuclear characteristics are also present in multi-lobulated cells, when the nucleoli are situated centrally within the separate lobules. Mitotic division is very seldom seen in Reed-Sternberg cells.

A clear area or 'hof' may occur in relation to the nucleus of those Reed-Sternberg cells which have a more basophilic cytoplasm. Yet this 'hof' is much less prominent than in the Reed-Sternberg-like cells occurring in infective conditions. Also in these latter cells, in contrast to the true Hodgkin Reed-Sternberg cell, the nucleolus is more often basophilic (Dorfman and Warnke, 1974).

Lacunar Cell

Figs. III.15m–o
Fig. V.19c

This is a large (25 μm or more) multilobulate cell, probably closely related to the Reed-Sternberg cell. It is characterized by the extensive cytoplasmic collapse seen in formalin fixed material, giving the 'lacunar' effect, from which the cell takes its name. Where the cytoplasm persists it is pale and almost 'water clear,' and may be extensive. The nucleus also differs from that of the Reed-Sternberg cell in that lacunar cells have a greater degree of nuclear lobulation, the nuclear membrane is finer and the nucleoli smaller. Intermediate forms between the Reed-Sternberg and lacunar cell occur in some cases. Closely packed lacunar cells present an unusual appearance which may cause difficulties in interpretation, and they are most easily recognized when occurring singly amonst packed small lymphocytes (Anagnostou et al, 1977).

The Giant Cell of Lymphocyte Predominant Hodgkin's Disease

This form of giant cell, described by Lukes and Butler (1966), is probably related to the classical Reed-Sternberg cell. It only occurs in the lymphocyte and histiocyte predominant form of Hodgkin's disease and Lukes (1971) has given it an unwieldy designation, 'L and H variant of the Reed-Sternberg cell'. The nucleus is large and delicately folded. The chromatin is finely dispersed and the nuclear *Fig. III.13b* membrane is less distinct, and the nucleoli smaller, than in true Reed-Sternberg cells. The cytoplasm is indistinct and may show some eosinophilia. These cells are liable to be confused with foreign body giant cells. In this respect it is helpful to remember that these 'L and H' variants have a very high nuclear cytoplasmic ratio, whereas foreign body giant cells, with their extensive cytoplasm, do not.

Mononuclear Hodgkin Cells

In any case of Hodgkin's disease there are variable numbers of atypical mono- *Figs. III. 13b, 14b, 15l* nuclear cells, which share some of the nuclear characteristics of the Reed-Sternberg cell. These cells have a distinct nuclear membrane, a vesicular nucleus and often a large central eosinophilic nucleolus. In contrast to the Reed-Sternberg cell, mitosis is not uncommon and, indeed, this is generally considered to represent the actively proliferating cell in Hodgkin's disease. The cytoplasm is often markedly basophilic and may display a juxta-nuclear 'hof'. This type of cell has often been referred to as the 'atypical reticulum cell' of Hodgkin's disease and was called the 'Hodgkin cell' by Moeschlin in 1951. It had previously been recognized by others, including Sternberg (1903), who regarded it as an intermediate stage *Figs. V.38b, 39b* in the development of the Reed-Sternberg cell. These Hodgkin cells usually outnumber Reed-Sternberg cells but are of limited diagnostic value because of the great difficulty in distinguishing them with certainty from reactive immuno-blasts, particularly if the latter are in any way atypical.

The salient characters of the different types of Hodgkin's Disease

The features of the lymphocyte predominant and nodular sclerotic types of Hodgkin's disease have already been discussed in previous chapters, and the lymphocyte depleted variety will be considered in the next section. The segregation of one type from another is arbitrary as there is a spectral range of appear-

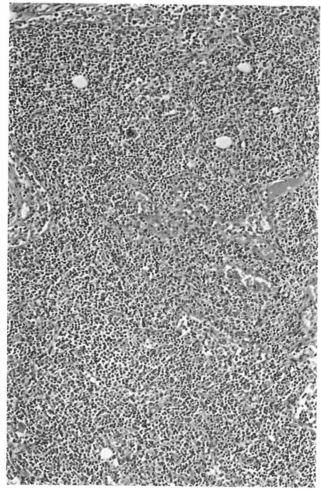

V.40a

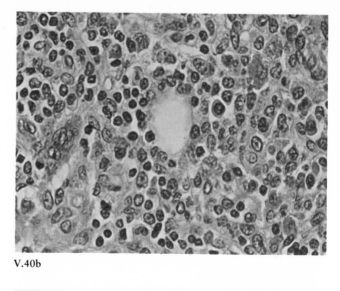

V.40b

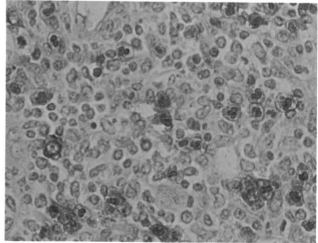

V.40c

V.40a-c Secondary Myelosclerosis

V.40a There is a polymorphic replacement of the node in which occasional giant cells can be made out, and it should be noted that the sinuses are unaffected.

V.40b The myeloid and erythroid metaplasia in apparent while a few magakaryocytes can be recognized; the eosinophil myelocytes are obvious.

V.40c The chloroacetate esterase reaction emphasizes the myeloid elements.

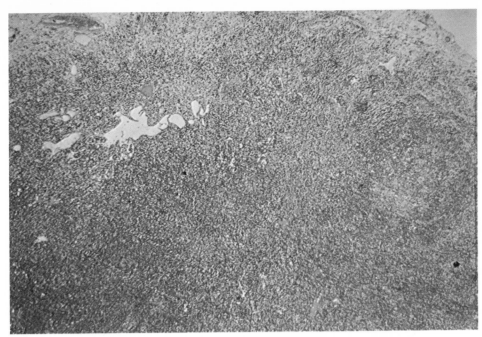

V.41a

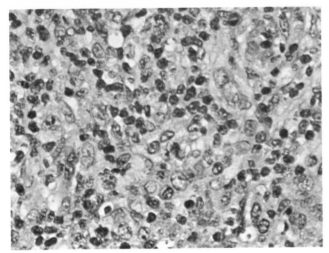

V.41b

V.41a-b   The Lymphadenopathy of Sjögren's Syndrome

V.41a   There is a diffuse but irregular replacement of the node, while the follicles have survived in the right hand side but are somewhat inconspicuous; the contraction due to the diffuse fibrosis has rendered the sinuses more apparent.

V.41b   The high power shows the character of the infiltrate; lymphocytes, plasma cells and eosinophils and large numbers of transformed lymphocytes or immunoblasts, but no specific giant cells. In spite of the fibrosis, fibroblasts are not obvious.

ances, though to some extent the nodular sclerotic form appears somewhat distinct from the other forms of the disease.

For example, comparing the lymphocyte predominant type with that of mixed cellularity, in the former lymphocytes are more numerous, while Hodgkin and Reed-Sternberg cells are less common, and necrosis and fibrosis are rare. Comparing the lymphocyte depleted and the mixed cellularity forms, in the former there is much more fibrosis, and both Reed-Sternberg and Hodgkin cells are more numerous, while, as the name suggests, the number of lymphocytes is diminished. Yet none of these distinctions are absolute, and different appearances may be seen in the same biopsy or the same patient. The character of the nodular sclerotic form, and the problem of the distinction between the cellular phase of nodular sclerosis and the mixed cellularity phase of Hodgkin's disease, have already been considered (chapter III).

Significance of epithelioid histiocytes in Hodgkin's disease

Another difficulty arises in classifying those cases of Hodgkin's disease in which clusters of epithelioid histiocytes are present. It is not uncommon to find histiocytes, including epithelioid forms, in typical cases of mixed cellularity Hodgkin's disease. Generally such histiocytes occur in small clumps or are scattered irregularly throughout the node. However, Reed-Sternberg cells and the other features of mixed cellularity Hodgkin's disease remain apparent; this corresponds to Cross' poorly differentiated histiocytic group of Hodgkin's disease (1969). On

Figs. V.39a–c

the other hand in the *epithelioid or lymphocytic and histiocytic type of Hodgkin's disease* (Lukes and Butler, 1966) which has been included in the *lymphocytic preponderant type* of the Rye classification, variable numbers of histiocytes, which are occasionally binucleate, occur diffusely or in aggregates throughout the node. Reed-Sternberg cells are difficult to find, but the lymphocyte predominant type giant cells are plentiful. There is usually no necrosis, and no increase of fibrous tissue. The lymphocytes are of small mature type, in contrast to the distorted nuclear forms of the small and medium sized lymphocytes that char-

Figs. V.39d,e

acterize the so-called Peedell-Lennert lymphoma or epithelioid-cell lymphogranulomatosis (see p. 92). Having made these precise distinctions, it must be confessed that the categorization of cases of Hodgkin's disease in which there are histiocytic clusters is far from easy and their natural history is uncertain.

It is a consequence of this merging of the morphological features of the various types of Hodgkin's disease, that their reported frequency is so variable in different centres. In essence there is sometimes doubt as to whether a proliferative change of one sort or another in a lymph node should be regarded as indicative of Hodgkin's disease, or not. Such doubts are enhanced when the material has been poorly prepared. Unhappily many pathologists, when uncertain, believe that it is safer to diagnose Hodgkin's disease rather than admit their doubts, whereas we believe that it is far more injurious to falsely diagnose Hodgkin's disease than to fail to recognize it. In the latter instance the error of omission will soon become apparent, whereas to submit a young adult with a minor reactive lymphadenopathy to the ardours of modern chemo- or radiotherapy, is indeed hazardous.

This liability to overdiagnose Hodgkin's disease is well displayed by a review of 600 cases submitted to Symmers (1968), with a histological diagnosis of Hodgkin's disease. The diagnosis could only be confirmed in 53% of these; 38% were reactive or inflammatory conditions and 9% were other primary or secondary malignant diseases or lymphoproliferative conditions.

It remains to consider three conditions in which there is a polymorphic lymphoid proliferation but in which lymphadenopathy is not ordinarily the presenting manifestation. Thus a lymph node biopsy would not usually be required for diagnosis but might be performed for clinical evaluation.

3d. There is a polymorphic infiltrate composed of lymphocytes, immunoblasts and large, often bizarre, lymphoid cells, some of which show complexly folded nuclei

Mycosis fungoides has, since the introduction of cell marker techniques, often been equated with Sézary's syndrome (p. 153). Nevertheless they are completely different clinically and histologically. Both involve the dermis and are predominantly T-cell manifestations, but this is equally true of lymphomatoid papulosus (Feuermann and Sandbank, 1972). In the erythrodermic phase of mycosis, the lymph nodes show the changes of dermatopathic lymphadenitis. This may also be present in the nodular phase, but once systemic involvement has occurred the morphological changes in the enlarged lymph nodes are as specific as those in the skin (Epstein et al, 1972; Rappaport and Thomas, 1974; Saxe et al, 1977).

Mycosis fungoides

The lymph node involvement in the early stage is paracortical (T-zone); later the whole node is replaced by a polymorphic infiltrate in which giant cells are prominent, interspersed with lymphoid cells, histiocytes and eosinophils. Thus it is not surprising that the appearances have been confused with Hodgkin's disease. The giant cells have large complex indented nuclei, rich in basi-chromatin, so that the nucleoli may be difficult to discern. There is a sharp nuclear membrane surrounded by a rim of acidophil cytoplasm. In addition to these giant cells, which are seldom seen except in mycosis fungoides, there will be the ordinary cerebriform cell seen in Sézary's syndrome and the smaller T-cell lymphocytes with their irregular twisted nuclei. In contrast to Hodgkin's disease there are many immunoblast-like cells, but no fibrocytes and no Reed-Sternberg or Hodgkin giant cells.

3e. There is a polymorphic appearance due to the occurrence of myeloid transformation (extramedullary hematopoiesis) in lymph nodes

Myelosclerosis ordinarily presents with gross splenomegaly and a leuco-erythroblastic anaemia. Though the lymph nodes may not be markedly enlarged they invariably show some degree of myeloid transformation. In both primary and secondary myelosclerosis, there is myeloid transformation of the whole node, associated with fibrosis of an unusual type in that there are multinucleate fibro-

Myelosclerosis

Fig. V.40

213

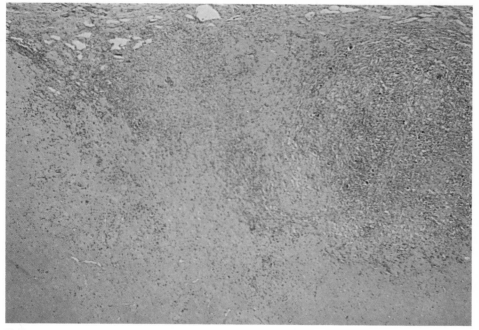

V.42a

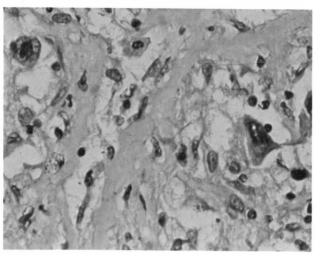

V.42b

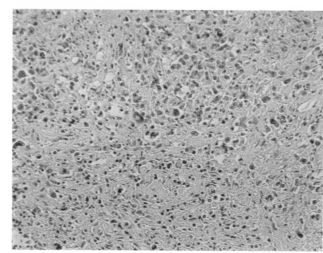

V.42c

V.42a-c   Hodgkin's Disease; Lymphocyte Depleted with Diffuse Fibrosis

V.42a   There is a diffuse fibrosis and in the areas where cells are present they are scanty and separated by collagen strands.

V.42b   Between the dense strands of collagen there are lymphocytes, some being transformed (immunoblasts), histiocytes and occasional eosinophils together with mononuclear Hodgkin cells; typical Reed-Sternberg cells can usually be found.

V.42c   The abnormal lymphoid cells, giant cells and histiocytes are isolated one from another by the massive fibrosis.

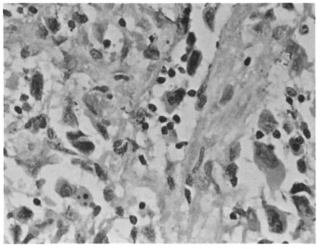

V.43a

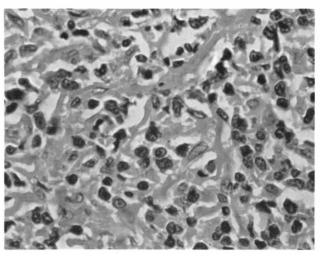

V.44a

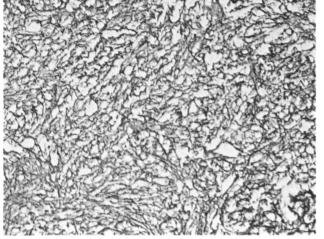

V.43b

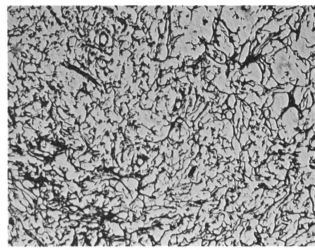

V.44b

V.43a-b   Diffuse Malignant 'Lymphoma' with Fibrosis

V.43a   Between the strands of collagen are a range of large pleomorphic bizarre cells, none of which have the specific characters of the Reed-Sternberg or Hodgkin cell. The other cells are small lymphocytes and fibroblasts. It is clearly a malignant neoplasm and almost certainly a sarcoma, but it is impossible to be more specific.

V.43b   The reticulin showing the close relationship of the fibres to the individual cells confirming that it is a lymphoreticular neoplasm, but it cannot be more precisely categorized than as a 'polymorphic reticulosarcoma' or 'large cell lymphoma', though the latter term infers a recognition of lymphoid origin.

V.44a-c   Malignant 'Lymphoma' with Fibrosis

V.44a   In this case the large tumour cells, separated by a diffuse hyaline fibrosis are clearly of lymphoid origin, but it is more difficult to be dogmatic as to the particular form.

V.44b   The reticulin pattern is similar to that of 43b but the network is rather looser suggesting that this is a stromal reaction, rather than that the tumour cells are desmogenic.

V.44c   Immunoperoxidase stain for immunoglobulin reveals a monoclonal reaction indicating that the tumour is of B-lymphocyte origin and can be classed as a plasma cell sarcoma.

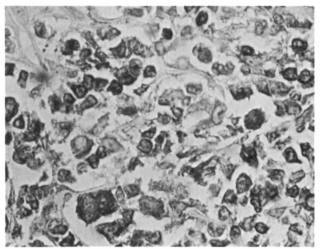

V.44c

cytes having some resemblance to osteoblasts. In addition there may be numerous megakaryocytes and histiocytic giant cells. The essential difference between primary and secondary myelosclerosis is that in the primary form there is an intrasinusoidal haemopoiesis whereas in the secondary form, occuring as a late result of polycythaemia or chronic myeloid leukaemia, there is ordinary replacement fibrosis and the haemopoiesis tends to occur extra-sinusoidally in the paracortical tissues.

3f. *There is a polymorphic infiltrate composed of lymphocytes, immunoblasts and plasma cells; fibrosis is often marked*

Sjögren's lymphadenopathy

There is no doubt that in a proportion of cases of *Sjögren's syndrome*, lymphoproliferative reactions may occur. In some cases there may be actual sarcomatous change, but it is certainly rare. The reports summarized by Anderson and Talal (1971) are not easy to interpret, but Zulman et al (1978) have provided an excellent review, while Lennert et al (1979) have displayed the histological features.

Fig. V. 41

The salivary glands show a change similar to the benign lymphoepithelial lesions (Cruikshank, 1965) but with rather more marked reactive follicles. The initial nonspecific change in the lymph node is also a reactive hyperplasia. In the late stages of the disease there may be a change from a polyclonal hyperglobulinaemia to macroglobulinaemia (IgM) with lymph node changes analogous to those in Waldenström's disease. Alternatively hypoglobulinaemia may develop in association with an unusual form of lymphoproliferation that has been confused with Hodgkin's disease. Follicles become inconspicuous and there is a diffuse cellular proliferation. A reticulin impregnation may reveal that the follicles have not been destroyed, but only obscured and that, though there is diffuse fibrosis of the paracortical tissue, the sinuses are unaffected. The proliferation consists of lymphocytes, plasma cells and eosinophils together with large numbers of transformed lymphocytes and immunoblasts, but no Reed-Sternberg cells (though some of the immunoblasts may recall the mononuclear Hodgkin cell). The other striking feature is that, in spite of the diffuse fibrosis, there is little evidence of fibroblastic proliferation. In fatal cases this fibro-immunoblastic proliferation occurs widely in the viscera. It may well be that in some cases a true sarcomatous change of lymphoid origin (immunoblastic sarcoma) develops. It is, however, not possible on the available evidence to be very precise as to what is meant by the 'pseudolymphoma' and 'reticulum cell sarcoma' that have been reported as occurring in Sjögren's syndrome.

4. The diffuse involvement is associated with reduced cellularity and fibrous replacement or infarction

4a. *Diffuse Lymph Node Involvement with Fibrosis*

The presence of extensive fibrosis, when it occurs in a somewhat nodular form, has been discussed in chapter III (p. 109). However, fibrosis may be disorganised *Fibrosis in chronic reactive lymphadenitis* and more diffuse in type, without the survival of isolated cellular nodules. In these circumstances residual cells are scattered more or less randomly throughout the fibrous tissue. This form of response, like the nodular varieties of fibrosis, may follow any *chronic reactive lymphadenitis* and is not infrequently seen in chronic dermatopathic lymphadenopathy and in Whipple's disease. There may on occasions be a marked desmoplastic response to a neoplasm, with relatively few identifiable malignant cells; metastatic carcinomatous involvement of axillary lymph nodes invaded by a scirrhous carcinoma of the breast often shows this change.

Many of the diffuse processes already described in this chapter may be associated with extensive fibrosis and reticulin formation. One of the most characteristic is the *lymphocytic depleted form of Hodgkin's disease with diffuse fibrosis*. A *Lymphocytic depleted Hodgkin's disease* whole range of intermediate phases may occur between the reticular variant, already described and this diffuse fibrotic variant. The account of this form of Hodgkin's disease given by Lukes and Butler in 1966 cannot be bettered: 'The *Fig. V.42* fibrosis varies in character and distribution. Most commonly it is loosely cellular, fibrillar in character and disorderly in distribution. At times it is cellular and fibroblastic. On occasions it is composed of compact hypercellular amorphous proteinaceous material that resembles precollagen. In general this type of fibrosis is hypocellular, disorderly in distribution and non-birefringent.' Lymphocytes are few, but diagnostic and bizarre Reed-Sternberg type cells, eosinophils, and plasma cells may be identified, randomly distributed within the fibrous tissue, or in small aggregates. Variable degrees of necrosis, with acute inflammatory features, occur commonly. There may be evidence of local scarring, but there is no tendency to form distinct collagen bands such as are seen in nodular sclerosing Hodgkin's disease. In some instances part of the node may be more cellular, and in such cases Reed-Sternberg type cells predominate, corresponding to the 'reticular form' of lymphocyte depleted Hodgkin's disease already described.

This variant of Hodgkin's disease is most commonly encountered following *Differentiation of lymphocytic depleted Hodgkin's disease from malignant lymphoma* therapy and in terminal cases; extensive fibrosis is known to occur in untreated cases, but there is no doubt as to the fibrogenic role of radiotherapy. The differentiation of this form of Hodgkin's disease from some of the large cell malignant lymphomas (pleomorphic immunoblastic sarcoma or polymorphic reticulosarcoma, (p. 176), may be difficult. However, in these tumours, when fibrosis is extensive, numerous bizarre malignant cells are usually still apparent, whereas in lymphocyte depleted Hodgkin's disease, particularly following therapy, it may be difficult to find diagnostic Hodgkin cells. Plasma cell sarcoma (p. 172) is usually associated with a diffuse loss of reticulin, or displacement of reticulin resulting in clumps or trabeculae of neoplastic plasmacytoid cells, often with a perivascular orientation. However, on occasions there may be extensive formation of reticulin, isolating individual cells. This can occur both in typical plasmacytoid immunoblastic sarcomas and in those lacking plasmacytoid fea-

Figs. V.43,44

·tures. The amount of reticulin formation and tissue fibrosis is very variable even in different areas of a single section, and does not appear to be related to the degree of cellular differentiation or to the presence or absence of demonstrable immunoglobulin. Sometimes the increase of reticulin and fibre formation may not be very obvious in ordinary stained preparations and only becomes apparent with the reticulin method. In other cases diffuse fine fibrosis is easily seen as strands of deeply eosinophilic slightly refractile material between the cells. Alternatively fibrosis may be very extensive, widely separating the neoplastic cells either individually, or in clumps. As a consequence of this rigid fibrous matrix the neoplastic cells may appear markedly angular in form, with sharply delineated cytoplasmic borders.

Many of these cases correspond to the 'fine compartmentalized fibrotic' type of sclerotic non-Hodgkin's lymphomata described by Bennett (1975), who emphasized that this form of diffuse fibrosis was only to be seen in the 'diffuse mixed' and 'diffuse undifferentiated' large cell types. This would conform to our experience, as would the fact that diffuse fibrosis in a particular cytological type of malignant lymphoma is a histological indicator of a more favourable prognosis.

Finally, a proportion of these tumours are of non-lymphoid origin, possibly of histiocytic type or of some other undefined mesenchymal cell. Such cases correspond to the dictyocytic reticulo-sarcomata of Robb-Smith (1938) and the reticulosarcoma of Mathé, Rappaport, O'Connor and Torioni (1975). The differential diagnosis from anaplastic carcinoma with desmoplasia has already been considered.

4b. *Diffuse lymph node involvement with massive necrosis or infarction*

Necrosis in Hodgkin's disease

Localized necrosis is a not uncommon occurrence in diseased lymph nodes, and has already been mentioned in relation to some of the reactive lymphadenopathies and Hodgkin's disease. Focal necrosis may be extensive in Hodgkin's disease of mixed cellular, or nodular sclerotic types, presenting as large necrotic areas bordered by degenerating cells in which the typical Hodgkin's cells may be discerned; such changes are illustrated in Fig. III.15d.

Fig. V.45

In lymphocyte depleted Hodgkin's disease necrosis usually occurs in grossly enlarged nodes, of which the major portion may be infarcted. In these circumstances the diagnosis may be difficult as the residual cells at the periphery of the lesion are very often poorly preserved and may be largely of reactive inflammatory type. Indeed diagnostic features of Hodgkin's disease may only be revealed by examining sections from several levels of the node, or from an adjacent smaller node in which infarction has not occurred.

Fig. V.46

While it may be difficult to establish any diagnosis in some infarcted nodes, the differentiation of lymphocyte depleted Hodgkin's disease from a large cell malignant lymphoma (immunoblastic sarcoma, polymorphic reticulosarcoma) may be well nigh impossible. The survival of a few bizarre malignant cells can provide the only clue.

218

The distinction of lymphocyte depleted Hodgkin's disease or immunoblastic *Necrosis in metastatic tumours* sarcoma from metastatic carcinoma or malignant melanoma may also present difficulties when infarction is extensive. Metastatic carcinoma cells bordering an area of necrosis often show degenerative features, and may be more atypical in nuclear morphology than the primary tumour. Such cells may have large multi-lobulate nuclei with prominent nucleoli and a vacuolated or sometimes eosino-philic, collapsed cytoplasm, resulting in a superficial resemblance to the Reed-Sternberg cell, which itself may show degenerative and bizarre features in areas of necrosis. In addition the occurrence of an inflammatory cell infiltrate bordering necrotic tissue may mimic the mixed cellular infiltrate associated with Hodgkin's disease. Metastases of a cryptic nasopharyngeal carcinoma to cervical lymph nodes constitute a particular problem in this respect.

However, it should not be forgotten that a reticulin impregnation may resolve many of these diagnostic difficulties in an infarcted lymph node. It is very rare for the reticulin network to undergo lysis in infarcted tissue, so the pattern of the node, invisible in the mass of necrotic tissue, may be displayed. Secondly the cytological character of the necrotic cells may be revealed by the argyrophilic staining, though no details could be made out by ordinary aniline dyes. Accord- *Fig. V.46* ingly a reticulin impregnation may facilitate a definite diagnosis of metastatic carcinoma (though the primary site may remain obscure), Hodgkin's disease or a malignant lymphoma.

Infective conditions may also result in extensive necrosis but usually there is *Necrosis in infective lymphadenitis* some residual evidence of the infective process if not of its precise identity. Thus it is always expedient to stain an infarcted lymph node for organisms, not forgetting that in addition to Gram, Ziehl-Neelsen and fungal stains, simple techniques such as toluidine or methylene blue may reveal organisms when the *Fig. II.13a* classical methods have failed. It should not also be forgotten that massive hae-morrhagic infarction is the characteristic lymph node reaction in anthrax (Albrink et al, 1960); while diffuse coagulative necrosis may occur in yersinial and myco- *Anthrax; Yersinia* bacterial infections, but in tularaemia, necrosis is more commonly focal as de- *Fig. V.47* scribed in earlier chapters. Furthermore in severe fulminating infections, when extensive necrosis is associated with a florid reactive hyperplasia, there may be confusion with a neoplastic process. This may be accentuated by nuclear atypia in the transformed lymphocytes, if these are also affected by the necrotic process and show degenerative changes.

Massive necrosis of lymph nodes has been described in certain forms of poly- arteritis nodosa (Churg and Strauss, 1961; Mark and Fehér, 1959; Symmers, *Necrosis in polyarteritis nodosa* 1978). Though it would be unusual for any form of polyarteritis to present as a lymphadenopathy yet a lymph node biopsy might be undertaken in an obscure case of pyrexia of unknown origin in the hope of providing a diagnosis. The recognition of the vascular lesions particularly in the hilum and capsule might provide the clue, but it should not be forgotten that arteriolar necrosis is usually present in drug hypersensitivity lymphadenopathy.

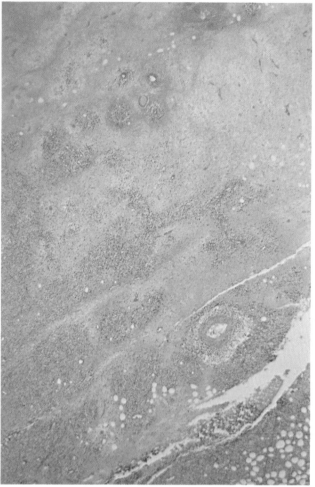

V.45

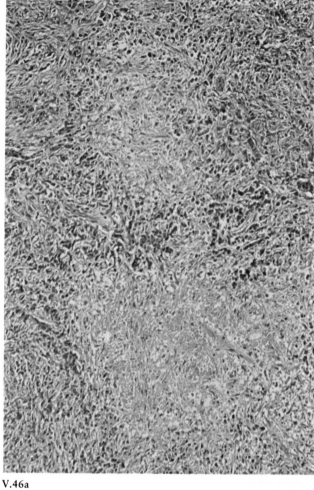

V.46a

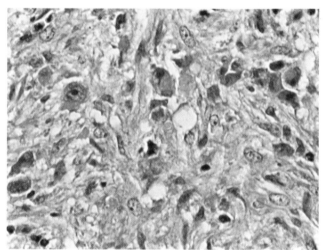

V.46b

V.45 Hodgkin's Disease Lymphocyte Depleted with Massive Infarction

There is extensive fibrosis and infarction. Diagnosis would depend on histological identification in areas of cellular survival, often in relation to blood vessels.

V.46a-b Immunoblastic Sarcoma with Massive Necrosis

V.46a In this malignant tumour there are large areas of necrosis, but enough surviving tissue to allow a diagnosis. It should be recognized that the cells bordering a necrotic area are often bizarre.

V.46b The high power view shows that the surviving cells beyond the zone of necrosis have the characters of an immunoblastic sarcoma.

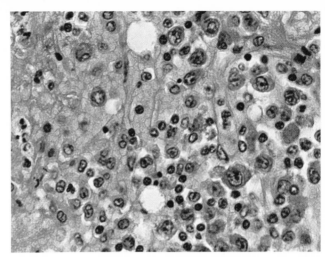

V.47b

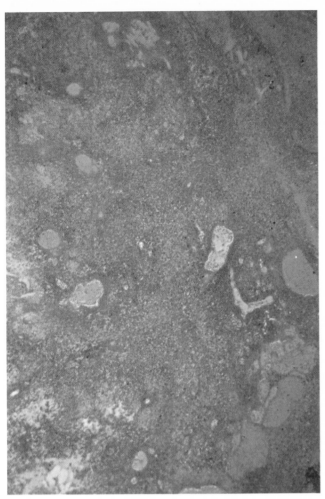

V.47a

V.47a-b   Infective Lymphadenitis with Extensive Necrosis; Anthrax

V.47a   There is massive haemorrhaic necrosis with loss of architectural detail and only occasional small foci of identifiable cells.

V.47b   The high power view shows that the residual cellular
area consists of lymphocytes, monocytes and many immunoblasts
some of which appear abnormally large and atypical. Anthrax
bacilli were demonstrated by gram staining of adjacent nodes
and the organism was cultured.

Lymphomatoid granulomatosis   Liebow and his colleagues (1972) in their detailed account of lymphomatoid granulomatosis emphasized that extensive necrotic lesions in lymph nodes were uncommon. It happens, however, that in two cases which we have seen with the typical pulmonary and nervous system changes, the lymph nodes, in addition to the lymphoproliferative lesions, had massive areas of necrosis associated with angeitis.

Infarction in venuous thrombosis   Finally, in addition to the various causes of lymph node infarction which have been described, it is well to remember that simple thrombosis of the nodal veins can be an inductive factor as Davies and Stansfeld (1972) showed.

In each case a definitive diagnosis can only be achieved by a critical analysis of the degree of disturbance of the normal lymph node architecture and the cytological characters of the cells, normal or abnormal, that are present. In the particular instance of an infarcted node, even a small area of well preserved tissue may provide the clue to the diagnosis and multiple sections should be taken to locate such areas.

In this book we have attempted to display the principles on which a diagnosis of the lesions in a lymph node biopsy may be achieved, in the hope that it will provide some assistance to histopathologists and perhaps enlighten their colleagues as to the difficulties which have to be faced. To some, this analytical approach may appear unnecessary, for it is true that on occasions, a pathologist, experienced in lymph node histology, may at a glance arrive at a diagnosis, apparently by inspiration, and might be unable to analyze how his conclusions were derived, just as it is difficult to explain the immediate recognition of a friend after a long absence.

On the other hand, the use of decision trees as identification keys for biological specimens is well established, though they can be misleading when carelessly used. It has not been possible to describe or illustrate every condition which may be found in a lymph node biopsy and with intention, the photo-micrographs have been drawn from the ordinary material submitted to a diagnostic pathologist, rather than selecting perfectly stained ultra-thin sections.

As Rupert Willis once remarked 'No pathologist lives long enough to become infallible in the field of lymph node diagnosis'. It is hoped that this volume may have helped to reduce this fallibility of judgement.

APPENDIX I

The Classification and Nomenclature of the Lymphadenopathies

'I have no objection to your giving names any signification which you please, if you will only tell me what you mean by them.'
Plato: Charmides

'Pluralitas non est ponenda sine necessitate.'
Occam, 1491

'It does not follow that there is but one single manner of arrangement that will necessarily be the "best", even if developed by rational minds.'
Van Neil, 1946

'The various classifications of lymphadenopathies have been most useful in the hands of those who have defined them and the propagation of these faiths have been met largely by failure.'
Rosenberg et al, 1961

'People's reasons for wanting a definition is to take care of the borderline case and that is what a definition, as if by definition, will not do.'
Nemerov, 1975

THE SEQUENTIAL ARRANGEMENT in this book has been in relation to lymph node characters seen under the microscope, in the hope that this would facilitate identification of the abnormality. In naming these conditions, the simpler nomenclatures adopted in various current classifications have been used. However, it is not possible to evade a review of the various nomenclatures and classifications of lymph node disorders that have been propounded with various objectives in view.

From Thomas Hodgkin to Dorothy Reed

The first clear clinical account of a primary lymph node disorder was given by Thomas Hodgkin in a paper 'On some morbid appearances of the absorbent glands and spleen' which he read in 1832. He did not carry out any histological studies, but some of his specimens have been preserved, and nearly a hundred years later were shown to have the microscopical characters of the condition that we associate with his name (Fox, 1926), while the superb drawings of postmortem dissections, which accompanied his presentation, still exist (Carswell, 1898; Dawson, 1968). The significance of Hodgkin's contribution was that he emphasized that a disease process could involve the lymph nodes and the spleen as a syndrome, at a time when the functions and inter-relation between these organs was unrecognized, just as it was of fundamental importance that Professor Hughes

Bennett (1845) thirteen years later showed that there was a condition in which there was a great increase in the leucocytes associated with enlargement of the spleen, liver and lymph nodes.

It was in 1856 that Samuel Wilks, who was to become an unofficial publicity agent for diffident Guy's physicians, described a number of cases similar to Hodgkin's and proposed an eponymic title, while Cornil (1855) had suggested the term lymphadenoma the year before, though it is usually attributed to Wunderlich (1856).

It is unnecessary to recount the priority wrangle over leukaemia between Hughes Bennett's supporters and Virchow, but in his book on tumours (1864/5), Virchow introduced the name 'lymphosarcoma' for non-leukaemic conditions, but included under this term, not only sarcomas of lymphoid tissues, but also Hodgkin's disease and a number of other conditions. Meanwhile Cohnheim (1865) described 'pseudo leukaemia', in which the histological characters were identical with those of leukaemia but without a leucocytosis, and Billroth (1871) proposed 'malignant lymphoma' for a group of lymphoid conditions, though he admitted that the term was difficult to define pathologically or clinically and had little merit except as a collective term. While the German pathologists were creating chaos in the lymphadenopathies by introducing more and more terms for ill-differentiated conditions, in Great Britain, where histo-pathology was still the concern of clinicians, endeavours were made to define clinico-pathological entities.

The main forum for clinical and pathological discussion was the Pathological Society of London, and on March 19th, 1878, there was a meeting devoted to leukaemia and lymphadenoma in which the opening paper was given by Wilks, but the major contribution was provided by Dr. W. S. Greenfield, at that time at St. Thomas's Hospital in the same post that Hodgkin himself had held. Bearing in mind the limitation of histology at this period, Greenfield gave a clear account of the microscopic features, emphasizing the destruction of the normal glandular pattern, the fibrosis and the presence of multinucleate cells, first noted by Billroth (1858) though Virchow (1864) usually gets the credit; however, as Rather (1972) and Ober (1977) have emphasized the awarding of the accolade is dependent on the criteria required for identification of a 'peculiar' Hodgkin giant cell. As to the nature of Hodgkin's disease, Greenfield felt that it was initially a local disease, 'an irritative overgrowth of some normal lymphatic tissue leading to similar implications of adjacent glands and then spreading to more distant areas. Clinically and anatomically there is little distinction at this stage from cancer. . . .'.

In 1881 Greenfield became professor of general pathology and clinical medicine at Edinburgh and during his thirty years tenure of the chair he had a profound influence on undergraduates and post-graduates. However, he published very little and it was only from one of his pupils, Stuart McDonald (1911), that the emphasis he placed on the essential histological characters of Hodgkin's disease was revealed.

At the end of the century the clouds of confusion began to lift in Germany. Virchow (1892) thundered that Cohnheim's pseudo-leukaemia was a 'misch masch' for all those cases which could not be included in any definite category, while Kundrat (1893) proposed that 'lympho-sarcoma' should not be used in the broad sense adopted by Virchow thirty years before but be restricted to a sarcomatous tumour involving lymphoid cells. However, Sternberg (1898) gave an account of thirteen cases of pseudo-leukaemia which he believed was a peculiar form of tuberculosis of lymphoid tissue (tubercle bacilli had been detected in eight of his cases); there is no doubt from his excellent description and illustrations that he was dealing with cases of Hodgkin's disease (he was one of the first to use Ehrlich's staining methods), and it is his account of the giant cell that accords him eponymic recognition.

In December 1901, Professor Sir Frederick Andrewes of St. Bartholomew's Hospital took part in a discussion on lymphadenoma in its relation to tuberculosis which disposed on histological and bacteriological grounds of Sternberg's idea that Hodgkin's disease was a form of tuberculosis. Andrewes' histological account and illustrations made it clear that Hodgkin's disease was a distinct histopathological entity; he spoke of hard and soft lymphadenoma and the illustrations of the hard variety correspond to nodular sclerosis, while the soft variety is clearly mixed cellularity. In the following year Miss Dorothy Reed (1902) studied eight cases of Hodgkin's disease and though unaware of Andrewes' report endorsed his findings; her drawings of the Hodgkin giant cell are superior to those of Andrewes showing the nuclear and nucleolar configuration admirably, but her drawings of the general pattern of the tissue change are much inferior; nor did she distinguish the nodular sclerotic or hard variety from the mixed cellular or soft form. Her clinical description was excellent while her discussion on the nature of Hodgkin's disease shows real insight, though it is impossible to say how much she was influenced by Welch's views: '.... macroscopically, the growth differs from malignant tumour in the absence of capsular infiltration and implication of adjacent tissues. We do not know of any malignant neoplasm, the metastases of which occur in only one form of tissue. Hodgkin's disease does not metastesize by cellular transplantation but by causing a proliferation in pre-existing lymphoid tissue apparently anywhere in the body. . . .'

Miss Dorothy Reed (1874–1964) was a member of Osler's 'golden' 1900 graduation class at Johns Hopkins, with Lawrason Brown, Curtis Burnam, Henry Christian, Clarence Farrar, Albion Hewlett, Warren Lewis, Glanville Rusk, Florence Sabin and John Bruce MacCallum, of whom Osler spoke as 'one of the most brilliant young men it has ever been my lot to teach'. Unhappily he succumbed to tuberculosis at the age of thirty.

Dr. Reed (later Mrs. C. E. Mendenhall) wished to become a paediatrician, but as there was no residency vacancy at Hopkins, she accepted Welch's offer to work in pathology, and after she had done some work on *Pasteurella (Yersinia) pseudo-tuberculosis*, he suggested she should investigate Sternberg's claim; Welch had worked with Cohnheim and when he came to Breslau, Welch suppressed the paper on lymphosarcoma that he had prepared for Professor Ernst Wagner. Dr. Reed's fossicking in pathology did not deflect her from her initial purpose and she made a successful career in paediatrics.

Longcope (1903) agreed with Dorothy Reed's view that Hodgkin's disease was a distinct clinical and pathological entity with a definite histological picture and this viewpoint was aided by Ziegler's monograph (1911), but there was dispute as to its nature. Was it an infection or a neoplasm or something midway between the two? Those who supported the neoplastic idea were unwilling to accept that Hodgkin's disease was a distinct entity but preferred to regard it as a varient of malignant lymphoma or lymphoblastoma which included, in Mallory's view (1914), 'lymphocytoma, lymphoma, lymphosarcoma, pseudoleukaemia, lymphatic leukaemia and Hodgkin's disease'.

However, new concepts were to arise which were greatly to influence ideas about primary lymph node disorders.

The ideas of Adami and Maximow. Reticulosis and Reticulosarcoma

In 1913 Adami suggested that it would be desirable to distinguish from true neoplasms a group of diffuse overgrowths, for which he proposed the unhappy term 'hyperblastosis'; these might be regarded as due to a disturbance of metabolic equilibrium, and (with considerable prescience) he continued, 'might possibly be combated eventually (certainly not today) along the lines of organotherapy' (Adami, 1918). He concluded by saying 'every transition is observable in this series between the development of overgrowths of fully differentiated tissue, non-malignant grades of anaplasia and diffuse malignant infiltrative growths'. Ewing (1928) was to expand and endorse this viewpoint.

Although the idea of the reticulo-endothelial system had been evolving from vital staining and the functional studies of Aschoff and his colleagues, it was not until 1924 that Aschoff presented a comprehensive account of the system. It was not surprising that classifications of disorders of the reticulo-endothelial system were proposed and the collective term 'reticulo-endotheliosis' was put forward by Schnittenhelm (1925) and Epstein (1925), to include the storage disorders, monocytic leukaemia, Hodgkin's disease and mycosis fungoides; these authors failed to recognize that Aschoff's concept was of a group of cells linked on a functional basis irrespective of their origin or histogenetic potentialities.

However, Maximow's idea of the pluripotentiality of the undifferentiated mesenchyme did provide just such a histogenetic background. Maximow's hypothesis (1927) was that throughout the adult connective tissue naturally including lymphoreticular tissue, there were inconspicuous undifferentiated mesenchymal or reticulum cells, which maintained the differentiation potentialities of the embryonic mesenchyme and under suitable stimuli could differentiate into haemic, phagocytic, fibrocytic or sinus lining cells. Under resting conditions in densely cellular tissue, such as a lymphnode, the mesenchymal or reticulum cells were difficult to make out, but in loose connective tissue the oval leptochromatic nuclei, lying in a faintly basophil synplasma spreading along reticulin fibres, could be recognized. Under stimulation the cell outline became obvious and the cytoplasm faintly acidophilic, while the vesicular nucleus enlarged and the nucleolus became prominent; karyokinetic division was common but it was a non-phagocytic cell and aniline dyes were stained very faintly. This is the reticulum cell with potentialities for differentiation along haemic, histiocytic or fibrocytic lines, in the process developing the cytological characters of the differentiated cell. Maximow believed that under pathological conditions the reticulum cell might undergo nuclear division without cytoplasmic separation and resulting in the mirror image Reed-Sternberg giant cells. He took the view that the small lymphocyte was an undifferentiated haemocytoblast which could 'revert' to a large lymphocyte from which monocytes and granulocytes were derived; it was of course accepted that the plasma cell evolved from the lymphocyte.

It seemed desirable to give this brief recapitulation of Maximow's ideas, which were based on detailed histology, as there is much confusion on the part of modern writers who do not appear to have read the original papers and believe that Maximow's reticulum cell was a histiocyte whereas it would probably be equivalent to cells identifiable as a transformed lymphocyte or an undifferentiated histiocyte. However, Maximow's reticulum cell had maintained, in the adult, pluripotent differentiation (i.e. to haemic, histiocytic or fibrocytic cells) whereas the small lymphocyte, from which the plasma cells were derived, had potentialities as multipotent haemic stem cells (haemocytoblast) with differentiation to monocyte or granulocyte. Recent studies of adult bone marrow and the introduction of the spleen colony assay technique have resulted in the recognition of pluripotent haemic stem cells (Cline and Golde 1979; Bessis 1979), thus confirming many of Maximow's observations; yet lymph node histopathologists, with the exception of Lennert (1978), appear to have ignored this work.

In accordance with Maximow's ideas, Tschistowitch and Bykowa (1928) proposed a classification of disorders of the lympho-haemopoietic organs embracing hyperplasias and infections, Gaucher's disease, leukaemia, myeloma, Hodgkin's disease and lymphosarcoma, subdivided in the first instance as to whether it was the parenchyma or the stroma that was involved. They suggested that 'reticulosis' should be used as a generic term for these conditions and two years later Uehlinger (1930) put forward another classification of the reticuloses. The term reticulosis was first introduced by Letterer (1924) in his description of a child with acute reticulosis of infancy (Letterer-Siwe disease) as he felt that the proliferated cells had close affinities with Maximow's reticulum cells and reticulosis was a suitable designation, analogous to leukosis, lymphadenosis etc; ten years later Letterer (1934) emphasized that he had used the term – the title of his original paper was 'Aleukaemische Reticulose' – to designate a proliferation of undifferentiated reticulum cells and not as a collective term, but by this time it was an 'in' word. This was, in the main, a consequence of the work of a group of investigators at St. Bartholomew's Hospital, London, supported by a grant given by a Mrs. T. E. Rose for research into lymphadenoma, from which her daughter had died. The team was under the general direction of Dr. Mervyn Gordon (1932) a distinguished bacteriologist and one of the earliest clinical virologists. Gordon excluded a whole range of micro-organisms as aetiological agents of Hodgkin's disease, but he believed that he had isolated a filtrable agent and devised a test for Hodgkin's disease which attracted considerable excitement at the time; a lymph node extract was inoculated intracerebrally into rabbits and in a positive result, the animal developed a peculiar form of ataxic paraplegia. The agent which Gordon used to call E. B. (for elementary bodies, not Epstein-Barr) was soon shown to be present in eosinophils and neutrophils and is now thought to have been a proteolytic enzyme derived from leucocytes (King, 1939). An interesting observation from this investigation was the recognition that patients with Hodgkin's disease showed cutaneous anergy to tuberculin and a whole range of other bacterial and fungal antigens.

Although the aetiological studies of this research team were as unrewarding as previous or subsequent work in this field, yet the histological investigations carried out by Miss Pullinger (1932) were to be of considerable importance. She restated with great clarity the essential pathological features of Hodgkin's disease, but recognized that there were other conditions, which had some of the microscopical features in common with true lymphadenoma, but in which the typical picture was incomplete. As examples of these she mentioned cases in which there was no increased fibrosis or eosinophilia, but the presence of numerous reticulum cells, a few being of the multinucleate Reed-Sternberg type, lying in a lymphoid stroma and there were other cases in which the predominant cell was an actively phagocytic histiocyte. Even more significant for a comprehension of the histogenesis of primary lymph node disorders was that Pullinger, having given an account of Maximow's concept of the pluripotentiality of the reticulum cell, wrote: 'It seems probable that a group of diseases of reticulum exists in which proliferation is followed by differentation into one or several of the possible cell progeny. Letterer's term reticulosis is more suitable than reticulo-endotheliosis and has the advantage that it allows of subdivision according to the predominant cell type, thus the major member of the group, lymphadenoma (Hodgkin's disease) becomes, if one prefers it, fibromyeloid reticulosis'. So it was that the histogenetic concept of reticulosis was stated in 1932.

Maximow's ideas also influenced European thought on the sarcomatous conditions of lymphoid tissue. Oberling (1928) proposed the collective term 'reticulosarcoma' for these tumours, which could then be qualified to indicate their particular cytology; he set out a classification of reticulosarcomata separated into differentiated or undifferentiated types and the former included myeloma, lymphosarcoma, sinus-lining tumours etc.

Roulet (1930, 1932) a pupil of Rössle's, who was critical of Aschoff's concept of the reticulo-endothelial system, described in two papers, a series of cases of malignant lymph node tumours that were distinct from lymphosarcoma. According to Roulet these tumours should be called 'Retothelsarkom' rather than reticulo-endothelial sarcoma as they were not derived from the sinus lining (littoral cells) but from cells accompanying the reticulin fibres, which Rössle had suggested should be called 'retothelium' (Maximow's undifferentiated reticulum or mesenchymal cell). Roulet described three types, an undifferentiated, and a differentiated form and forms associated with leukaemia and Hodgkin's disease. Roulet's papers were criticized both on concept and nomenclature and retothelsarcoma never gained any popularity. However his basic concept, which was very similar to that of Oberling, was widely accepted and Ahlström (1933) included in his classification a polymorphic retothelsarcoma.

In America a rather different course had emerged. In the first instance in 1925 Brill, Baehr and Rosenthal described a new clinico-pathological entity, though in retrospect isolated cases could be identified in earlier writings. At first it was called 'Splenomegalia lymphatica hyperplastica' and believed to be a relatively benign condition, but in their next paper (1927), as some of the cases had undergone sarcomatous change, they felt it must be regarded as a malignant condition from the start and renamed it 'Follicular lymphoblastoma'. Numerous other reports appeared and by 1932 the Mount Sinai group had described nineteen cases and it was possible to get a clear picture of the clinico-pathological features. The average age at onset was 42, with a slight male preponderance, there was usually generalised lymphadenopathy, and splenomegaly with a considerable liability to serous effusions, but few other symptoms, slight anaemia and lymphopenia. At the time of the reports seven of their cases had died, the longest surviving eleven years and the average was 5.75 years, while those still alive had been under observation for at least five years, with one for fourteen years. There was no doubt that a proportion of the cases underwent sarcomatous change but the frequency was uncertain at that time, though it is known now to be about 10%. Not only were the clinical features of what was sometimes called Brill-Symmers disease clear but also the histology. There was extreme enlargement and increase in number of the follicles due to a uniform proliferation of large lymphocytes or 'lymphoblasts' surrounded by a rim of small lymphocytes; and similar follicular structures occurred in non-lymphoid tissue (bone-marrow, liver, dermis, loose connective tissue etc.). When sarcomatous change took place, there was cellular atypia and the follicular structures were disrupted with infiltration into the surrounding tissue while the patient became gravely ill and soon succumbed.

This detailed clinico-pathological account of 'follicular lymphoblastoma', as it was seen in the early 1930's, is presented on account of the emphasis placed on the presence or absence of nodularity in the more recent classifications of lymph node disorders.

Opposing views: Fluid Lymphoma versus Clinical Entities

In the field of classification Ewing (1928) endorsed Adami's ideas that the diffuse overgrowths or progressive hyperplasias were distinct from malignant neoplasms. He wrote: 'The discussion of lymphoma in general, necessarily includes the consideration of various processes, some of which are chiefly inflammatory, some neoplastic, and others intermediate in position. Extensive tumour-like hyperplasia of lymphoid tissue occurs in the following scheme of clinical conditions: (1) simple lymphoma; (2) leukaemia, lymphatic and myelocytic, in its various phases; (3) pseudo-leukaemia; (4) Hodgkin's disease; (5) lymphosarcoma. The complexities of the subject of lymphoid tumours depend chiefly upon the lack of knowledge of etiology and partly upon the lack of accurate anatomic classification. It seems to the author that some advantage would result from rigid application of simple anatomic principles in the classification of these processes even at the risk of carrying the anatomic distinctions too far.'

The classification adopted by the American Lymph Node Registry, which was described by Callendar (1934) clearly followed Ewing's proposals, as there was segregation according to the type of cell (lymphocytic, granulocytic, reticulum cell etc) and the type of proliferation: (I) Reactive; (II) Leukaemic proliferative neoplasm; (III) Aleukaemic proliferative neoplasia; (IV) Malignant. In Canada, Waugh (1937) in an admirable paper on the inter-relationships of various systematic haematopoietic processes set out clearly which conditions he would regard as hyperplastic, which sarcomatous and which intermediate, though for this group he put forward the etymologically unreasonable term 'kataplasia' which is sometimes found in Japanese writings (Tanaka, 1973).

On the other hand, Warthin was the leader of what one might call the 'fluid lymphoma' school, which was to confuse the field of lymphadenopathies for nearly thirty years, by producing mandala-like diagrams in which any lymph node disorder might become transformed into any other; in a paper on 'The genetic neoplastic relationships of Hodgkin's disease, aleukaemia and leukaemia' (1931), he wrote: 'Hodgkin's disease is a neoplasm and related genetically to the lymphoblastomas of which both the aleukaemic and leukaemic forms are identical pathologically; and mycosis fungoides is likewise a neoplasm belonging to the same generic group. The essential difference between these different clinical forms consists in different degrees of dedifferentiation and subdifferentiation and the organ or tissue primarily involved. Transition forms exist between all of these groups and one type may be transformed into another.'

It would seem that in America at this time little interest or understanding had been shown in the European concept of reticulosis, though there were occasional papers such as that of Goldzieher and Hornick (1931) in which several cases of a systematized proliferation of primative lymphoid cells were designated as 'reticulosis', though there is no doubt that 'reticulo-endotheliosis' was at that time the more popular generic term. However Dameshek (1933) presented a

masterly review of 'Aleukaemic reticulosis' in which he distinguished the proliferative diseases of the cells of the reticulo-endothelial system, including Hodgkin's
disease amongst these, from the true neoplastic lesions, giving as an example the
reticulum cell sarcoma of Ewing (1928).

In 1938 Robb-Smith wrote a paper on the classification of the lymphadenopathies under the title of 'Reticulosis and Reticulosarcoma: a histological
classification' which was an extension of Pullinger's ideas and was based on the
large amount of lymphnode material which had accumulated during the Rose
Research lymphadenoma project. There was a clear distinction between the
reactive conditions, the progressive hyperplastic or lympho-proliferative conditions (reticulosis) and the sarcomatous conditions (reticulosarcoma), the terms
being used in a collective sense, with adjectival qualifiers related to the predominant cells involved in each described condition. The individual cell types were
characterized morphologically. In the case of the reticuloses, it was emphasized
that in the lymphoreticular tissue (this was the first use of this anatomical term)
when there was a cellular proliferation in one of the three anatomical compartments – the follicles, the sinuses or the intrafollicular area, which at that time
was called the medulla but is now designated the paracortical or thymic dependent
area, it would be mirrored in other involved tissues; for example a generalized
follicular proliferation would not only affect the follicles of lymphoid tissue and
the malpighian bodies of the spleen, but would also induce follicle-like proliferations in the hepatic periportal tissue, bone marrow, dermis etc. and there was
homologues of the other two compartments both in nodal and extra-nodal tissue.
The histology of the various types of reticuloses and reticulosarcomata were
described, the majority being conditions already well known, e.g. lymphoid follicular reticulosis (follicular lymphoblastoma), the haemic medullary reticuloses
(the leukaemias), reticulum-celled medullary reticulosis (histiocytosis X), storage
reticulum-celled medullary reticulosis (lipidoses), fibro-myeloid medullary
reticulosis (Hodgkin's disease); in addition there were one or two not so familiar,
such as lymphoreticular medullary reticulosis (Hodgkin's paragranuloma,
lymphocytic predominant Hodgkin's disease) histiocytic medullary reticulosis
(malignant histiocytosis). The reticulosarcomata were also subdivided according
to the predominant neoplastic cell and mention was made of the trabecular
variant (nodular sclerotic lymphosarcoma, Bennett and Millet, 1969) and that the
lymphoblastic reticulosarcoma might manifest itself in a medullary (diffuse) or
follicular form; the latter might arise in lymphoid follicular reticulosis and criteria
for distinguishing the hyperplastic from the blastomatous change were set out.

As this was a heuristic classification, there was no attempt at clinical correlation; with the support of the Lady Tata Memorial Trust, an Oxford Lymph Node
Registry was established to which material was sent for opinion and a careful
follow up maintained. Reports of the follow-up and clinico-pathological correlation of the first 1,000 cases and of 3,000 cases was published in 1947 and 1964.

The general reaction to the classification in Europe was that it was interesting.

As Bodley Scott said (1951) . . . 'it avoids what the late Professor Whitehead called the fallacy of oversimplification', while Willis (1960) wrote: 'Complicated histopathologic subdivisions, like that of Robb-Smith, which praiseworthy though it may be as an attempt to clarify a confused subject, obscures the essential unity of the whole group of lymphoid neoplasms. Many of the variants of structure given different names by Robb-Smith may be seen in one tumour. What is wanted is not more but less complexity in our histogenetic concepts.'

The classification was largely ignored in the United States, for in 1938 with World War II imminent, pathologists were concerning themselves with other matters than the lymphadenopathies. At least two very significant advances in the care and understanding of lymph node disorders were a direct consequence of the war. The initiation of chemotherapy of Hodgkin's disease with nitrogen mustard arose from the naval disaster in Bari harbour when the S.S. John E. Harvey, loaded with a hundred tons of mustard gas, exploded, and the significance of the late effects of mustard gas on the haemopoietic tissues of the survivors was recognized (Rhoads, 1946). The requirement that biopsy material from U.S. servicemen should be centralized at the Armed Forces Institute of Pathology in Washington provided, in the lymphatic tumour registry, a large number of specimens for study.

However, the first reviews of lymph node disorders came from civilian hospitals and renewed the dispute between the 'clinical entity' and 'fluid lymphoma' schools initiated by Warthin in the thirties. Gall and Mallory (1942) reported a series of over 600 cases of lymphoma which they classified as lymphocytic, lymphoblastic, stem-cell, clasmatocytic, Hodgkin's lymphoma and Hodgkin's sarcoma. Although Ewing in 1913 in a paper on the endotheliomata suggested the term reticulum cell sarcoma as a designation for a syncytial sarcoma, it was Gall and Mallory in this review who proposed the use of reticulum cell sarcoma to describe poorly differentiated malignant neoplasms, either of stem cell or histiocytic origin.

It should be appreciated that, following Oberling (1928), reticulosarcoma had been widely used by latin pathologists (German countries preferred Rössle's term retothelsarkom) as a generic term for all malignant tumours of lymphoid and haemopoietic tissue; tumours could be further qualified (e.g. syncytial, dictyocytic, lymphoblastic, histiocytic, etc) to characterise a particular form of malignant tumour. Japanese pathologists, following Akazaki's example (1943), also used reticulosarcoma as a generic term and occasionally reticuloma, though this latter never gained popularity. The conclusions of Gall and Mallory were that 'The value of this (cytologic) classification has been put to the test of clinical correlation and, although considerable overlapping was observed, as would be expected in so closely related a group of diseases, sufficiently constant differences were found in the age of onset, duration of the disease, maximal frequency of involvement of various organs and the degree of radio-sensitivity to delineate a series of different clinical syndromes and it has been shown by multiple examinations at significant time intervals that the cytologic type is remarkably constant, although a few cases show a progressive failure of differentiation as the disease progresses'. On the other hand, Custer and Bernhard (1948) in a study of 1300 cases said: 'Radiologists and clinicians, even many experienced pathologists, prefer to regard the subgroups as separate entities. Thus a differential diagnosis between Hodgkin's disease and reticulum cell sarcoma, or between lymphosarcoma and chronic lymphatic leukaemia, would seem to make a great deal of difference; actually it makes little or none. They are all malignant mesenchymal tumours which vary only in degree and type of differentiation'. Custer and Bernhard found 'a striking fluidity in histologic pattern with transitions and combinations that could best be interpreted as indicating a single neoplastic entity having a number of variants'. In a later paper (1960) they stated that in over 35% of cases there was a significant change in the histological character of the malignant growth.

Far more influential was the publication of Jackson and Parker 'Hodgkin's Disease and Allied Disorders' in 1947, the same year in which the review of the first 1000 cases of the Oxford Lymph Node Registry appeared (Robb-Smith, 1947). Jackson and Parker gave a clinico-pathological review of about 800 cases of primary lymph node disorders of which over a third were Hodgkin's disease, a little less than a third each of lymphoid leukosis and reticulosarcomata and a small group of giant follicle lymphoma and plasmacytoma.

The main interest of their work was their approach to Hodgkin's disease, which on histological grounds they divided into three types, paragranuloma, granuloma and sarcoma and showed that each had a different natural history. In 1934 Gow had reported that 'mononuclear reticulosis' had a much better prognosis than typical lymphadenoma. This was one of the conditions which Pullinger (1932) had separated from Hodgkin's disease, on the basis that there was no fibrosis or eosinophilia but instead there was scattered proliferation of reticulum cells in a lymphoid stroma. Two years later Rosenthal (1936) discussed 'the significance of tissue lymphocytes in the prognosis of lymphogranulomatosis' and proposed that Hodgkin's disease should be divided into three types according to the proportion of lymphocytes, reticulum cells or fibrosis and that the predominantly lymphocytic type had a better prognosis. Soon after this Jackson (1937) had described the histological features of their paragranuloma as 'early Hodgkin's disease' and Robb-Smith (1938, 1947) characterised Gow's 'mononuclear reticulosis' as lymphoreticular medullary reticulosis, but felt that both histologically and clinically it was distinct from Hodgkin's disease.

In their monograph Jackson and Parker gave a detailed account of Hodgkin's paragranuloma which had a very much better prognosis than their cases of Hodgkin's granuloma corresponding to classical Hodgkin's disease. The histological feature of paragranuloma was 'a diffuse infiltration of the nodes by lymphocytes which may be so great that an erroneous diagnosis of lymphocytoma is easily made. Buried within this mass of lymphocytes are found nevertheless the typical Reed-Sternberg cells for which a careful search must be made. Reticulum cells often containing phagocytosed debris are present in varying numbers'. This description corresponds precisely to that of lymphoreticular medullary reticulosis save that a further criterion of the latter condition is an absence of increased reticulin or collagen.

However, Parker and Jackson included in paragranuloma, nodes in which were found 'aggregates of reticulum cells resembling the lesions in Boeck's sarcoid with plasma cells and eosinophils' which conformed to Robb-Smith's Peedell's disease or Lennert's lymphoma, while they also accepted some degree of fibrosis. It is fairly clear that it was these cases that made up the 25% of paragranuloma that turned into Hodgkin's granuloma; as they put it, 'It may be argued that these cases of Hodgkin's paragranuloma that fail to change into Hodgkin's granuloma represent indeed an entirely different disease'. Hodgkin's granuloma corresponded essentially to classical Hodgkin's disease, but Hodgkin's sarcoma, which was comparatively infrequent, was very different; the patients were older, the primary site was often in the abdomen and the prognosis was very grave and though they said that some cases of Hodgkin's granuloma evolved into sarcoma, no figures were given and it seems probable that the majority of cases of Hodgkin's sarcoma were in reality 'large cell malignant lymphoma' (pleomorphic immunoblastic sarcoma, polymorphic reticulo-sarcoma) and a few cases which now would be classed as lymphocytic-depleted Hodgkin's disease.

Apart from their studies on Hodgkin's disease, Jackson and Parker discussed the clinical and pathological features of giant follicle lymphoma, myeloma, leukaemia and reticulosarcoma and there is no doubt that their book had a valuable influence, as they emphasized the distinct clinico-pathological features of the various lymphadenopathies. Yet Custer and Bernhard (1948) were maintaining their thesis of fluidity in histological pattern and case reports appear of patients who started with Hodgkin's disease, which turned into a lymphosarcoma and finally developed chronic lymphatic leukaemia (Lame, 1953). If, as was maintained, this chameleon-like activity was occurring in over a third of all cases, any attempt at precise histological diagnosis of lymph node disorders was a waste of time, provided the biopsy excluded a secondary carcinoma or an inflammatory condition. It was this idea of histological instability that encouraged the use of the meaningless portmanteau term 'lymphoma' or 'malignant lymphoma' to embrace a variable group of lymph node disorders some of grave prognostic significance, others chronic and relatively benign.

Parker and Jackson deplored this approach and wrote: 'The term "lymphoma" or "malignant lymphoma" is not infrequently used to cover this group of disorders. This we believe to be a mistake (we ourselves have so erred), for these terms connote to some a specific disease while to others they are vague and meaningless. We further believe that it is wrong and misleading to group all these conditions under one general term (as is so often done), just as it would be wrong to include without further definition under "pneumonia" those cases of pneumonia due to viruses, those due to pneumococci and other bacteria, and those due to unknown agents. Fortunately, we can properly speak of the "pneumonias". We cannot, in our opinion, speak with equal propriety and clarity of "the lymphomas".'

Videbaek, (1949) in a paper from Denmark, 'Do Malignant Lymphomas Represent Varying Differentiation of the Same Growth?' observed: 'The introduction of the American term malignant lymphoma to designate the group comprising lymphogenous leukaemia, lymphosarcoma, reticulum cell sarcoma, follicular lymphoma, and Hodgkin's disease expresses the feeling of helplessness in the face of a group of disorders characterized especially by enlargement of the lymph nodes and a fatal course'.

On the other hand some clinicians found a precise histological diagnosis of value in prognosis and a significant influence was the introduction of effective chemo-therapeutic agents, as critical clinical trials were instituted, and it was desirable that there should be reasonable precision as to the conditions being treated. It is interesting that this resulted in a change in therapeutic terminology; as instead of speaking of a five or ten years survival, the response to treatment was assessed as complete or partial remission or failure.

In 1951, the Faculty of Radiologists organized a symposium on 'The Reticuloses' in which the pathological review was presented by Professor W. St. C. Symmers, who gave a valuable account of the European concept of reticulosis, classifying them as benign, potentially malignant and malignant including sarcomata.

Sir Ronald Bodley Scott dealt with the clinical aspects in which he said 'I am becoming more and more convinced that there are, within this group, several distinct morbid processes – each with a different clinical course. Although at present most of them are eventually fatal, precise histological diagnosis allows a more accurate and confident prognosis', and there was a discussion opened by Professor McWhirter on the relative merits of chemo-therapy and radio-therapy in localised Hodgkin's disease.

It was about this time that Galea (1952) reviewed 400 cases of Hodgkin's disease and a hundred cases of lympho-reticular medullary reticulosis in the Oxford Lymph Node Registry in the hope of determining the factors that were associated with an improved prognosis. In general the findings with lymphoreticular medullary reticulosis agreed with those of Jackson and Parker's paragranuloma; young adults with localized disease and a long disease-free interval without the steady progression as in Hodgkin's disease, but a late liability for intrathecal involvement with paraplegia while about a fifth of the cases might develop a reticulosarcoma after ten to fifteen years, though in contrast to Parker and Jackson, if histological criteria were strict, there was no transformation into Hodgkin's disease.

In the Oxford Lymph Node Registry, Hodgkin's disease proper was subdivided into three types – cellular, sclero-cellular where fibrosis was quite prominent and sclerotic where there were comparatively few cells; sclero-cellular included both nodular sclerosis and some cases of mixed cellularity, while the sclerotic type corresponded closely to the Rye lymphocytic depletion type. In addition two variants of Hodgkin's disease had been recognized – Peedell's disease in which there was a diffuse epithelioid proliferation with eosinophils and very little fibrosis (which corresponds fairly closely to Lennert's lymphoma – Robb-Smith, 1978) and a diffuse cellulo-fibrotic type occuring at the higher age groups. Both these variants, which together only totalled 8% of all cases of Hodgkin's disease, had a slightly better prognosis than the typical Hodgkin's disease, but not so good as lympho-reticular type of reticulosis (analogous to lymphocytic predominant Hodgkin's disease, but considered to be a distinct entity). There was an impression that the prognosis in the sclero-cellular form was slightly better than the other two histological variants but Galea's statistical analysis failed to confirm this, nor was there any evidence that the predominance or diminution of any particular cell type in Hodgkin's disease proper had any prognostic influence; instead it was apparent that the major factor determining prolonged survival was the extent of disease at the time of diagnosis, cases with disease localized to a single site having four times the expectation of prolonged survival over those with two sites involved. Peters (1950) had already emphasized the great improvement in survival if adequate treatment could be given to patients with localised disease and she wrote 'In the light of present knowledge, the diagnosis of Hodgkin's disease should not be regarded with despair and the patient treated as incurable'; other radiotherapists were quick to follow her example with equally gratifying results.

Dr. Peter's insistence that Hodgkin's disease was initially a local disorder, was important not only from the therapeutic approach, but also because it reinforced the growing view that the concept of a single disease, lymphoma, usually generalized, with variable clinical and histological manifestations was wrong and it was important to distinguish both histologically and clinically the different types of lympho-proliferative or sarcomatous disorders.

It was about this time that a number of English pathologists (Harrison, 1952; Lumb, 1954; Jelliffe and Thomson, 1955; Symmers 1958; Dawson and Harrison 1961) described a condition which was called benign or nodular Hodgkin's disease or reticular lymphoma, that had a lobulated or pseudo-follicular appearance with lymphocyte preponderance and relative absence of fibrosis, and corresponded to Rosenthal's (1936) L-R type of lymphadenoma or the nodular variant of the lymphocyte predominant Hodgkin's disease of the Rye classification. There was some discussion as to the relationship of these overlapping conditions to Jackson and Parker's Hodgkin's paragranuloma and to Hodgkin's disease proper but the majority view regarded them all as Hodgkin variants which was endorsed by Lennert's (1953) study from Frankfurt. However Poppema, Kaiserling and Lennert (1979) have reopened the question of their segregation on cytological and epidemiological grounds.

Tapping the Riches of the AFIP Lymphoma Tumour Registry

Two important papers appeared in 1956. Smetana and Cohen (1956) reviewed the Hodgkin's material in the lymphatic tumour registry of the U.S. Armed Forces Institute of Pathology. Out of 437 cases they accepted 388 of which 9% were paragranuloma, 79% granuloma, 1% sarcoma and 11% unspecified; a fifth of the granuloma group showed considerable sclerosis and at seven years had a marginally better prognosis than the granuloma group as a whole, but much worse than in paragranuloma. In 1969, Smetana re-examined the forty patients that had survived twenty years. There were only 3% of the Hodgkin's granuloma group alive, whereas the vast majority of the paragranuloma cases were still alive, although the figures in the two papers show some discrepancy. Smetana had not found any evidence of transformation from paragranuloma to granuloma and indeed was doubtful as to their pathogenetic identity in spite of their morphological similarity.

It was also in 1956 that Rappaport, Winter and Hicks studied a group of 253 cases of follicular lymphoma from the Armed Forces Institute of Pathology as they felt that there was confusion between reactive follicular hyperplasia and the lymphomatous condition which itself showed considered cytological variability. They emphasized the morphological differences between the reactive and follicular nodule and divided their follicular cases into five cytological types:* – lymphocytic well-differentiated type I [part of small cleaved]; lymphocytic poorly differentiated ('lymphoblastic') type II [part of small and large cleaved and small cleaved]; mixed type (lymphocytic and reticulum cell) type III [part of small and large cleaved and non-cleaved]; reticulum cell type IV [part of large cleaved and large non-cleaved] and Hodgkin's type V. They admitted that the Hodgkin's type was quite distinct, on the basis of age, clinical presentation, and prognosis and that there was no evidence of cases changing from Hodgkin's type to one of the lymphoid follicular forms or vice versa; indeed the type V corresponded to the lobular form of benign Hodgkin's disease mentioned earlier, which would be included in Lukes' nodular form of lympho-histiocytic predominant Hodgkin's disease.

Rappaport and his colleagues recognized that the other four types were different from the majority of cases of malignant tumours of lymphoid tissue as regards age of onset, clinical presentation and prognosis and that a proportion of the cases changed from a follicular to a diffuse sarcomatous pattern; this was much more frequent in types III and IV, which in general had a worse prognosis. It was a pity that this careful study had to be made on members of the armed services as the age of onset was abnormally low (they noted that their series were ten years younger than other published studies); also as their survival figures were based for the most part on a five year interval, when only two thirds of the cases

---

* The square-bracketed terms correspond to the Lukes and Collins nomenclature

were traced, they failed to display the striking differences between follicular lymphoma and truly malignant lymphoid tumours. Rappaport and his colleagues 'found no evidence that follicular lymphoma necessarily originates in the centre of reactive follicles – it is possible and even likely that these structures represent newly formed follicles that have undergone malignant transformation'; nevertheless their illustration and description of the cleaved cell (centrocyte) could not be bettered – 'their nuclei varied considerably in shape with angulated and indented forms predominating . . .'; indeed discussing the abnormal lymphoid cells found in the peripheral blood they mention that the nucleus is partially or completely divided by a characteristic cleft (so-called 'notched nuclear cells' of Anday and Schmitz, 1952, which had been recognized in leukaemia by Isaacs, 1939). Their conclusions were that 'We do not regard follicular lymphoma as a separate and distinct disease entity but as a variant of diffuse lymphoma of corresponding cellular composition. It is conceivable that formation of follicle-like nodules may represent an attempted imitation of a normal pattern, in other words, an attempt at differentiation such as we find in other malignant tumours. . . . Since progression occurs from the follicular into the diffuse form, never the reverse, follicular lymphoma may be considered a stage that in some instances precedes the diffuse lymphoma. The duration cannot be predicted with any degree of certainty in an individual case. Therefore it would not be accurate to call it either a "benign" variant of lymphoma or to regard it as an early form of the disease. . . . Most authors still regard follicular lymphoma as a well-defined clinical and pathological entity. In contrast the present study represents an attempt to integrate the malignant lymphoma of the follicular type with the generally accepted cytological classifications of malignant lymphomas, adding the term 'follicular' or 'nodular' whenever this appears indicated by the prevailing architectural pattern', and they end by setting out a classification (Table 6) which was to be the basis of the 'Rappaport Classification'.

Table 6

Classification of Malignant Lymphoma
(Rappaport, Winter and Hicks,* 1956)

	Diffuse	Nodular (follicular)
1. Lymphocytic type, well-differentiated		
2. Lymphocytic type, poorly differentiated		
3. Mixed type (lymphocyte and reticulum cell)		
4. Reticulum-cell type		
5. Hodgkin's type		

* In the 1966 Rappaport classification (The Washington AFIP), Reticulum-cell type is divided into histiocytic and undifferentiated lymphoma, and Hodgkin's type into Hodgkin's paragranuloma, granuloma and sarcoma.

It is unfortunate that the authors in this admirable descriptive paper, excellently illustrated, in their very proper endeavour to distinguish reactive hyperplasia from follicular lymphoma, succeeded to some extent in discouraging the concept of follicular lymphoma as a clinico-pathological entity, so that it was necessary to 'rediscover' its clinical specificity and germinal centre origin thirteen years later (Lennert and Niedorf, 1969; Kojima, 1969).

Of course there were many clinicians and pathologists who would not accept the Rappaport concept of diffuse or follicular lymphomas and continued to provide good clinico-pathological accounts of follicular lymphoma (Robb-Smith, 1947, 1948, 1964; Sluiter, 1956) while Wright (1956) maintained its germinal centre origin.

The death knell of the fluid lymphoma school was sounded at New Orleans in 1957 when Edward Gall, and Henry Rappaport, 'after three years of fiery debate and negotiation' (Gall 1962) took part in a seminar on diseases of lymph nodes and spleen organised by the American Society of Clinical Pathologists. They presented an agreed classification which was very similar to that of Rappaport, Winter and Hicks, but their terminology had become more complex; for instance what Robb-Smith had called lymphoid follicular reticulosis was now to be designated 'Malignant lymphoma, lymphocytic poorly differentiated, follicular (follicular lymphoma type II)' but much of this tautological verbiage disappeared as the classification became more widely used.

Even more significant was the fact that on the basis of the cases presented Gall and Rappaport were prepared to recognize nine distinct types of primary lymphadenopathy, eight reactive lymphadenopathies as well as storage disorders and metastatic growths but it was somewhat disconcerting that only 47% of the thousand participating pathologists correctly diagnosed precirculated slides of Hodgkin's disease and many of the other conditions were mis-diagnosed as Hodgkin's disease; this is very similar to Symmers' (1968) experience under slightly different circumstances ten years later.

About this time a number of different classifications of lymph node disorders were put forward by Lumb (1954), Harrison (1956), Marshall (1956) and Custer (1960); some of these, such as that of Marshall, recognized that there was a type of cellular proliferation distinct from that seen in malignant lymphomas, but indulged in mental gymnastics to squeeze them into the category of neoplasms, speaking of 'tumours of reticular tissue with limited and unlimited spread' (Harrison) or 'multifocal benign neoplasms with progressive extension but without evidence of malignancy' (Marshall), while other systematists evaded the problem.

In 1961 Lennert presented a masterly account of the reactive lymphadenopathies and in 1964 Robb-Smith provided a comprehensive review of the lymphadenopathies based on the analysis of a follow-up of 3000 cases in the Oxford Lymph Node Registry, which included a comparison of the various classifications then in use. In 1963 Rappaport completed the fascicle on tumours of the haematopoetic system in the Atlas of Tumour Pathology of the U.S. Armed

Forces Institute of Pathology although it was not actually published until 1966. It is a superbly illustrated histological account of the whole range of lympho-reticular disorders, from the leukoses to the reticulosarcomata and includes progressive hyperplastic conditions but Rappaport upheld the lymphoma view-point and failed overtly to recognize the distinctions between progressive lympho-proliferation and truly destructive malignant neoplasms.

The classification Rappaport (Table 6) used was that of his follicular lymphoma paper, but following Mallory (1942) and Gall (1956), he replaced reticulum cell malignant lymphoma by two categories – undifferentiated and histiocytic – and added an unclassified group, while all the categories were divided into diffuse or nodular types; Hodgkin's disease was classed as paragranuloma, granuloma and sarcoma.

The Rye Conference and after

Contemporary with the publication of the Rappaport fascicle, was the work of Robert Lukes and his colleagues on Hodgkin's disease (Lukes, 1963; Lukes and Butler, 1966; Lukes, Butler and Hicks, 1966). They studied the Hodgkin's material of the Armed Forces Institute of Pathology which had already been reviewed by Smetana and Cohen (1956), and accepted 377 cases.

Lukes and Butler first grouped the cases according to the Jackson and Parker scheme and found that 91% were Hodgkin's granuloma which was similar to Smetana's analysis; however, when they examined critically 14 cases of granu-loma with sclerosis which had a better prognosis in Smetana's series, they not only confirmed this, but found that these patients had distinct clinical features and the nodes had a characteristic histology which they called nodular sclerosis. It corresponded, in fact, to the hard form of lymphadenoma illustrated by An-drewes in 1902, but Lukes et al emphasized that in addition to the structural feature of nodules of lymphadenomatous tissue surrounded by encircling bands of collagen, the giant cells were unusual, as there was a lacuna-like clear space in the cytoplasm surrounding the nuclei which were often hyperlobulated.

In all, Lukes and Butler (1966) defined six variants of Hodgkin's disease – (1) and (2) Lymphocytic and/or histiocytic predominance which might be nodular or diffuse. This corresponded to Jackson and Parker's paragranuloma, but to it Lukes transferred from the Jackson granuloma group, the nodular form corre-sponding to the Hodgkin's variety of Rappaport's follicular lymphoma (1956). Histiocytic predominance included the Peedell-Lennert lymphoma etc. (3) No-dular sclerosis which was the important new category. (4) Mixed cellularity which corresponded to the residuum of Jackson and Parker's Hodgkin's granu-loma. (5) Diffuse fibrosis in which there was irregular fibrosis, paucity of lym-phocytes but Reed-Sternberg cells were prominent and (6) Reticular in which there was a fine widespread fibrosis and with few lymphocytes and numerous Reed-Sternberg giant cells, which were often bizarre in character.

This classification attracted considerable interest on account of the good prognostic correlation, although nodular sclerosis was the only new category and the only one with particular clinical features. However the classification was felt to be too complex and at a conference on 'Obstacles to the Control of Hodgkin's Disease' held at Rye, New York in September 1965, a simplification – the Rye classification (Lukes et al, 1966) – was recommended for international adoption in which there were only four categories – (1) Lymphocyte predominance (embracing Lukes and Butler diffuse and nodular lymphocytic and/or histiocytic Hodgkin's disease (2) Nodular sclerosis; (3) Mixed cellularity (unchanged from Lukes and Butler) and (4) Lymphocytic depletion (embracing Lukes and Butler's reticular and diffuse fibrosis). Cross (1969) later proposed a somewhat different histological classification whose intricacy did not appear to be justified by any gain in clinical correlation.

At the Rye conference, a classification of clinical staging of Hodgkin's disease was also proposed (Rosenberg, 1966) but this had been modified and at the present time the staging procedure agreed at a work-shop in Ann Arbor in April 1971 (Carbone et al, 1971) has been generally accepted for Hodgkin's disease, though modified for other lymphomas (Moran et al, 1975).

Prospective and retrospective studies have shown good correlation between the Rye histological types and prognosis etc. (Butler 1971, 1973), though in various trials experienced pathologists only agreed as to the type in about two thirds of individual slides (Keller et al, 1968; Lukes, Gompel and Nezelof, 1966; Coppleson et al, 1970; Crum et al, 1974). Furthermore in various reported series the proportion of nodular sclerosis ranged from 12% (Cross, 1969) to 73% (Kadin et al, 1971), but how much this was due to case selection or histological interpretation is impossible to determine as none of these series have been related to population incidence; certainly there has been a tendency to include cases lacking nodular sclerosis, but with lacunar cells, as the cellular phase of nodular sclerosis (Strum and Rappaport, 1970; Lukes, 1971; Kadin et al, 1971; Patchefsky et al, 1973), though Butler (1975) and many other pathologists are much stricter in their diagnostic requirements.

The outcome of the Rye conference was a widely accepted histological classification of Hodgkin's disease, but the other primary lymphadenopathies were still in confusion, which was not resolved at the International Symposium on Lymphology held at Zurich in July 1966. Karl Lennert and Robert Lukes had been invited to discuss the classification of malignant lymphomas from the European and American viewpoints.

Lennert (1967) explained that he could only present his own classification. He accepted the idea of three categories of lymphadenopathies – reactive, sarcomatous and progressive hyperplasias which he preferred to call autonomous hyperplasias; he emphasized the importance of recognizing that lymphocytes could be transformed to 'blast' forms by phytohaemagglutinins, and the value of special stains, including enzymic and histochemical methods and electron microscopy.

In the light of this he believed that the follicular lymphoma was derived from cells of the germinal centres, which he called germinoblasts and germinocytes and that it was possible to identify plasmablastic and immunoblastic sarcomas distinct from the stem cell lymphomas, but he appeared unwilling to accept the use of reticulosarcoma as a collective term and there was confusion as to whether the term reticulum cell was being used in Maximow's pluripotential sense or for a cell differentiated along histiocytic lines.

Lukes (1967) gave a paper which he had already delivered as a keynote address in Japan two years earlier, entitled 'The evolution of a modern classification' in which he admitted that 'though the majority of United States pathologists generally agree on the definition of malignant lymphoma as a malignant neoplasm of lymph node derivatives, beyond that there is no agreement'. Lukes followed Gall (1955) in recommending the discontinuance of 'reticulum cell sarcoma' though accepting the terms stem cell and histiocytic sarcoma and he upheld the view of Rappaport et al (1956) that follicular lymphoma was not a lymphoma of germinal follicles but an expression of the tendency of lymphoma cells to aggregate in nodular fashion; currently immunologists would not regard these two concepts as distinct. He endorsed Gall and Rappaport's 1958 classification save that he omitted the mixed type of malignant lymphoma and felt that Hodgkin's disease should be classed according to the grouping which he and Butler (1966) had proposed; he suggested that greater attention should be paid to the haemic and immunoglobulin changes in lymph node diseases.

The Immunological Approach to non-Hodgkin's Lymphoma

Just over a year later, in October 1967, there was an international conference on leukaemia and lymphoma at Ann Arbor with a large number of notable addresses. Robert Good* and Joanne Finstad (1968) discussed the 'Association of lymphoid malignancy and immunologic functions' in which they presented the concept of the relationship of B- and T-cells to lymphoid malignancy; and Dameshek integrated these observations with his ideas on immunoproliferative disorders, the transformation of lymphocytes on antigenic stimulation to 'blast' forms (Dameshek's immunoblasts) and he suggested that lymphoid neoplasms could be regarded as growth aberrations of immunological competent cells (immunocytes).

Lukes spoke on 'The pathologic picture of the malignant lymphomas' giving essentially the same paper supporting the Rappaport classification, which he had delivered in Zurich fifteen months before, but in the discussion, Hayhoe asked whether, in view of Good's suggestion that lymphomas could be divided into those that were thymic dependent or bursa equivalent dependent, would it not be possible to prepare a classification displaying this? Dr Lukes replied 'Dr Good

---

* At the Rye conference in September 1965, Cooper, Peterson, Gabrielsen, and Good (1966), had presented a paper in which they suggested that both experimental and human lymphocytic malignancy might be classified according to the site of initial involvement, either the thymic dependant or immunoglobulin production areas, but according to the published report, the paper elicited no discussion.

and I may be closer together than is thought, in that the poorly differentiated lymphocyte appears to be what Germany's Karl Lennert believes is related to the germinocyte, one of the follicular centre cells and therefore related to the central lymphoid tissue. One of the types of histiocytic lymphoma also appears to be related to his germinoblasts which are also follicular centre cells'. Incidentally it was at this conference that the term 'non-Hodgkin's Lymphoma' was first used (Aisenberg, 1968).

While these philosophical disputations were proceeding, a practical problem was being attacked at the Institut Gustave-Roussy, Villejuif, near Paris – to provide a satisfactory histopathological definition of Burkitt's tumour, the African child-hood malignant lymphoma which Denis Burkitt had characterized ten years earlier. Almost all the lymphoma aficionados participated and an enlightened reading of the preface to the WHO monograph reveals the difficulties that Cos Berard and the other editors faced (1969). The resultant was an outstanding success, for not only did they provide an admirably illustrated account of Burkitt's tumour itself, but also of a whole range of conditions with which it might be confused.

Lennert (1971, 1973) amplified his views as to the germinal centre origin of follicular lymphoma in Milan in 1971 and at Nagoya later in the same year, when he emphasized that he regarded this condition as a clinico-pathological entity and regretted that his views did not conform to Rappaport's concept. It was at this joint U.S. – Japanese Nagoya meeting that Lukes and Collins (1973) accepted Lennert's ideas on follicular lymphoma and integrated the immuno-topographical concept (Robb-Smith, 1974) into the categorization of the lympho-mata. Much more significant from a diagnostic point of view they emphasized the specific cytological characters of the follicular cells, cleaved and non-cleaved, which no other histopathologist had done before, although the nuclei of leuk-aemic cells in follicular lymphoma had been noticed to be notched or have a cleft (see p. 238). Kojima et al (1973) on the basis of electron microscopic studies endorsed the views of Lennert, Lukes and Collins, but Dorfman (1973), in an excellent histopathological account, was unconvinced and deplored any changes in terminology or classification. Consequent on the work of Jaffe et al (1974), Dorfman accepted the germinal origin of follicular lymphoma and made some confirmatory studies of his own (Levine and Dorfman, 1975).

There was a third lymphoma conference in 1971, though it attracted much less attention than that at Nagoya. It was held at the U.S. National Cancer Institute and concerned the comparative pathology of haemopoietic and lympho-reticular neoplasms in a wide range of species, such as blue mussels, cut-throat trout, hog-nose snakes, harbour seals and owl monkeys. Krueger (1977) com-pared these animal tumours with analogous conditions in man.

The Nagoya conference made it clear that Japanese pathologists accepted the concept of progressive hyperplastic lymphadenopathies (reticulosis, cataplastic or preblastomatous lesions) as distinct from truly malignant reticulosarcomata (Akazaki, 1973; Tanaka, 1973). There was also a discussion on immunoblastic lymphadenopathy which did not appear in the conference monograph but was mentioned by Lennert (1972) in Vienna in March 1972, where he called the condition 'lymphogranulomatosis X'. Recently Lennert et al (1979) have pointed out that their first cases were seen in 1947, while Flandrin (1978) recalled that he had described some in 1972; Gams et al (1968) had displayed the interrelationship between this form of lymphadenopathy and those known to be drug induced. It was at this Vienna meeting that Lennert put forward what he called a 'traditional' classification of lymphomas which were classed as (1) Reticulosarcoma; (2) Lymphosarcoma divided into lymphocytic and lymphoblastic (including the Burkitt tumour); (3) Germinoblastic (follicular lymphoma) which could eventually evolve into a germinoblastic sarcoma; each was sub-divided as to whether it was a tumour or associated with a leukaemic blood picture. He also discussed immunoglobulin assay and found that many of the large cell malignant lymphomas which would ordinarily be classified as reticulosarcomas or histiocytic lymphomas had a high IgM content and so should be classed with lymphoid tumours, something which he had mentioned at Zurich in 1966. In October 1972 Lennert and his colleagues (Stein et al, 1972) pursued the matter in a paper on 'Malignant lymphomas of B-cell type' in which they concluded that as many reticulum cell sarcomas are IgM producers, they should be classed as 'lymphatic not reticulocytic' in origin and the classification of reticulum cell sarcomas should be revised.

It was in Freiburg in September 1972 that Lukes and Collins (1974) first outlined their functional approach to the classification of malignant lymphomata; this was very similar to their later accounts (see Table 7), but it is difficult to be sure what it was they said in 1972, as the published account refers to papers which did not appear until the following year.

It was also in 1972 that Cottier et al proposed a standardized system of reporting lymph node morphology in relation to immunological function; their nomenclature was simple and non-commital and the cell types were well illustrated yet the actual recording procedure was extremely complex, as it was largely based on lymph node changes associated with congenital immunodeficiencies.

In 1973 and 1974 there was an eruption of progress and polemics in the immunological approach to the lymphadenopathies. In January 1973, Smith et al presented evidence that in a case of mediastinal malignant lymphoma of the Sternberg type, the lymphoid cells could be of T-cell origin, but they did not discuss the morphology of the tumour cells. Later in the year Brouet et al (1973) and Broome et al (1973) showed that the cerebriform cell which Lutzner and Jordan (1968) had described in Sézary's Syndrome was also T-cell derived.

In June 1973 a workshop on the classification of non-Hodgkin's lymphoma was held in Chicago and though no proceedings were published, some of the contributions are known. Lukes gave a demonstration of a new form of malignant lymphoma which he called 'a malignant convoluted lymphocytic lymphoma', occuring in children in association with a mediastinal mass; the striking feature was the convoluted nuclear pattern and he believed the tumour was of T-cell origin. The work had been done in association with Maurice Barcos, but it would not be formally presented until 1974 (Barcos and Lukes, 1975), though it had already been discussed by Smith et al (1973) and would be described in detail by Lukes and Collins (1974, 1975). Lennert realized that Lukes' convoluted nuclear cells corresponded to the cells in a particular type of malignant lymphoma, which his group had been studying, and found that the cells gave a focal paranuclear reaction for acid phosphotase; this reaction had been recognized by Leder (1965) in cases believed to be very primitive erythraemia though many of the children had large thymic masses.

In Chicago Lennert et al (1974) spoke on 'New criteria for the classification of malignant lymphoma' which he repeated at a meeting in Prague in August 1973. He discussed chronic lymphatic leukaemia, follicular lymphoma, lymphocytic lymphosarcoma and lymphoplasmacytoid immunocytomas, but the most significant section dealt with the so-called 'reticulosarcoma' ('histiocytic malignant lymphoma') which was an extension of the Vienna and Lancet papers of the previous year and was amplified in a later paper (Stein, Kaiserling and Lennert, 1974). Lennert used detailed cytochemical, immunochemical and electron microscopic methods on a series of malignant tumours which he considered conformed morphologically to the reticulum cell sarcoma or histiocytic malignant lymphoma of American pathologists and found that the majority of these tumours had the characters of immunoblastic or plasmablastic sarcomas of B-cell origin and were not derived from reticulum cells or histiocytes.

These observations were fully endorsed by others but, once again, confusion arose over the use of 'reticulum cell' either in Maximow's sense of a pluripotent cell or as a synonym for a histiocyte as used by Rappaport and others. Lennert's semantic difficulties are apparent in two papers, spanning a decade, in which he discussed 'reticulosis' (1964, 1974). He quotes Oberling (1928) but, like Robb-Smith (1938), Oberling used reticulosarcoma as a collective generic term. Gall and Mallory (1942) who introduced the term reticulum cell sarcoma into the classification of malignant lymphoma, in their table, showed it in inverted commas as a bracketed designation covering the stem cell and clasmatocytic malignant lymphomas, a viewpoint endorsed by Rappaport (1964); it was probably Rhoads (1928) who first suggested that the reticulum cell was derived from a phagocytic cell, whereas Ewing (1928) made it clear that he regarded it as less mature than the lymphocytes from the germinal centres or pulp cords, Taylor (1974, 1976) using the immunoperoxidase techniques on a series of malignant tumours diagnosed by Robb-Smith as various types of reticulosarcoma, found that of the poorly differentiated tumours, it was possible to demonstrate intracellular monoclonal immunoglobulins in about two thirds with the presumption that they were of B-cell origin, while there were also a small number of tumours giving a positive reaction for muramidase inferring a relationship to the histiocyte; accordingly Taylor suggested that the reticulum cell has been used as a designation for both the histiocytic cell group and the transformed lymphocyte.

Following the enzymic histochemical studies of Müller-Hermelink et al (1974), Lennert (1975) accepted that there were four types of reticulum cell – histiocytic, fibroblastic, dendritic, and interdigitating, and that there could be 'true' reticulo-sarcomas corresponding to these four cell types. So far he (1978) was only able to recognize the histiocytic type, but Motoi et al (1978) using Taylor's muramidase technique and Leder's chloracetate esterese reaction, identified a range of lymph node tumours as of histiocytic origin.

The London Conference and the Classification Epidemic

At the end of September 1973, there was the notable non-Hodgkin's lymphoma symposium in London. The principle papers on classification were given by Lukes and Collins (1975) and Lennert, Stein and Kaiserling (1975) but as usual it is difficult to determine what had been presented at the conference and what was added subsequently.

Table 7

Functional Classification of Malignant Lymphoma
(Lukes and Collins, 1975)

I. U-cell (undefined cell) type

II. T-cell types
   1. Mycosis fungoides and Sézary's syndrome
   2. Convoluted lymphocyte
   3. Immunoblastic sarcoma of T-cells

III. B-cell types
   1. Small lymphocyte (CLL)
   2. Plasmacytoid lymphocyte
   3. Follicular center cell (FCC) types (follicular, diffuse, follicular and diffuse, and sclerotic)
     a) small cleaved
     b) large cleaved
     c) small non-cleaved
     d) large non-cleaved
   4. Immunoblastic sarcoma of B-cells

IV. Histiocytic type

V. Unclassifiable

Lukes and Collins' classification (Table 7) was almost identical with that published after the Freiburg meeting. They explained that they used the adjective functional, not in the sense that the classification reflected the functional activity of the tumour cells but rather that there was a possibility of morphological identification of malignant cells which were the counterparts of the B- and T-lymphocytes in various phases of development; in addition there were categories in the classification for undefined, unclassifiable and histiocytic types of malignant lymphomata. Each tumour type was well illustrated with a clear description of the morphological character of the individual cells, including the T-cell convoluted lymphocyte. Butler et al (1975) gave a preliminary report on its practical application.

Lennert and his colleagues (1975) presented an analytical study of a series of cases using electron microscopy, histochemistry and immunoglobulin assays as well as ordinary staining methods. They identified and illustrated six morphological types:

Table 8

Cytological and Functional Classification of Malignant Lymphoma
(Lennert, Stein and Kaiserling, 1975)

1. Chronic lymphocytic leukaemia

2. Diffuse germinocytoma (malignant lymphoma, lymphocytic, intermediate)

3. Germinoblastoma (follicular, follicular & diffuse, diffuse, sclerotic), which can show a transition into germinoblastic sarcoma

4. Immunoblastic sarcoma of the B-cell type (until now: reticulosarcoma)

5. Lympho-plasmacytoid immunocytoma, which can be the substrate of macroglobulinaemia Waldenström and can show a mixed cellularity (lymphocytic and histiocytic)

6. Lymphoblastic (paraleukoblastic) sarcoma and leukaemia, which are, at least in most cases, probably neoplasias of germinoblasts.

Lennert suggested that a study of the functional properties of lymphoma cells, such as they had presented, offered a possibility for developing a scientifically based classification. Although there were ideological differences, these two classifications were basically very similar and could, as Hansen and Good (1974) showed (Table 9), be superficially equated quite easily; but both Rappaport (1977) and Nathwani (1979) have emphasized their fundamental differences. In both cases the axis was cytological and there was no attempt to provide a meaningful clinical grouping; nevertheless this physio-morphological approach received strong support from Gérard-Marchant (1974) and others.

However it would seem that at the symposium the view was expressed that

Table 9

Comparison of the Functional Classifications of Non-Hodgkin's Lymphoma
(Hansen and Good, 1974)

Lennert	Lukes and Collins
I. Undefined (not B or T) stem cell, (?) precursor cell (?)	
II. B-cell (lymphocytic) types	
1. Chronic lymphatic leukemia	1. Small lymphocytic type chronic lymphatic leukemia
2. Lymphoplasmacytoid immunocytoma	2. Plasmacytoid lymphocytic
3. Germinal center cell tumors	3. Follicle center cell tumors (follicular, diffuse, sclerotic)
a. Diffuse germinocytoma b. Germinoblastoma (follicular, diffuse, sclerotic)	a. Cleaved follicle center cell tumors

c. Germinoblastic sarcoma
d. Paraleukoblastic (B-lymphoblastic) sarcoma including Burkitt's lymphoma
	b. Noncleaved follicle center cell tumors
	  1. Small (Burkitt)
	  2. Large

4. Immunoblastic (reticulo-) sarcoma, B-cell type	4. Immunoblastic (reticulum cell) sarcoma, B-cell type
III. T-cell (lymphocytic) types	
1. Sézary syndrome	1. Sézary syndrome
2. ? Lymphoblastic sarcoma (acute lymphoblastic leukemia), T-cell type	2. Convoluted lymphocytic (acute lymphoblastic leukaemia), T-cell type
3. Chronic lymphatic leukemia, T-cell type	3. Small lymphocytic type (chronic lymphatic leukemia), T-cell type
IV. Reticulohistiocytic, M-cell types	
1. Reticulosarcoma, M-cell type	1. Histiocytic
V. Unclassifiable	

both these classifications were premature and it was recommended that Rappaport's should continue to be used for the time being.

The most important clinico-pathological paper was probably that of Spiro et al (1975) on follicular lymphoma, which fully confirmed the observations of the Mount Sinai group half a century before, that this was a nosological entity with a characteristic natural history and morphology, rather than simply a variant of malignant lymphoma as Rappaport et al (1956) had seen it.

Two months after the London conference, Lukes and Collins (1975) presented their classification to the American Cancer Society in New York, but the details, as published, corresponded to that of the 1972 Freiburg meeting rather than the London proposals (for example under T-cells, immunoblastic sarcoma and Hodgkin's disease are shown with a question mark) and the photo-micrographs were not so good as those in the British Journal of Cancer paper.

In March 1974, the International Academy of Pathology held a meeting in San Francisco when the 'long course' was devoted to the 'Reticulo-endothelial system, function, reactions, and neoplasia' at which Dorfman presented a 'working classification' (Dorfman, 1974 Table 10) which was published in the *Lancet* the following June and incorporated into the Academy monograph (Rebuck, Berard and Abell, 1975).

He described it as a compromise between those of Rappaport and Lukes and the classification proposed by Farrer-Brown et al at the 1973 Chicago meeting (Berard and Dorfman, 1974), but there was no indication of the content of the various categories nor the morphological character of the cells. It followed Rappaport in that the prime axis was the follicular or diffuse nature of the proliferation; while Rappaport's five diffuse categories were increased to nine and there was provision for a composite lymphoma, and whether or not there was sclerosis.

Table 10

'Working Classification' of Non-Hodgkin's Lymphoma
(Dorfman, 1974)

Follicular lymphomas*
(follicular or follicular and diffuse)   Small lymphoid . .   . .   Mixed small and large lymphoid   Large lymphoid . .   . .
Diffuse lymphomas*
Small lymphocytic (SL)(CLL)   SL with plasmacytoid differentiation   Atypical small lymphocytic   Convoluted lymphocytic (thymic)   Large lymphoid (pyroninophilic)   Mixed small and large lymphoid   Histiocytic   Burkitt's lymphoma   Mycosis fungoides   Undefined   * Composite lymphomas, comprising two well-defined and apparently different types of lymphoma within the same tissue and lymphomas associated with sclerosis, are suitably designated.

Two months later Bennett, Farrer-Brown et al (1974) published in the *Lancet*, a modification of the classification they had presented at the 1973 Chicago workshop (Table 11); there were no details as to the contents or character of the various categories, which were similar to those put forward by Dorfman, but the major and significant difference was that the primary axis determined whether the tumour was of a low- or high-grade malignancy. It seemed that this classification had been accepted as workable by a number of British hospitals taking part in a collective lymphoma enquiry, and a retrospective survey (Bennett, 1975) has confirmed its usefulness.

It was also in the *Lancet* that the first report of the Kiel classification appeared (Table 14). It arose in the following manner: after the London symposium, a group of European pathologists were asked if they could work out a new classification and terminology and so the European Lymphoma Club was founded. After a session with Lukes and 'intensive discussion and joint studies of a large number of microscope slides', the members of the club met at Kiel in May 1974, when they considered a draft prepared by Lennert (1974; Table 12) which was a considerable expansion of his London paper and divided the lymphomata into low and high grade malignancy. It was comparable with the 1966 Rappaport classification but incorporated the newer ideas on immunocytology and topography which Robb-Smith (1974) had advocated earlier in the year. The members approved the principles but amended the terminology and this version was ac-

Table 11

Classification of Non-Hodgkin's Lymphomas
(Bennett, Farrer Brown, and Henry – 1974)

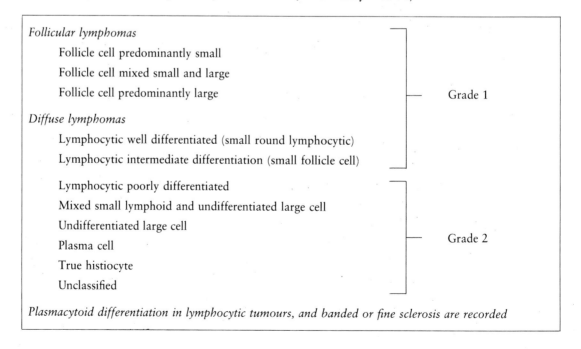

Follicular lymphomas
    Follicle cell predominantly small
    Follicle cell mixed small and large
    Follicle cell predominantly large — Grade 1

Diffuse lymphomas
    Lymphocytic well differentiated (small round lymphocytic)
    Lymphocytic intermediate differentiation (small follicle cell)

    Lymphocytic poorly differentiated
    Mixed small lymphoid and undifferentiated large cell
    Undifferentiated large cell
    Plasma cell — Grade 2
    True histiocyte
    Unclassified

Plasmacytoid differentiation in lymphocytic tumours, and banded or fine sclerosis are recorded

cepted at a meeting in Amsterdam on July 7 1974; the *Lancet* report (Gérard-Marchant et al, 1974) provided a useful commentary on the principles which had been adopted in the preparation of the classification (Lennert, 1978).

Table 12
Lennert's Classification for the European Lymphoma Club May 1974

Low-grade malignant lymphomas	*High-grade malignant lymphomas*
Lymphocytomas B-cell types: CLL hairy-cell leukemia T-cell types: Sézary syndrome (and mycosis fungoides?) Others *Immunocytoma* (lympho-plasmacytoid) lymphoplasmacytic lymphoplasmacytoid polymorphic *Germinocytoma* (diffuse) *Germinoblastoma* follicular follicular and diffuse diffuse nonsclerotic sclerotic (Bennett's type)	*Germinoblastic sarcoma* *Lymphoblastic sarcoma;* including ALL B-cell types: Burkitt's tumor non-Burkitt's tumor T-cell type: convoluted type of Lukes undefined unclassifiable *Immunoblastic sarcoma*

Three weeks after the appearance of the Kiel proposals, the *Lancet* published a witty suggestion from Kay (1974) for a classification of non-Hodgkin lymphoma classifications (Table 13) which effectively silenced any further would-be systematists.

Table 13
Kay's Classification of Non-Hodgkin's Lymphoma Classifications (1974)

Well-defined, high-grade, oligosyllabic

Poorly differentiated, polysyllabic ⎰ diffuse / circumlocutory / with dyslexogenesis

Unicentric ⎰ derivative / neologistic

Multicentric, cycnophilic (Gk. κυκνοξ=swan)

Cleaved and convoluted types ⎰ Rappaport (non-Lukes) / Lukes (non-Rappaport)

In September 1974, at a conference on 'Conflicts in childhood cancer', Barcos and Lukes (1975) presented their formal account of the convoluted T-cell mediastinal tumour in children, a subject under discussion since 1973 and described in detail by Lukes and Collins in 1974. Although the convoluted cell could usually be shown to be of T-cell type, yet it had become apparent that the Sternberg leukosarcoma might be associated with B- or T-cells (Stathopoulos et al, 1974), and a convoluted or non-convoluted cell malignant lymphoma (Nathwani et al, 1976), while half the cases of childhood T-cell acute lymphatic leukaemia did not have mediastinal involvement (Williams et al, 1978) and convoluted cell malignant lymphoma was not uncommon in adults (Rosen et al, 1978).

The Search for a 'via media'

After all the hurly-burly of the previous year, it is hardly surprising that 1975 was devoted to reflection and assessment of the contending proposals. Lennert and Lukes and their colleagues published their classifications in detail, while there were review articles by Mathé et al (1975), Braylan, Jaffe and Berard (1975), and Diebold (1975), the latter including a variant classification of his own.

Lennert (1975) and his colleagues presented the Kiel Classification, with excellent illustrations and descriptions of the cell types, at a congress in Vienna in August 1974 (Lennert, 1975), and at the International Congress of Haematology in London in 1975 (Lennert et al, 1975).

As a whole the Kiel classification is straightforward, the nomenclature much simpler than that of Lukes and Collins or some of the neo-Rappaport variants which encourage the use of confusing abbreviations such as DMWDLL, NHL/D &NHL, T-IBS or LRMPS. It does not claim to be 'functional', but recognition of immunoglobulin synthesis, as an indication of B-cell derivation, is important in its taxonomy; however the Kiel classification proper, as against Lennert's (1978) modifications, did not accept the terms B- and T-cell in the nomenclature. There is a division into lymphomas of low- and high-grade malignancy and the former are said to correspond to Robb-Smith's (1964) progressive hyperplasias, but the Kiel low grade includes the diffuse centrocytic type which would be classed as a sarcoma by Robb-Smith; it is clear that Lennert (1978) is not happy at including it in this grade, for as he says '. . . it lies at the lower limit of all low-grade malignant lymphomas, but is significantly poorer than the prognosis of the others'.

At a meeting of the European Lymphoma Club held in Paris in February 1975, it was agreed to add plasmacytic lymphoma (extramedullary plasmacytoma) to the low-grade lymphoma and to subdivide the immunoblastic malignant lymphoma into those with plasmablastic and/or plasmacytic differentiation and those without such differentiation, which would include T-cell immunoblastic lymphoma. It was presumed that tumours formerly diagnosed as reticulum cell

Table 14

Kiel Classification of Non-Hodgkin's Lymphomas compared with Rappaport's Classification
(Gérard-Marchant et al, 1974)

Kiel classification	Rappaport equivalent
Low-grade malignancy	
Malignant lymphoma (ML) – lymphocytic (CLL and others)	M.L. well-differentiated lymphocytic – diffuse
M.L. – lymphoplasmacytoid (immunocytic)	{ M.L. lymphocytic type with dysproteinaemia / Lymphoproliferative diseases with dysproteinaemia
M.L. – centrocytic	M.L. { well / poorly } Differentiated lymphocytic { nodular / diffuse }
M.L. – centroblastic-centrocytic follicular* / follicular* and diffuse / diffuse*	M.L. (poorly differentiated lymphocytic / mixed-cell histiocytic – / lymphocytic / histiocytic – nodular) { nodular / diffuse }
High-grade malignancy	
M.L. – centroblastic	{ M.L. – histiocytic – nodular or diffuse / M.L. – undifferentiated
M.L. – lymphoblastic Burkitt type Convoluted-cell type Others	M.L. – undifferentiated Burkitt's lymphoma { M.L. poorly differentiated lymphocytic – diffuse? / M.L. undifferentiated – non-Burkitt?
M.L. – immunoblastic	M.L. histiocytic – diffuse

* With or without sclerosis. M.L. = Malignant lymphoma

sarcomas or malignant lymphomas, histiocytic type, are either malignant immunoblastic or centroblastic lymphomas and that if a histiocytic tumour exists apart from the group of malignant histiocytosis, it should not be included in the 'malignant lymphomas'; however, as was mentioned earlier (p. 246), in Lennert's later papers (1975, 1978), he accepts the existence of histiocytic and fibre producing tumours in lymphoid tissues though calling them 'true reticulosarcomas'.

One of the consequences of the proposals and counterproposals on the classification of the lymphomata was that clinicians and statisticians, who had been reasonably contented with the Rappaport scheme, were now thoroughly confused and alarmed at the plethora of new groupings and unfamiliar terms that showered upon them. The lymphoma section of the International Cancer Congress held in Florence in October 1974 had a Tower of Babel atmosphere as data was presented under disparate nomenclatures and groupings. A year later, in the hope of resolving these differencies, the U.S. National Cancer Institute convened a conference of clinicians and pathologists at Airlie House, Warrenton, Virginia, in September 1975. The various classifications which have been discussed here were considered, but it soon became apparent that there was no agreement possible on the terminology for a unique classification (Biomedicine: editorial, 1975), while the clinicians revealed their concern and urged an early resolution of the current confusion and called for a universally acceptable classification to replace the Rappaport classification. Rappaport (1976) defined the qualities to be required of such a classification as 'clinically useful, scientifically accurate, reproducable, easily taught and readily learnt'. Aisenberg (1977) remarked on another occasion: 'It seems to me that pathologists are getting into difficulties in the area of non-Hodgkin's lymphomas. Not only do we clinicians have trouble in understanding pathologists, but at times they seem unable to understand each other.'

In the spring of 1976, as a consequence of the Warrenton débâcle, the National Cancer Institute agreed to organise a retrospective review of biopsies from over a thousand cases of non-Hodgkin's lymphoma with an adequate follow up; these would be classified according to the various systems both by their originators and by other pathologists familiar with lymph node histopathology. The results would be analyzed in great detail both from the point of clinical usefulness and histological reproducibility in the hope that this might provide the basis for the creation of a new classification as satisfactory as was that of Rappaport for nearly twenty years. The pathologists' reviews were completed by the latter half of 1978 and conferences were held in Stanford, California, in June 1979, and January 1980; the outcome of this study will be discussed at the end of this essay (p. 262).

The World Health Organisation classification (Table 15) of neoplastic diseases of haematopoietic and lymphoid tissues (Mathé et al, 1976) appeared just in time to be one of the contenders in the National Cancer Institute study; it had been under discussion since 1961 and it is admitted that the classification proposals 'still lack agreement in several areas'. It embraces a far broader group of conditions than is ordinarily included under non-Hodgkin's lymphoma, though the demarcation line of this group is far from clear. In the WHO list the primary division is between systemic diseases, which embraces the leukaemias and analogous conditions, and tumours which includes Hodgkin's disease. The coloured illustrations are excellent and there is a short description of each named condition, but the cytological account of the individual cell types is quite inadequate. It would not be difficult to question the logic behind certain of the arrangements and nomenclatural principles, but the test of any classification is whether or not it is helpful in some particular way and this remains to be seen. It did not receive a very warm reception. Dorfman (1977) described it as 'lamentably retrogressive', Lennert (1978) wrote 'there is no reason to assume that this classification will find the world wide reception that a WHO classification should have'; while Chelloul et al (1976) were hardly complimentary. Nevertheless Mathé (1977, 1978) has shown, at least in his hands and those of his colleagues, that the categories are meaningful and facilitate thereapeutic selection and consequent prognosis.

Table 15

World Health Organisation Classification of Neoplastic Diseases of the Haematopoietic and Lymphoid Tissues (Mathé et al, 1976)

I. SYSTEMIC DISEASES

A. ACUTE LEUKAEMIAS AND RELATED DISEASES
1. Acute lymphoid leukaemia
2. Acute myeloid leukaemia
3. Acute monocytoid [monocytic] leukaemia
4. Malignant histiocytosis
5. Acute erythraemia (di Guglielmo)
6. Erythroleukaemia
7. Megakaryocytoid [megakaryocytic] leukaemia
8. Acute panmyelosis
9. Acute leukaemia, unclassified

B. CHRONIC LYMPHOID LEUKAEMIA AND OTHER LYMPHOPROLIFERATIVE DISEASES
1. Chronic lymphoid leukaemia
2. Primary macroglobulinaemia (Waldenström)
3. Myeloma
4. Plasma-cell leukaemia
5. Heavy-chain diseases
6. Sézary's disease
7. Chronic lymphoproliferative disease, unclassified

C. CHRONIC MYELOID LEUKAEMIA AND OTHER MYELOPROLIFERATIVE DISEASES
1. Chronic myeloid leukaemia
2. Variants of chronic myeloid leukaemia
   (a) Neutrophilic leukaemia
   (b) Eosinophilic leukaemia
   (c) Basophilic leukaemia
3. Chronic erythraemia (Heilmeyer-Schöner)
4. Polycythaemia vera (Vaquez-Osler)
5. Idiopathic thrombocythaemia
6. Myelosclerosis with myeloid metaplasia
7. Chronic myeloproliferative diseases, unclassified

D. CHRONIC MONOCYTOID LEUKAEMIA AND SYSTEMIC HISTIOCYTOID DISEASES
1. Chronic monocytoid [monocytic] leukaemia
2. Histiocytosis X

E. UNCLASSIFIED LEUKAEMIAS
1. Hairy cell leukaemia

F. OTHERS
1. Malignant mastocytosis

II. TUMOURS

A. LYMPHOSARCOMAS
1. Nodular lymphosarcoma
2. Diffuse lymphosarcoma
   (a) Lymphocytic
   (b) Lymphoplasmacytic
   (c) Prolymphocytic
   (d) Lymphoblastic
   (e) Immunoblastic
   (f) Burkitt's tumour

B. MYCOSIS FUNGOIDES

C. PLASMACYTOMA

D. RETICULOSARCOMA

E. UNCLASSIFIED MALIGNANT LYMPHOMAS

F. HODGKIN'S DISEASE
1. With lymphocyte predominance
2. With nodular sclerosis
3. With mixed cellularity
4. With lymphocyte depletion

G. OTHERS
1. Eosinophilic granuloma
2. Mastocytoma

Discussions and Reviews

Many symposia may be enjoyable and profitable to the participants while the published proceedings are often disappointing, but fortunately there are exceptions and a non-Hodgkin lymphoma conference (Jones and Godden, 1977) held at San Francisco in October 1976 was one of these. It opened with a somewhat over-critical, but none the less useful, review by Dorfman (1977) of the various classifications; he proposed to make his own 'working classification' (1974) even more complex by providing for plasmacytoid differentiation and epithelioid inclusions in all types of diffuse lymphoma and by dividing the lymphoblastic lymphoma into convoluted and non-convoluted forms; there are no reports of its use in other centres. The outstanding section of the conference for histopathologists was a round-table discussion on the details of the various classifications under the chairmanship of Dr. Berard (1977) in which Rappaport, Lukes, Dorfman, Berard, Seligmann and others took part; it clarified much of the confusion, differences, and agreements between the various systematists and made apparent why it was that there was no successful outcome to the Warrenton meeting in the previous year. Seligmann (1977), discussing the question of immunological classifications, made the profound observation, 'It is obvious that an immunological classification cannot be satisfactory for clinical purposes. Any immunological classification should be combined with a morphological one and there is an urgent need for a workable and reproducable pathological classification.'

Lukes and Collins (1977) have reviewed a combined series of nearly 400 cases from their respective institutes and are satisfied that their original hypothesis was justified and their classification is histologically workable, but it would seem that they are more concerned with the biological aspects of their functional classification that its immediate practical value in prognosis and therapeutic selection. In a paper read in Chicago in April 1977, Lukes et al discussed the results of their multiparameter studies in a large series of cases of lymphomata which has been steadily broadened (Lukes et al, 1978; Taylor, 1979; Taylor et al, 1979) in subsequent papers. There is no doubt that marker techniques have enhanced the ability to identify with greater precision the character of lymphoid cells, but how much this contributes to an understanding of the nosology of the condition associated with the lymphoma is still uncertain. Lukes and Parker (1978) in their review of immunological and cytochemical studies of lymphoreticular neoplasms conclude; 'Identification of the cytologic types of lymphoma and clinical-morphologic entities permits investigation of the basic biologic mechanisms and ultimately it will lead to the design of more fundamental biologic approaches to therapy.' Pinkus and Said (1978) used a similar range of techniques in a smaller series from Boston, but were more cautious in their conclusions, suggesting that such studies 'may aid in formulating an accurate classification and possibly may have prognostic significance'.

An international colloquium in Paris in June 1977 (Mathé, Seligmann and

Tubiana, 1978) revealed that too many papers were being read and there were too few round-table discussions of the 1976 San Fransisco type. Mathé again discussed the WHO classification but added little to what he had said two years before. Kristin Henry (1978) gave a well illustrated account (including electron micrographs) of cell types used in their classification for the collective 'national lymphoma investigation'; the account was later published in book form (Henry, Bennett and Farrer-Brown, 1978); which revealed that there had been further changes in their classification which must render comparability difficult. This group has a particular interest in tumours of the plasma cell series, and a critical but informed attitude to histiocytic tumours. For a wide ranging cytological account, including ultrastructure, of malignant lymphoid cells, it would be difficult at the present time, to better the cytological analysis provided by Rilke et al (1978). Lukes could only repeat what he had said a short time before and Lennert found himself in a similar position, but he was able to report a small study in reproducability in which he found that, with experienced observers, there was really very little to chose between the classifications of Rappaport, Lukes and Kiel, but marginally (or statistically) Kiel had a slight advantage. Lennert also pointed out that the relative frequency of the various types of lymphadenopathy submitted to the Kiel lymph node registry over the eight year period 1965/73 had varied very little; even more remarkable, the relative proportions were strikingly similar to the proportions of the population incidence calculated for the Oxford area in 1938/47 (Robb-Smith, 1947).

Table 16

Comparison of the Proportional Incidence of Lymphadenopathies in the Kiel and Oxford Areas
(Lennert 1978; Robb-Smith 1947)

	Kiel Lymph Node Registry 1965/73	Oxford Lymph Node Registry 1938/47
Hodgkin's Disease	44%	47%
Lymphocytic and Lymphoplasmacytic	22%	24%
Centroblastic/Centrocytic	12%	8%
High grade Malignancies including centrocytic lymphoma	22%	21%

There have been a number of studies assaying the value of the Kiel classification in relation to prognosis and Brittinger (1978) reported the findings of his group at this Paris meeting; there was good separation of the various low grade malignancies, but little or no differences amongst the high grade varieties, while centrocytic lymphoma was closer in character to the high than the low grade. Delbruck (1978) examined the five year survival of over 200 cases and found that 67% of the low grade survived five years but only 23% of the high grade. Meugé (1978), in a rather larger series from Bordeaux, found that the low grade had a mean survival of 4.5 years, the high grade only 7 months. It is unfortunate that analogous figures are not available for the other classifications, since the National Cancer Institute study is of a rather specialized type.

At the conclusion of one of the Paris sessions O'Connor and Sobin (1978) provided a conversion table of the various classifications to allow translation from one to another and so facilitate international comparisons; unhappily there is considerable disparity between O'Connor and Sobin's table and that prepared by Henry et al (1978) for a similar purpose; this would suggest that it is more important to consider the content of the various categories than their descriptive title; it is this content which has not been revealed in many of the 'fringe' classifications.

Galton et al (1978) read a very significant paper on the 'Clinical spectrum of lymphoproliferative diseases' at a Lymphoma and Leukaemia conference in New York in the latter part of 1977. Discussing the clinical and pathological manifestation of lymphoid disorders, he emphasized that there could be a solitary mass of lymphoid tissue which might remain localized or if it underwent malignant change, would infiltrate, spread locally and perhaps metastasize widely. On the other hand there were many lymphoproliferative conditions – good examples being chronic lymphocytic leukaemia or follicular lymphoma – in which there was a generalized dissemination at initial presentation which appeared to be achieved by a process somewhat analogous to physiological recirculation with a homing mechanism for particular sites or tissues. Malignant change in a monoclone in one of these sites might result in metastatic dissemination, but on occasions there could be a generalized malignant dissemination throughout the lymphoreticular tissue which would seem to be a consequence of a form of recirculation, with, in addition, metastases to other organs. Galton also discussed the progression from a lymphoproliferative condition to a truly malignant one. This topic was dealt with by Robb-Smith (1976) in Sydney; while Lennert et al (1979) have reviewed in great detail the premalignant lymphadenopathies, and a Lancet editorial (1979) considered the broader biological implications of this phenomenon. It was the failure of appreciating the distinction between a naturally generalized disorder such as follicular lymphoma as against the local spreading character of Hodgkin's disease that justified Rosenberg's (1977) observation that 'for many pathological sub-groups of non-Hodgkin's lymphoma, the Ann Arbor staging procedure is seriously defective in identifying prognostic factors or in selecting treatment'.

Early in 1978 Lennert, in association with his colleagues, produced a superb monograph, 'Malignant lymphomas other than Hodgkin's disease', which is not only a fitting companion to the earlier volume on lymph node cytology and lymphadenitis which he contributed to the mighty Henke-Lubarsch Handbuch seventeen years ago, but in itself is a milestone in lymph node research. Lennert recalls that the first account of these conditions in the Handbuch consisted of seven pages in Carl Sternberg's (1926) review of blood diseases. Now we have a richly illustrated volume of nearly a thousand pages, embracing the morphology and functional analysis of lymphoreticular tissue, together with a masterly account of the natural history and histopathology of the majority of the proliferative and malignant lymphomas, using a slight modification of the Kiel classification, which mentions B- and T-cells which are 'not sanctioned' in the official classifications of the European Lymphoma Club (Table 17). It is an exciting experience to read this book and a comfort to be offered a resolution of many difficult problems.

Table 17

Modification of the Kiel Classification of Non-Hodgkin's Lymphoma
(Lennert et al, 1978)

I. Low-grade malignancy

†*M.L. lymphocytic*
 Chronic lymphocytic leukaemia, B-cell type
 Chronic lymphocytic leukaemia, T-cell type
 Hairy-cell leukaemia (?)
 Mycosis fungoides and Sézary's syndrome
 T-zone lymphoma

†*M.L. lymphoplasmacytic / lymphoplasmacytoid* (lymphoplasmacytoid immunocytoma)

†*M.L. plasmacytic* (plasmacytoma*)

†*M.L. centrocytic*

†*M.L. centroblastic/centrocytic*
 Follicular
 Follicular and diffuse
 Diffuse
 with or without sclerosis

II. High-grade malignancy

†*M.L. centroblastic*
 Primary
 Secondary

†*M.L. lymphoblastic*
 B-lymphoblastic, Burkitt type and others
 T-lymphoblastic, convoluted-cell type and others
 Unclassified

†*M.L. immunoblastic*
 with plasmablastic / plasmacytic differentiation (B)
 without plasmablastic / plasmacytic differentiation (B or T)

---

*Only extramedullary plasmacytoma   †*M.L.* = malignant lymphoma

A useful paper presented at a meeting of the Japanese Pathological Society in November 1978, described a careful investigation of observer disagreement between more and less experienced Japanese histologists, and was compared with

Byrne's (1977) analogous study in America. Suchi and his colleagues (1979) also determined the frequency of the different types of malignant lymphoma in their country and found that as a whole, T-cell lymphomas were more common in Japan than in Europe or America, while there was an irregular geographical distribution in Japan itself. This was confirmed and amplified at a Symposium on T-cell malignancies held in Tokyo a year later (Shimoyama and Watanabe 1979).

This emphasizes that any proposals for an international classification of lymphomas must take cognisance of regional variation.

It is to be hoped that this period of introspection and analysis is drawing to a close; a valuable critical review by Mann, Jaffe and Berard (1979) concludes that 'the malignant lymphomas exhibit a multiplicity of histologic and cytologic patterns; approaching these tumours with a functional perspective allows one to develop a conceptual understanding of this morphologic diversity'. Gertrude Stein somewhat more succinctly said: 'A difference to be a difference must make a difference.'

Nathwani (1979) has written an excellent but critical review of the various classifications discussed in the last few pages, in which he points out the difficulties in precise comparison since most of the systematists have different criteria for the tumour types though they may carry identical or apparently identical names. He concludes that what is required is a 'morphologic classification which clearly defines homogenous-type groups', but leaves somewhat obscure what constitutes such a group. Nathwani ends by proposing a compromise working classification in which the prime axis determines whether the tumour is diffuse, or follicular and/or diffuse, which is then subdivided into fifteen different catagories, though William of Ockham might be doubtful about some of the methodology.

It was hoped that it might be possible to conclude this somewhat prolix discussion by presenting a classification which was simple, meaningful for clinicians and pathologists and universally acceptable, but this is still an *ignis fatuus*.

The N.C.I. Working Formulation

The analysis of The National Cancer Institute's non-Hodgkin's Lymphoma study is still proceeding, and it has been agreed that nothing should be published until the draft report has been approved by the participants; so it is only possible to give a brief account of this major endeavour.

This study, as was mentioned earlier, involed a review of a little over a thousand lymph node biopsies of cases of 'non-Hodgkin's lymphoma' which had been under follow up for at least three years. The slides available were the ordinary routine preparations which were to be examined by twelve pathologist – six being the originators of one of the classifications under consideration, and the other six were histopathologists with a special interest in lymph node disorders. Proformas with precise categorization had been prepared for each of the classifications, i.e. Rappaport, Kiel, Lukes and Collins, Dorfman, National Lymphoma Investigation (NLI of Bennett, Farrer-Brown and Henry), WHO. The pathologist associated with a particular system was only required to collocate the biopsies on that system, whereas the six 'control' pathologists were expected to classify them by all six systems; furthermore, all the pathologists were to re-examine and categorize a random twenty per cent of the slides to assess internal reproducability. The analysis of this mass of histological reports, integrated with a twelve-page clinical summary for each patient, was undertaken by a team of biostatisticians under the general direction of Professors Saul Rosenberg, Hoppe and Brown, together with Dr. Costan Berard; this has resulted in each participant receiving, so far, six volumes of data weighing over seven kilograms.

Two meetings of the investigators have been held at Stanford, California; in June 1979 and January 1980. At these meetings there have been discussions on the principles of the enquiry, and details of the analysis both from the point of view of the relationship of clinical manifestation and prognosis to the histological categories of the various classifications, as well as their inter-relationship, the degree of reproducability and inter-pathologist agreement. In addition, the pathologists as a group concerned themselves with terminology, morphological criteria and the possiblility of producing a compromise conjoint classification. It soon became obvious that any compromise was out of the question, but consideration was given to a grouping in which the prime axis was prognosis, divided into conditions of low, intermediate and high grade malignancy which were then categorized on morphological criteria. It was felt that this approach had possibilities as it was likely to be of clinical value and did not preclude the use by pathologists of a more detailed classification employing a different analytical approach. At the second meeting, at which unfortunately only one of the European pathologists could attend, additional clinical data was available, and Professor Rosenberg submitted for consideration a draft classification on the lines of that discussed the previous June; consequent on this the pathologists recommended the introduction of a 'working formulation of non-Hodgkin's Lymphoma for clinical usage' (Table 18); those who were not present at the meeting have agreed to support this curiously titled schema, though it has been emphasized that it would probably only be used in conjunction with some of the existing classifications. It would be unreasonable to make a judgement on this 'formulation' until an agreed document is available which would provide definitions and guidance as to what is, or is not to be included in each of the ten categories. It should not be difficult to use this schema if restricted to the main headings which correspond closely with the categorization adopted in this book. Unhappily, attitudes either enthusiastic or sententious are being adopted, and it would be well to recall that, when Michael Faraday was asked what was the use of his experiments in magnetism (which resulted in the dynamo), he retorted 'What is the use of a new born babe?'

Clearly, a classification such as the 'Formulation' will not satisfy all needs, nor

261

Table 18

A Working Formulation of Non-Hodgkin's Lymphoma for Clinical Usage
(U.S. National Cancer Institute Non-Hodgkin's Lymphoma Study, 1980)

LOW GRADE	HIGH GRADE
A. *Malignant Lymphoma* *Small Lymphocytic* consistent with chronic lymphocytic leukaemia plasmacytoid	H. *Malignant Lymphoma* *Large cell, immunoblastic* plasmacytoid clear cell polymorphous epitheloid cell component
B. *Malignant Lymphoma, follicular* *Predominantly small cleaved cell* diffuse areas sclerosis	I. *Malignant Lymphoma* *Lymphoblastic* convoluted cell non-convoluted cell
C. *Malignant Lymphoma, follicular* *Mixed, small cleaved and large cell* diffuse areas sclerosis	J. *Malignant Lymphoma* *Small non-cleaved cell* Burkitt's follicular areas
INTERMEDIATE GRADE	
D. *Malignant Lymphoma, follicular* *Predominantly large cell* diffuse areas sclerosis	
E. *Malignant Lymphoma, diffuse* *Small cleaved cell* sclerosis	MISCELLANEOUS
F. *Malignant Lymphoma, diffuse* *Mixed, small and large cell* sclerosis epitheloid cell component	Composite Mycosis Fungoides Histiocytic
G. *Malignant Lymphoma, diffuse* *Large cell* cleaved cell non-cleaved cell sclerosis	Extramedullar Plasmacytoma Unclassifiable Other

should it be expected so to do. It is essential to define the purpose of any taxonomic endeavour, and this review has displayed how these objectives have changed over the years. Basically, a medical classification may categorize aetiological agents or pathogenesis, to facilitate diagnosis and therefore therapy and prognosis, or these latter facets may be the prime objective. However, there is always a danger that these pragmatic approaches will be supplanted by a classification displaying some philosophical system, which is satisfying to its originator and supporters, but which appears almost purposeless to critical onlookers. It was Isiah Berlin who spoke of the danger of 'going to sleep on some comfortable bed of unquestionable dogma.'

Details of technical methods in lymph node diagnosis

THE DIAGNOSIS OF LYMPHOMA and leukaemia is dependent upon histological and cytological criteria, in association with a knowledge of the clinical condition of the patient.

Many of the morphological features are subtle, and sometimes can only be appreciated in thin sections of the highest quality, perfectly stained. These desirable high standards may not always be possible for the diagnostic pathologist in a busy routine department, but proper tissue preparation, fixation, processing, embedding, sectioning and staining are possible and these form the foundations for the diagnosis of a lymph node biopsy.

To facilitate diagnosis the pathologist may use special histochemical and immunohistochemical methods. The application of these methods has already been discussed in the text but the technical details are described in more detail in this Appendix.

The Appendix is arranged as follows:

    A. Simple Stains and Histochemistry

    B. Immunological Surface Markers

    C. Immunohistochemistry

A. Simple Stains and Histochemistry

Tissue sampling

It was emphasized in chapter I that the site and method of biopsy is the prerogative of the surgeon. Ideally surgeon and pathologist should act in concert to select the largest most abnormal-appearing lymph node and ensure its removal, intact if possible. Small thin blocks of the node should be fixed as soon as samples have been taken for microbiology, frozen section, electron microscopy, imprints and immunological studies.

Fixation

Ten per cent buffered formalin solution is the usual fixative in most institutions; it provides good morphology and is relatively foolproof. Fixation for 12–48 hours is recommended; if blocks are small, as they should be, 24 hours is adequate. Formalin should be buffered (pH 7.0) with sodium phosphate or acetate; marble chips are not recommended, for buffering is slow and calcium carbonate may deposit in the the tissue.

Fixatives containing mercuric chloride (e.g. Zenker's) give better nuclear detail. The B–5 fixative variant has been in use for several years at the University of Southern California section of haematopathology with excellent results; sodium acetate maintains a near neutral pH, and the staining reactions are similar to tissues fixed in neutral buffered formalin.

B–5 Fixative

Solution A:	Mercuric chloride	6 gms
	Anhydrous sodium acetate	1.25 gms
	Hot distilled water	90 ml
	Store at 4°C	

Solution B: 10% Buffered formalin

Add 1 ml of solution B to 9 mls of solution A immediately prior to use; fix thin blocks for 2–4 hours (not longer), rinse and transfer to 70% ethyl alcohol for storage prior to dehydration and impregnation. Mercury crystals must be removed prior to staining with the aid of iodine followed by sodium thiosulphate solution. **Buffered formal-acetone** is the preferred fixative for cytochemical methods, and is prepared as follows:–
Dissolve 20 mg $Na_2 HPO_4$ and 100 mg $KH_2 PO_4$ in a mixture of 45 ml acetone, 30 ml water and 25 ml formalin (40 formaldehyde). The final pH should be about 6.6 Store at 4° – 10°C.

Bone marrow examination

Traditionally bone marrow diagnosis has been based upon the cytology of cell smears prepared from needle aspirates of the marrow cavity. Assessment of marrow cellularity and the proportions of the different cell types can only be an approximation.

In 1972 Lukes and Tindle described a method of preparing thin sections of marrow aspirates:– particles of marrow removed at orthodox sternal aspiration are flushed into EDTA (Ethylene diamine tetraacetic acid) solution and thence into B-5 fixative. Within 24 hours the sediment is filtered through a fine (50μm) wire mesh,* the red cells passing through, and the particles remaining. The particles are collected together with a knife, embedded in 20% agar at 46°C, hardened in 5% formalin, and processed through alcohol and xylol and embedded in paraffin. Serial sections are cut and stained with haematoxylin and eosin, and the immunoperoxidase methods. The use of Giemsa or PAS stains may aid cellular identification while their spatial arrangement in the marrow can be readily appreciated.

Fixation for Electron microscopy

Dice tissue into 1–2mm blocks with a new razor blade. Fix at 4°C in 4% glutaraldehyde or in Graham and Karnovsky fixative: (4% formaldehyde, 5% glutaraldehyde in 0.1 molar cacodylate buffer at pH 7.2).

---

* Catalogue No. 6207 Mesh 120. United Surgical Co. How Medica. Largo, Florida 33540

Processing: Dehydration, Clearing, Impregnation, Embedding

Automatic processing machines may be employed; the manufacturer's recommendations should be followed. Particular attention should be given to maintaining 'fresh' reagents in the various baths; avoiding contamination of absolute alcohol with water and of xylol with alcohol. Timing of exposure to each bath is important; delayed weekend or holiday runs, prolonging some stages, are to be avoided. Temperature of the paraffin baths should be held at 60°C or less; prolonged heating above 60°C will induce poor morphology, and will denature antigens rendering immunohistological techniques useless. All these procedures are well discussed by Bowling (1967, 1976).

Sectioning

Thin sections (4μm or one lymphocyte thick) are desirable. Cooling of the block (Freon or Arctic sprays) facilitates the cutting of thin sections. However, as the block warms it will expand and microtome settings at 4μm may yield 6–8μm sections.

Staining procedures

Haematoxylin and eosin staining serves as the basic method in this book and is used for surgical pathological diagnosis in most institutions. In general, any variant of the ordinary method, e.g. Lie et al (1971), will give adequate lymph node staining, with the proviso that staining with both haematoxylin and eosin components should not be too intense, otherwise fine nuclear and cytoplasmic details may be obscured; azo-eosin has advantages as a counterstain.

Details of certain stains that we have used with advantage are described in the next few pages, but in addition it is useful to refer to some standard methods that can illuminate particular problems of lymph node histology.

For reticulin preparations, the method of Gordon and Sweets (1936) is adequate in most instances, but where the results are unsatisfactory finer preparations may be achieved by Robb-Smith's (1937) modification of Foot and Menard's method.

Goldner's modification (1938) of Masson's Trichrome stain is probably the most effective of the trichrome methods for lymph node histology and though intended to be used after Bouin or Susa fixation, works well after formalin. Kramer and Windrum's (1955) metachromatic method is reliable for the display of basophils and mast cells and the procedure of Fite et al (1947) is excellent for demonstrating lepra bacilli. Metalophil cells can easily be stained specifically in frozen sections using the Del Rio-Hortega (1921) techniques, but there are no really reliable methods for paraffin sections, though with persuasion, good results can be obtained with Marshall's (1948) technique or that of Black and Spear (1958).

Giemsa Stain*

Reagents: 10ml stock Giemsa solution†
40 ml distilled water

Method: 1. Stain deparaffinised sections for 1 hour in diluted Giemsa solution.
2. Differentiate in (a) 1% glacial acetic acid; 3 quick dips; (b) 95% alcohol until blue colour no longer runs off the slide.
3. Check differentiation under microscope and stop differentiation in absolute alcohol.
4. Take from absolute alcohol, through several changes of xylol to mounting medium.

*Modified from the method of Lennert (1961)
†Giemsa stock solutions are available from many suppliers; results may differ according to source. Lennert recommends Merck of Darmstadt.

Riu's Stain for Smears and Imprints

Reagents: Solution A: Dissolve 0.18g eosin yellow and 0.07g methylene blue in 100ml methanol, filter and store in a dark bottle (stable at room temperature for six months).

Solution B: Dissolve 0.7g methylene blue, 0.6g azure 1, 6.25g KH_2PO_4 and 2.6g $Na_2HPO_4 \cdot 12\ H_2O$ in 500ml distilled water, mix and stand at room temperature for 24 hours. Adjust the pH to 6.4 with sodium hydroxide or hydrochloric acid. Filter (Stable at room temperature for six months).

Method: 1. Cover air-dried smears with solution A for 30 seconds.
2. Add a mixture of two volumes of solution B to one volume of solution A, mix well by agitation and stain smears for 90 seconds to 2 minutes.
3. Rinse in distilled water, dry and mount.

Results: Resembles other Giemsa-type stains, except a slight blue tint, and red cells are stained yellow-red. Excessive amounts of heparin may slightly interfere with staining.

Sudan Black B Stain for Smears or Frozen Section

Reagents: Alcoholic phenol phosphate buffer: Dissolve 32g crystal phenol in 60ml of absolute ethanol, add 0.6g $Na_2 \cdot HPO_4\ 12\ H_2O$ and make up to 200ml with distilled water.

Stock Sudan Black B solution: Dissolve 0.3g Sudan Black B in 100ml of ethanol. Make up to 200ml with alcoholic phenol phosphate buffer. Mix well.

Sudan Black B stain: Add 60ml stock Sudan Black B solution to 40ml of alcoholic phenol phosphate buffer solution. Mix well and filter before use.

Method: 1. Cut unfixed material on cryostat or use formalin fixed sections. Fix smears in cold formal-acetone solution for 30 seconds. Wash with tap water and dry.
2. Stain smears in Sudan Black B stain for 30 minutes to 1 hour at room temperature.
3. Wash with 70% ethanol for 2 minutes, followed by tap water for 2 minutes. Dry in air.
4. Counterstain with buffered 1% neutral red for 10 minutes. (For frozen section, use Harris' hematoxylin.) Rinse with water, dry, mount in glycerine jelly.

Results: Positive staining appears as distinct dark brown granules in cytoplasm of the mature and immature granulocytes and many 'myeloblasts'.

Peroxidase Stain for Monocytes and Granulocytes in Smears or Frozen sections

Reagents: Solution A: 0.3gm benzidine base in 99ml ethanol. Add 1 ml of saturated solution of sodium nitroprusside. Mix well.

Solution B: Add 0.3ml of 3% hydrogen peroxide to 25ml of distilled water. Use this solution immediately after preparation.

Method: 1. Cut frozen sections of formalin fixed material; smears should be fixed in formal – alcohol (40% Formalin 10ml, absolute alcohol 80ml, distilled water 10ml)
2. Cover smears with solution A for 2 minutes.
3. Add solution B (half volume of A) to smear, mix, and stain for 3–5 minutes.
4. Rinse in distilled water.
5. Counterstain with a Giesma stain or with 1% buffered neutral red at pH 5.0.
6. Wash with water, dry and mount.

Result: Structures with enzyme activity stain a dark brown.

* Benzidine and many of its derivatives are recognized as carcinogens. Several alternative substitute systems are available (cf. p. 281).

Cytochemical Methods

The majority of cytochemical methods useful in distinguishing different types of lymphoid cells can only be used on smears or frozen sections (Li et al, 1972). The accompanying table (Cramer, 1979) sets out the distinctions that can be made, while the technical details follow.

Table 19

Cytochemical procedures for the distinction of T-cells, B-cells and Monocytes

	NSE	ACP	MGP	Gluc	PAS	CAE
T-Cell	$+^1$	$++^2$	$- \to ++^3$	$++$	$- \to ++^4$	$-$
B-Cell	$-$	$-^5$	$- \to ++++^3$	$-$	$- \to ++^6$	$-$
Monocyte	$+++^7$	$+++^8$	$- \to +$	$-$	$- \to ++^9$	$\pm^{10}$

NSE = nonspecific esterase; ACP = acid phosphatase; MGP = methyl green-pyronine; Gluc = β-glucuronidase; PAS = Periodic Acid Schiff; CAE = chloroacetate esterase.

[1] Focal positivity, possibly confined to T-cells.
[2] Focal possibly confined to T-cells, prominent in T-cell ALL and convoluted lymphoblastic T-lymphoma.
[3] Generally positive in dividing cells (e.g. immunoblasts), strongly positive in protein-secreting cells (e.g., B-immunoblasts).
[4] Among T-cells – Sézary cells characteristically show beaded positivity.
[5] B-lymphocyte usually negative, but plasma cells positive.
[6] Among B-cells – those secreting carbohydrate containing IgA or IgM characteristically positive.
[7] Diffuse positivity, fluoride resistant in histiocytes, labile in monocytes.
[8] Diffuse staining, generally tartrate labile, partly resistant in histiocytes, resistant in 'hairy cells.'
[9] Debris often positive, glycogen positive in any of these cell types.
[10] Of particular value in distinguishing mast cells and granulocytes, for these are strongly positive. Sudan black B is also a valuable sensitive indicator of early granulocyte maturation.

Nonspecific Esterase Stain for Smears and Frozen Sections. (Mueller et al, 1975; Higgy et al, 1977)

Reagents: Pararosaniline solution: Dissolve lg of pararosaniline in 25ml of warm 2N hydrochloric acid solution. This solution should be filtered when cool and kept at room temperature. 'Hexazotize' by mixing equal volumes of this solution and a 4% sodium nitrite solution for one minute before use.

Alpha-naphthyl butyrate solution: Dissolve 100mg of α-naphthyl butyrate in 5ml ethylene glycol monomethyl ether. Keep at 4°–10°C before use.

Method: 1. Fix sections or smears with cold buffered formal acetone for 30 seconds. Wash with water and dry in air.

267

2. Incubate smears or sections in staining reagents in the following proportions at room temperature for 45 minutes

	cover slips	slides
Phosphate buffer (M/15, pH 6.3)	9.5ml	50.0ml
Fresh 'hexazonium pararosaniline'	0.05ml	0.2ml
α-naphthyl butyrate solution	0.5ml	2.0ml

This solution should be filtered before use.

3. Rinse in water, counterstain with 1% methyl green solution for 2 minutes (or Mayer's hematoxylin).

4. Rinse in water, dry, mount in synthetic mounting medium.

Result: Enzyme activity is dark yellow-brown and is mainly located in the cytoplasm of monocytes and histiocytes. Focal paranuclear staining with NSE has been reported in T-lymphocytes, initially in mice and subsequently in man. The reaction is not present in activated T-cells. Its specificity for T cells is not established.

Nonspecific Esterase with Fluoride Treatment

Reagents: As for non specific esterase.

Methods: As for nonspecific esterase, except for #2.

2. Incubate smears or sections in the following incubating medium at room temperature for 45 minutes:

	cover slips	slides
90mg NaF/60ml phosphate buffer	10.0ml	50.00ml
Fresh 'hexazonium pararosaniline'	0.05ml	0.2ml
α-naphthyl butyrate solution	0.5ml	2.0ml

This solution should be filtered before use.

Results: Monocytes are nonspecific esterase positive, but fluoride sensitive.

Macrophages and sinusoidal lining cells are fluoride resistant.

Acid Phosphatase and Tartrate-resistant Acid Phosphatase for Smears (Li et al, 1970; Catovsky et al, 1978)

Reagents: Fixative (methanol-acetone mixture): Add 10ml methanol to 90ml of 60% acetone in 0.03M citrate buffer. Adjust pH of this solution to pH 5.4 with 1N NaOH or HCl. Keep at 4°–10°C before use. (Stable for at least one month).

Pararosaniline solution: Dissolve 1g of pararosaniline in 25ml of warm 2N hydrochloric acid. This solution should be filtered when cool and kept at room temperature. 'Hexazotize' by mixing equal volumes of this solution and a 4% sodium nitrite solution for one minute before use.

Substrate solution: Dissolve 10mg naphthol-AS-BI phosphoric acid in 0.5ml N-N-dimethyl formamide, and dilute to 100ml with 0.1M acetate buffer (pH 5.0–5.2) to 100ml. Keep at 4°–10°C before use. (Stable for two months.)

Incubating medium: To 40ml of substrate solution add 0.25ml of 'hexazonium pararosaniline'; filter. Tartrate containing medium is prepared by adding 300mg of L-(+)-tartaric acid and 0.25ml of 'hexazonium pararosaniline' to 40ml of substrate solution. Adjust pH of this solution to pH 5.0–5.2 with concentrated NaOH. Filter and use immediately.

Method: 1. Fix smears with buffered cold methanol acetone mixture for 30 seconds. Wash briefly with distilled water. Air dry.

2. Incubate smears in incubating medium with or without tartaric acid at 37°C for 45 minutes.

3. Wash with water; counterstain with Mayer's hematoxylin.

4. Wash with water, dry and mount, in glycerine jelly.

Results: Acid phosphatase activity appears as discrete purplish to dark red granules in the cytoplasm of the blood cells. Presence of tartrate in the incubating medium inhibits enzyme activity in all types of blood cells. The neoplastic cells of leukaemic reticuloendotheliosis (hairy-cell leukaemia) have tartrate resistant acid phosphates activity.

Comment: Focal paranuclear acid phosphatase staining has also been described as a characteristic of T-lymphocytes. The method is difficult to standardise. For optimal results smears should be dried and left to stand at least 24 hours prior to fixation and staining. Incubation with staining medium for longer than the recommended time may also produce focal staining of B-cells.

Methyl Green-Pyronine Stain (modified from D'Ablaing et al, 1970)

Reagents:

Methyl green (G.A.–Chroma Gessellschaft)	1.0g
Pyronin (G.A.–Chroma Gesellschaft)	0.8g
Distilled water	320.0ml
Glycerine	80.0ml

Procedure for Preparing Stain:
1. Mix thoroughly the glycerine and distilled water.
2. Add methyl green and shake until the dye dissolves.
3. Add pyronin and shake until the dye dissolves.
4. Add 1ml liquid phenol and shake vigorously.
5. Add 5 drops of 1% acetic acid, shake thoroughly, adjust the pH to 4.2 with 0.2M Tris buffer.
6. Allow to stand for approximately 2 hours.
7. Staining solution is ready to use, and keeps indefinitely at room temperature.

Note: The stain should be decidedly blue in a thin film; if it is purplish red it is unsuitable.

Procedure for Staining:
1. Fix slides for 10 minutes in Zenker's solution. Wash briefly in running tap water.
2. Blot dry and place in the Methyl Green-Pyronin stain.
3. Stain overnight.
4. Take out and blot GENTLY on filter paper.
5. Slide in and out of butyl alcohol.
6. Slide in and out of xylol.
7. Mount in synthetic mounting media or Fisher's Permount (pinene polymer).

β-Glucuronidase for Blood and Bone Marrow Smears, Imprints, and Frozen Sections
(Yam et al, 1968)

Reagents: Naphthol-AS-BI-B-D-glucuronide solution: 7mg substrate in 0.5ml N,N-dimethyl form-amide; dilute to 100ml with 0.1 N acetate, at pH 5.2. Keep 4°–10°C before use.

Pararosaniline Solution: Dissolve 1g of pararosaniline in 25ml of warm 2 N hydrochloric acid. This solution should be filtered when cool and kept at room temperature. 'Hexazotize' by mixing equal volumes of this solution and a 4% sodium nitrite solution for one minute before use.

Method   1. Fix fresh smears or sections with buffered formal-acetone solutions for 30 minutes at 10°C. Wash with distilled water and air dry.
2. Incubate smears or sections in the following mixture for 90 minutes in a water bath at 37°C:

Naphthol-AS-BI-BD-glucuronide solution	10ml
'Hexazonium pararosaniline'	0.05ml

3. Wash in water. Counterstain with Meyer's hematoxylin 5–15 minutes – or methyl green 1–5 minutes. Dry mount in synthetic mounting media

Periodic Acid Schiff Stain

Reagents: Periodic acid solution: Dissolve 1g periodic acid in 100ml of distilled water and store in dark and at room temperature. This solution is stable for several days.

Schiff's solution: Dissolve 1g of basic fuchsin in 200ml of boiling distilled water. Shake and cool to 50°C. Filter and add to the filtrate 20ml of 1N hydrochloric acid. Cool further to 20°–30°C and add 1g of anhydrous sodium bisulphite with gentle mixing. Keep this solution in the dark for 2-3 days. Add 2g activated charcoal and shake for several minutes. Filter, keep the filtrate in the dark at 4°–10°C. This solution keeps well for several months. *If the filtrate is not crystal clear and colourless, repeat the charcoal, shake and filter.*

Diastase solution: Dissolve 500mg malt diastase in 50ml saline. Use immediately after preparation.

Method: 1. Fix smears or sections with absolute methanol for 10 minutes at room temperature, decant methanol, dry smears in air. Fixed paraffin sections should be dewaxed and taken down to water.
2. Add periodic acid solution to smears or sections for 10 minutes at room temperature. Rinse in distilled water and dry, if diastase treatment is desirable, place smears in diastase solution at 37°C for one hour. Rinse in distilled water and dry.

Results:

3. Stain with Schiff's solution at room temperature in the dark for 30 minutes.
4. Wash with running water for 10 minutes, dry, and counterstain with haematoxylin.
5. Wash, dry, mount in synthetic mounting medium and examine.

Results: Positive PAS stain is indicated by a diffuse pinkish colour in the cytoplasm of the granulo-cytes and granular and pinkish in the megakaryocytes, lymphocytes and erythroblasts (on smear). 'Normal' erythroid precursors in section do not stain with PAS.

Note that the PAS tartrazine modification may be preferred in some instances, the yellow background of this stain serving to enhance the contrast of the red PAS-positive material.

Chloroacetate Esterase Stain for Neutrophilic Granulocytes in Smears Frozen Sections or Fixed-Sections (Yam et al, (1971)

Reagents: Fresh 4% sodium nitrite solution.

New fuchsin solution: Dissolve 1g of new fuchsin in 25ml of warm 2N hydrochloric acid. This solution should be filtered when cool and kept at room temperature. 'Hexazotize' by mixing equal volumes of this solution and a 4% sodium nitrite solution for one minute before use.

Naphthol-AS-D-chloroacetate solution: Dissolve 10mg naphthol-AS-D-chloroacetate in 5.0ml N-N-dimethyl formamide. Keep at 4°–10°C before use.

Method: 1. Fix smears or sections with cold buffered formal-acetone for 30 seconds. Wash with distilled water and dry. Take paraffin sections to water.
2. Incubate fixed smears or sections at room temperature for 10 minutes in staining reagents in the following proportions (*without filtration*).

Phosphate buffer (M/15, pH 7.4)	9.5ml
'Hexazonium new fuchsin'	0.05ml
Naphthol-AS-D-chloroacetate solution	0.5ml

3. Wash in running water, counterstain with Mayer's hematoxylin, blue in alkaline tap water or dilute ammonia water.
4. Rinse in tap water, dry, clear in xylol if necessary, mount in synthetic mounting medium.

Results: Enzyme activity is seen as bright red-orange granules in the cytoplasm of mast cells and neutrophilic granulocytes. Eosinophils are negative.

Comment: All solutions except the fresh sodium nitrite solutions are stable for at least one month after preparation. The sodium nitrite solution may be kept at 4°–10°C for one week without affecting the cytochemical stain for chloroacetate esterase.

This method gives satisfactory results on fixed embedded tissues or frozen sections, but if a mercuric chloride-based fixative has been used, do not attempt removal of mercury pigment with iodine; this will inactivate the enzyme.

B. Immunological Surface Marker Methods

Immunological methods for B- and T-cell identification represent an extension of experimental immunology into the field of clinical pathology and diagnosis. These methods have undoubtedly contributed to current understanding of the nature of the lymphocyte and its neoplasms. Their role in diagnosis, if any, is not yet established. For this reason these methods will only be discussed here in general terms.

Surface Marker Studies – General Observations

Reports on the use of surface marker methods in the study of lymphocytic leukaemias and lymphomas are now very numerous. In general the findings are in broad agreement with those presented in the first part of the book. There are some discrepancies; many relate to technique; others relate to differences in classification. These have been discussed fully in a series of reviews (Taylor, 1977, 1978, 1979). See Table I, p. 17.

From all these studies chronic lymphocytic leukaemia has emerged as principally a B-cell disease, and acute lymphocytic leukaemia as a disease of nonmarking (null) cells. However some cases of acute leukaemia had T-cell markers; these were usually associated with a high white count, tissue masses and convoluted cell morphology. Rarely cases of acute leukaemia displayed B-cell markers (Burkitt-like leukaemia). Monoclonal circulating small lymphocytes were identified in some cases of B-cell lymphoma. Follicle centre cell lymphomas, with follicular or diffuse patterns (including Burkitt's lymphoma) reacted as B-cell tumours. Immunoblastic sarcoma (here regarded as approximately equivalent to reticulum cell sarcoma and 'histiocytic' malignant lymphoma) sometimes showed B-cell markers, sometimes T-cell markers, rarely a mixture of T- and B-cell markers, and in a proportion of cases no markers were detectable. 'Reticulum cell sarcoma' and 'histiocytic malignant lymphoma' gave similar results, though in a small proportion of these tumors, histiocytic markers were seen.

Practical Problems and Difficulties in Interpretation

Lymphocyte Separation Procedures. Since many of the methods are performed on separated living lymphocytes in suspension, it is important to use a separation procedure which will give the least bias in terms of selecting either T- or B-lymphocytes. The most commonly used method, the Ficoll-Hypaque density gradient technique, allows reasonable lymphocyte separation, with little T- or B-cell bias from peripheral blood, at least when the yield is greater than 70%. This method has generally been found to work well. Enrichment of peripheral blood monocytes by this method has proved a problem in some studies. It is essential to prepare smears or cytocentrifuge slides of the separated lymphocytes to allow differential counts to be made, in order to define in conventional morphological terms the cell population present.

The E-Rosette Phenomenon: Spontaneous Non-Immune Rosettes with Sheep Red Cells. The formation of spontaneous non-immune rosettes with sheep red cells (E-rosettes) has become an established technique for the identification of normal human T-lymphocytes. Applied to neoplastic lymphocytes, a positive E-rosette test has been taken as evidence of T-cell origin for certain of the leukaemias and lymphomas. However, the great variation of reported scores of 'normal' peripheral blood T-cells from different laboratories (ranging from 10%–70%) suggests that cautious interpretation is required.

Practical Considerations and Factors Influencing the E-Rosette Test. It is now obvious that diverse factors may influence the values obtained in the performance of the E-rosette test, not the least of which is the experience of the investigator or technician involved. Variations in the practical details of the performance of the test are also of great importance: for example, the ratio of lymphoid cells to sheep red cells, the ultimate overall concentration of cells, the temperature, the length of time allowed for the rosettes to form, and the mode of preparation for visual counting, whether in suspension by cytocentrifugation (variable force of centrifugation), or by smearing and rapid air drying. E-rosettes are notoriously fragile and unstable, and rough handling may reduce the score significantly.

Regarding the time factor, results suggest that the E-rosette score begins to plateau out when two or more hours are allowed for formation of rosettes at 4°C. That the incubation time is of crucial importance in assessing the E-rosette score is supported by a suggestion that short incubation methods detect only a proportion of T-cells (strong reactors), while more prolonged (overnight) incubation gives an assessment of total T-cell number. Rosette formation may also be influenced by other experimental manipulations. The performance of the test in group AB serum, or in the presence of Ficoll, or after incubation overnight in foetal calf serum, have all been claimed to enhance rosette formation to some degree (in the University of Southern California series the presence of Ficoll produced an average – and consistent – elevation of the score by 3–5 per cent).

The arbitrary nature of the lymphocyte/red cell reaction, between lymphocytes and red cells of different species, is further illustrated by the observation that a proportion of human lymphocytes form spontaneous non-immune rosettes with mouse red blood cells. This observation itself is not remarkable, except that the lymphoctyes forming rosettes with mouse red cells appear to be human B-lymphocytes, not T-lymphocytes.

The percentage E-rosette score of peripheral blood lymphocytes is markedly reduced in a number of disease states, particularly malignancy (lymphoid or other), either in response to therapy, or because of extensive spread of tumour, or for unknown reasons. Therapy with cytotoxic drugs results in reduced E-rosette scores, though prednisone alone appears to have little effect. It may be important, therefore, to ensure that control groups are not receiving any form of treatment nor suffering from any chronic disease. Acute infections cause transient alterations. There is a reduction in T-cell numbers with age, a finding most clearly revealed by determining the absolute lymphocyte counts, for the proportion of T-cells falls less obviously. The importance of calculating the absolute numbers of T- and B-cells, rather than considering only percentage scores as is the usual practice, cannot be overemphasized.

Conclusion

The reported variations in technique and the biological variation inherent in lymphocyte populations from different patients of various ages with diverse diseases, makes it essential to base interpretation upon an age-matched control population. It is also useful to control the test with pooled frozen lymphocytes (stored in aliquots in liquid nitrogen) once or twice weekly.

The B-Cell C₃ Receptor

The use of a red cell sensitised with antibody (IgM) and complement (C_3) as an additional determinant of B cell function has been widely reported. This is termed the EAC rosette method, and has been adapted for use on frozen tissue sections, as well as with cell suspensions. Alternatively, fluorescent labelled anti-C_3 antisera may be used to detect the C_3 receptor on cell surfaces. The Zymosan-C method, utilizing spontaneous binding of complement components to Zymosan beads, offers advantages in sensitivity, ease of performance and consistency.

The C_3 receptor occurs independently of the Fc receptor, and not all B-lymphocytes carry the C_3 receptor. It has been suggested that C_3 receptor-bearing cells are particularly found in follicle centre areas of lymph nodes. The previously accepted view, that all C_3 receptor-positive cells are B-lymphocytes, has been questioned by the observations that at least some neoplastic T-cells, and probably some normal T-cells, also form EAC rosettes.

An additional confusing factor is the possibility that the E component of the EAC reagent may react with E-rosette-forming cells (if sheep red cells are used).

The Fc Receptor and Surface Immunoglobulin as a B-Cell Marker

Three principal methods are available for the detection of Fc receptors of lymphocytes: adsorption of antigen/antibody complexes, adsorption of aggregated immunoglobulin (fluorescein or I^{125} labelled), adsorption of sheep (or other species) erythrocytes sensitised with specific IgG antibody (EA rosettes). The immunoglobulin class used in all of these methods must be IgG, as the lymphocyte Fc receptor appears specific for the Fc component of complexed or bound IgG. Free IgG will not attach to the Fc receptor; it must be aggregated or complexed with antigen. Theoretically, therefore, in assays of lymphocyte surface immunoglobulin, test antisera which do not contain any Ag/Ab complexes, or any immunoglobulin aggregates, should not bind to the Fc receptor. However, in practice most antisera do contain variable or trace amounts of complexed and/or aggregated antibody, and this may be an important source of error in assessing SIg by immunofluorescence methods. The problem of unwanted Fc binding can be avoided by the use of Fab fragments of antibody, which lack the Fc component but retain the variable portions of the light and heavy chain that determines antibody specificity.

The possibility of receptors for IgA and IgM is not excluded. IgM receptors certainly occur in some T-cells (T μ-cells) while other T-cells express a receptor for IgG (T γ-cells), thus diminishing the value of this test as a discrimination between B- and T-cells. Monocytes of course possess an avid Fc receptor, and significant Fc receptor activity has been reported in a variety of other normal and neoplastic cells (granulocytes, intestinal epithelium, carcinoma cells, etc.).

The aggregated immunoglobulin procedure appears to be the optimum procedure for B-cells, and the EA rosette procedure is best for histiocytes.

Surface immunoglobulin of B-lymphocytes may be detected by direct or indirect immunofluorescence methods using antisera against human immunoglobulin components (anti-κ, anti-λ, anti-γ, anti-α, anti-μ and anti-δ). Triple washed viable cells are examined in suspension, and the percentages determined by counting 200 or more cells. The use of a panel of antisera permits an assessment of clonality (monoclonal populations exclusively one light chain and one heavy chain though partial exceptions to this generalization do occur). Incubation of cells at 37°C may be necessary to induce shedding of Fc receptor-bound serum immunoglobulin. Fab reagents may be used to obviate nonspecific binding of antisera. The value and limitations of these methods are well discussed in the papers of Aiuti et al (1974), Lukes et al (1978) and Taylor (1979).

C. Immunohistochemistry

The identification of lymphoid neoplasms as of B-cell origin rests largely upon the demonstration of surface immunoglobulin in suspensions of lymphoma cells, as described in the preceding section. These methods, however, do not take account of the morphology of the immunoglobulin-producing cells. The established histological landmarks, upon which diagnosis is usually based, are thereby ignored.

Staining of Immunoglobulin in Tissue Sections

Generally, the immunofluorescence technique has been used for the demonstration of cytoplasmic immunoglobulin in tissue sections, but the method suffers several serious disadvantages for the morphological pathologist:

1. The histological and cytological detail is poor and cells are not immediately recognizable by orthodox morphological criteria

2. There is a requirement for specialized microscopy (ultra-violet light source)

3. The method demands fresh or specially processed tissue

4. Preparations are impermanent and rapidly fade upon examination

5. Tissue and cellular auto-fluorescence may obscure specific staining in tissue sections

The application of immunoperoxidase techniques to paraffin sections of formalin or Zenker-type fixed tissues avoids these disadvantages.

The morphological results of immunoperoxidase methods applied to formalin or Zenker-type fixed paraffin-embedded tissues are excellent, equivalent to any good H & E section, and the cytological features of the immunoglobulin-containing cells are directly comparable to the morphological criteria used in the identification of normal cells and in the diagnosis of lymphoma. In addition, preparations are permanent, and the method can be applied retrospectively to paraffin embedded tissues stored for ten or more years. This facilitates the study of the less common lymphomas, and material from different centres.

The specificity and sensitivity of the immunoperoxidase method applied to formalin-fixed, paraffin-embedded tissue has been proven by a study of tissues from more than 100 cases of myeloma in which the immunoperoxidase typing of the cytoplasmic immunoglobulin showed close correspondence with the serum paraprotein type determined independently.

Methods

Several variations of the immunoperoxidase method have been described, each using the enzymatic activity of horseradish peroxidase with a chromogenic substrate as a visual marker. Currently available methods have been reviewed elsewhere (Taylor, 1978). Those methods most commonly employed are illustrated in the accompanying diagram (Diagram 6).

Diagram 6

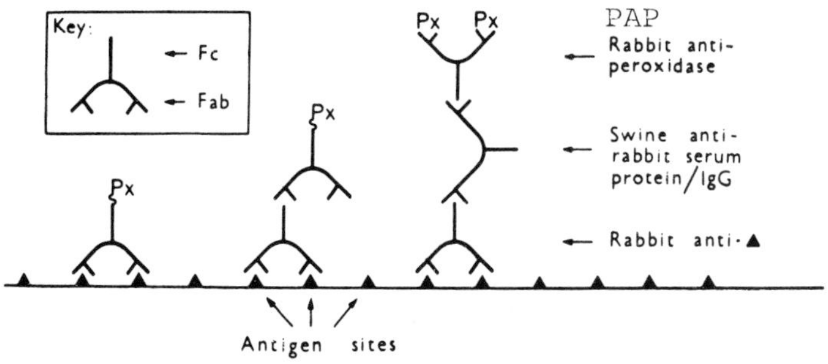

Immunoperoxidase techniques: direct conjugate procedure (left), indirect conjugate or sandwich procedure (centre), PAP (peroxidase-anti-peroxidase) method (right). The details of demonstrating ▲ antigen in tissue sections are set out in the text.

Peroxidase conjugated antibody methods, by direct or indirect techniques, are strictly analogous to comparable immunofluorescence methods. In the direct method (left of Diagram 6) the antibody/peroxidase conjugate has specificity directed against the antigen under study. In the indirect method (centre of Diagram 6) a primary antiserum having specificity against the antigen is applied initially, followed by a peroxidase/antibody conjugate from a second species, directed against the immunoglobulin components of the primary antiserum. This indirect, or sandwich method has certain advantages in that it is more sensitive than the direct method, is more versatile by substitution of primary antisera against a wide variety of antigens, and can be subjected to additional control of specificity by replacing the primary antiserum by other antisera of the same origin but irrelevant specificity.

The PAP (peroxidase anti-peroxidase) method (right of Diagram 6) was designed particularly to circumvent some of the disadvantages inherent in conjugation procedures, in which there may be denaturation of antibody, inactivation of enzyme, aggregation of unlabelled or partly labelled antibody, residual free enzyme, and residual free unlabelled antibody. Clearly free antibody, or antibody conjugated to inactivated enzyme, will bind competitively with active conjugate so reducing sensitivity, while denatured antibody, free enzyme, and aggregates will contribute to nonspecific staining. The PAP method has an additional advantage of enhanced sensitivity. The technique depends upon the addition of an excess of swine anti-rabbit immunoglobulin to bind the rabbit immunoglobulin of the PAP immune complex (consisting of rabbit antibody to horseradish peroxidase and horseradish peroxidase antigen) to the primary rabbit anti-Δ antibody.

The basic immunoperoxidase techniques were modified for application to formalin or Zenker-type fixed paraffin-embedded tissues in contrast to the usual mode of application to frozen sections of unfixed tissue. Two advantages accrued from this change: retrospective studies became feasible, and excellent morphological detail was obtainable.

Modes of Application of Immunoperoxidase Procedures

Immunoperoxidase procedures have been used for the detection and demonstration of cell surface antigens, intracellular antigens, and antigens distributed in the extracellular space of tissues. The detection of antigen in different localizations (e.g. cell membrane vs. cell cytoplasm) is dependent upon the mode of exposure of the cell population to the immunoperoxidase system. For example, living cells exclude immunoglobulin from the cytoplasm and any antiserum applied to viable cells in suspension will detect surface antigens only. Following fixation, varying degrees of penetration into cells (or into tissue sections) occurs, determined by the nature of fixation, the extent of disruption of the cell membrane, and the molecular size of the largest component of the immunoperoxidase detection system.

Cell Smears or Imprints

Fixed cell smears (using buffered formal acetone) have been used for demonstration of cytoplasmic antigen by both immunofluorescence and immunoperoxidase methods. There is good evidence that in such a system surface antigens (e.g. surface immunoglobulin) are also detectable and may be confused with cytoplasmic antigens.

Tissue sections

Tissue sections have been used for the demonstration of intracellular antigens and antigens distributed in the extracellular spaces or upon basement membranes. Cell surface antigens (such as surface immunoglobulin) present in small amounts are not well visualised in sections, even when unfixed cryostat sections are used.

This is due to the high level of specific 'background' staining of immunoglobulin in the extracellular fluids.

The morphological detail obtained by immunoperoxidase methods applied to cryostat sections is little better than with immunofluorescence. It is the compatibility of immunoperoxidase methods with formalin fixation and paraffin embedding, and with a variety of histochemical counterstains, that provides the greatest advantage of the immunoperoxidase procedure. Thus in formalin paraffin sections stained for cytoplasmic antigens (such as immunoglobulin or lysozyme) the detailed cytological features of antigen-positive and antigen-negative cells can be appreciated (see chapter I), and the different cell types can be recognized by the usual morphological criteria. This is of special value in the study of distribution of certain antigens (e.g. hormones, enzymes, and immunoglobulins) within the cells of normal tissues, within the neoplastic cells thought to be derived from them, and in certain other pathological states of excessive or diminished production of a hormone or other cell product.

Background Staining

The demonstration of antigens by immunoperoxidase procedures depends upon the development of contrast between the staining of the antigen and its surroundings.

1. Specific background staining may result from the presence of the antigen in varying concentrations throughout the material under examination. For example, in examining fixed bone marrow sections from multiple myeloma the neoplastic plasma cells stain intensely for immunoglobulin, as does the serum in which the marrow is bathed, producing diffuse heavy background staining of a specific type. Diffusion of antigen from intracellular sites prior to fixation, or following inadequate fixation also contributes to this type of staining. Similarly any degree of inflammatory infiltrate, tissue necrosis, or autolysis may produce diffusion of antigen. Prompt rapid fixation is therefore indicated.

2. Non-specific background staining may be of several varieties. Significant unwanted staining may occur because of the presence of antibodies of unwanted specificities within the antiserum used; this really is a form of unwanted specific staining and includes the naturally occurring animal antibodies reacting against human tissue components. This type of staining is best reduced by careful attention to the mode of preparation of the antiserum used. The presence of small amounts of nonspecific antibody may be countered by exploiting the differences in titre between the specific (wanted) antibody activity, and the antibodies of unwanted specificity, and diluting the antisera until only the wanted specificity is detectable. This provides part of the basis for chequer board (chess board) titrations to determine the optimum antibody concentrations for use in any system applied to tissue sections. In multiple layer methods each separate stage must be separately titrated against the other antibody stages, and an optimum

concentration selected for each. The result is somewhat subjective and is determined by selecting the concentrations which give the greatest useful contrast between specific positive staining and background of all types. This will not usually occur at the greatest intensity of positive staining, or at the greatest concentration of antibody due to steric inhibition effects at high concentrations (prozone).

In cell surface studies the optimum concentrations for antibodies is determined by a slightly different end point, selecting the dilution beyond which further two-fold dilution produces no additional fall in the percentage of positive cells for several dilution factors (plateau end point) (Preud'homme and Labaume, 1975).

3. Nonspecific staining occurring as a result of binding of a non-immunological type may be reduced by adopting the PAP method or enzyme bridge method, so avoiding the use of conjugated antisera which may contain denatured immunoglobulin, aggregated immunoglobulin, or free label. A tendency of PAP preparations to form aggregates upon storage can be controlled by high speed centrifugation prior to use.

Such staining can be further reduced by exploiting the fact that in a multilayer system the first protein added will show maximal nonspecific binding. Thus, if a 'neutral' immunoglobulin (i.e. one not reacting nor interfering with the specific antiserum) is added prior to the specific antiserum most of the sites of nonspecific binding will have been occupied by the initial immunoglobulin application. The rationale and success of this procedure has been demonstrated by Burns (1978). A similar approach employs antisera made up and diluted in a 'neutral' serum (Sternberger, 1974). This technique can markedly reduce background staining, but will not entirely abolish it owing to the reversibility of this type of bonding.

4. Binding of antisera through the Fc fragment, rather than through the specific antibody determinant, occurs in studies of lymphocyte cell surface antigens using viable cells in suspension, and may lead to erroneous interpretations. The binding of specific antisera to cell surface Fc receptors may be combated by the use of Fab fractions of immunoglobulin (F[ab']$_2$-divalent, or Fab-monovalent) derived by digestion, (Fc component removed – Nakane, 1975) in lieu of whole antibody as the specific antiserum. In multiple layer methods all of the antibodies used must be Fab fractions for any benefit to be obtained. Fc binding does not appear to be a problem in studies of fixed embedded tissues.

Control and Standardization

A system dependent upon the detection of antigen by specific antibody is only as good as the antibody or antibodies employed in the methodology. Preud'homme and Labaume (1975) have made the point that, 'we have (with one exception) never found truly monospecific commercial conjugates'. While it is true that many commercially available reagents give apparently specific reactions when assayed by precipitation diffusion techniques, it must be remembered that techniques for studies of surface immunoglobulin are considerably more sensitive than immunodiffusion, and may reveal the presence of unwanted specificities that may not be detectable by the former method. Similarly, immunoperoxidase procedures such as the PAP method, with its exquisite sensitivity, may detect trace specificities in tissue staining, requiring the use of antisera at higher dilutions.

The ultimate control for this nonspecific staining lies in utilizing highly purified antisera. Clearly, however, the degree of purification possible in different laboratory situations varies, and if the standards of Preud'homme and Labaume were to be demanded by all investigators, then much useful work would cease. Thus some compromise is necessary and there is no doubt that valid work can be carried out with commercially available reagents providing the need for careful control and interpretation is realised.

The most useful controls are known positives and known negatives. Controls are readily available for cytoplasmic immunoglobulin studies, in that myeloma cell populations are usually demonstrably monoclonal for κ and for λ, and for heavy chain classes. Every study should also include controls omitting the primary antiserum and substituting the primary antiserum by immunoglobulin from the same source and species, but directed against an irrelevant specificity; e.g. rabbit anti-human lysozyme or rabbit anti-human albumin antibodies provide good controls for rabbit anti-human immunoglobulin antisera, and rabbit antisera against the various human immunoglobulin components (anti-κ, anti-λ, anti-γ, anti-α, anti-μ, etc.) provide intrinsic controls one against the other.

Blocking controls, using antisera of like specificity but derived from a different species, are of value in some instances and result in diminution, but never complete abolition, of specific staining on subsequent addition of the primary labelled antibody. Of more direct value is a control system using antiserum preabsorbed against the specific antigen, following which marked reduction of specific staining should be observed. It is important to remember that the absorbing antigen may contain the same impurities as were present in the immunising antigen and may thus absorb out both wanted and unwanted specificities, giving an overall impression of monospecificity when in fact several specificities are present.

Technical Procedure

The sequence of steps in the procedure for the conjugate and the PAP methods are summarised on page 280.

Antisera and Conjugates

Only by careful personal supervision of the preparation, purification, and absorption of all the antisera can an investigator be sure of the quality of the reagents employed. In many circumstances this is a limiting step and appropriate antisera are purchased. Working dilutions are determined by chequer board titrations as already described. The dilutions given in the tables serve in our laboratories, but may differ with different reagents, different fixation procedures, etc.*

Substrates – Chromogens

The chromogen employed must be specific for peroxidase, producing a stable coloured product with a well-defined visible absorption spectrum clearly seen by light microscopy. It should be compatible with counter-staining procedures and should not be leached out by dehydration and mounting methods. Additionally, it should not inhibit the peroxidase enzyme nor denature it. It should be non-toxic and non-carcinogenic, widely available and inexpensive.

Immuno-peroxidase procedure for demonstrating cytoplasmic immunoglobulin in paraffin sections:

Indirect peroxidase conjugate method
1. Paraffin sections are dewaxed in xylol and brought to alcohol.
2. Block endogenous peroxidase with methanol containing 0.3% hydrogen peroxide 30 min.
3. Normal swine serum $^1/_{20}$ 10 min.
4. Rabbit antiserum to human immunoglobulin components* 30 min.
5. Peroxidase-conjugated swine anti-rabbit serum IgG $^1/_{20}$ 30 min.
6. Diaminobenzidine reaction, counterstain with haematoxylin, dehydrate, and mount in DPX (Kirkpatrick and Lendrum. Polysterene 20g, tricresyl phosphate 15ml, xylol 80ml) or Permount

The reactions are carried out in tris buffer (pH 7.6), with washes after stages 3, 4, and 5 in tris saline (dilution of tris buffer $^1/_{10}$ in normal saline).
For muramidase (lysozyme) substitute anti-muramidase antibody for anti-immungobulin in step 4.

Peroxidase-anti-peroxidase (PAP) immune complex method
1. Paraffin sections are dewaxed in xylol and brought to alcohol.
2. Block endogenous peroxidase with methanol containing 0.3% hydrogen peroxide 30 min.
3. Normal swine serum $^1/_{20}$ 10 min.
4. Rabbit antiserum to human immunoglobulin components[1] 30 min.
5. Swine anti-rabbit serum protein $^1/_{20}$ 30 min.
6. PAP $^1/_{100}$ 30 min.
7. Diaminobenzidine reaction, counterstain with haematoxylin, dehydrate, and mount in DPX

The reactions are carried out in tris buffer (pH 7.6), with washes after stages 3, 4, 5 and 6 in tris saline (dilution of tris buffer $^1/_{10}$ in normal saline).

---

[1] Dilutions according to chequer board titration; e.g. in conjugate procedure: anti-κ, anti-λ $^1/_{50}$, anti-γ, anti-α, anti-μ $^1/_{30}$; in PAP procedure: anti-κ, anti-λ $^1/_{2000}$, anti-γ $^1/_{400}$, anti-α, anti-μ $^1/_{300}$.

* Most of our antisera were obtained from Dakopatts A.S., Copenhagen (U. K. distributors—Mercia Diagnostics, Sandown Road, Watford, Herts; U.S.A. distributors—Dako Corporation, 22F North Milpas, Santa Barbara, California 93103). Sets of titrated immunoperoxidase staining reagents for a wide range of antigens, including immunoglobulins, hormones, CEA, and tissue specific antigens are becoming available from Dako and from Immulok, 1019 Mark Avenue, Carpinteria, California 93013, U.S.A.

Diaminobenzidine (DAB, 3, 4, 3^1, 4^1 tetra-amino-biphenyl hydrochloride), used with the method of Graham and Karnovsky (1966), (i.e. 6 mg of diaminobenzidine with 0.01% hydrogen peroxide in 10ml. of tris buffer), fulfills most of these criteria except that it is a potential carcinogen. It should therefore be used with full precautions. The reaction with DAB produces a crisp brown colour which does not fade and which contrasts well with haematoxylin or haematoxylin-eosin counterstains. Other substrates are available; the Graham alphanaphthol pyronine reaction (Lilley, 1965) produces a pink to red colouration but is less satisfactory than the DAB procedure in that the reaction product is alcohol-xylol soluble, a problem also encountered with 4-chloro-1-naphthol (blue-black) and 3-amino-9-ethylcarbazone (red).Hanker and Yates (1977) have recommended 'PPD-PC' (p-phenylene diamine dihydrochloride pyrocalitrol) which gives a blue end product.

Antigens demonstrable

An ever increasing variety of antigens have been demonstrated using immunoperoxidase methods and fixed embedded tissues. They include immunoglobulin light and heavy chains, J chain, secretor piece, lysozyme (muramidase), lactoferrin, transferrin, ferritin, albumin, α^1-antitrypsin, gastrin, parathormone, HCG, α-foetoprotein, estrogen, testosterone, haemaglobin A and F, carcino-embryonic antigen, hepatitis B surface antigen, rabies virus, toxoplasma, etc. The list grows almost exponentially. (Sets of reagents are available for many of these, see footnote on p. 280.)

Table 20

Immunoperoxidase – applications in Haematopathology

Immunoglobulin & J chain
1. Distinction of reactive process from lymphoma
   – lymphoplasmacytoid, plasmacytoma, B-cell immunoblastic sarcoma, follicle center cell lymphoma
2. Marrow plasmacytosis, reactive versus myeloma
3. Differential diagnosis of anaplastic tumour
4. Classification of sub-types of lymphoma
   Maligant lymphoma, lymphocytic, well differentiated – lymphoplasmacytoid
   B- and T-cell immunoblastic sarcoma

Lysozyme
1. Histiocyte marker in reactive and neoplastic states
2. Marker of myeloid cell maturation
3. Stains Auer rods in acute myeloblastic leukaemia

Other Antigens
Ferritin, lactoferrin, transferrin, haemoglobin A, haemoglobin F

Potential
Powerful investigative tool
   – cell antigens, including any enzyme
   – 'hormones' and hormone receptors – erythropoietin, thymopoietin
   – viruses – Epstein-Barr virus
Teaching

Table 21
Results of Immunoperoxidase Studies – Typical examples of Diagnostic Categories

	κ	λ	γ	α	μ	δ	J chain	Mx[1]
Reactive plasma cells	+ + + +[2]	+ + +	+ + + +	+ +	+ +	+	+	−
Reactive granuloma (histiocytes)	±	±	±	−	−	−	−	+ +
Multiple myeloma[3]	+ + + +	±	±	+ + + +	±	±	+	−
Waldenström's disease[3] (lymphoplasmacytoid)	±	+ + + +	±	±	+ + + +	±	+	−
B-cell immunoperoxidase sarcoma[3]	+ + + +	±	+ + + +	±	±	±	+	−
T-cell immunoblastic sarcoma	±	±	±	−	−	−	−	+
Histiocytic sarcoma	±	±	±	±	±	±	−	+ + +
Follicular lymphoma	± +	±	± +	±	±	±	+	−
Chronic lymphocytic leukaemia	−	−	−	−	−	−	−	−
Anaplastic carcinoma	±	±	±	−	−	−	−	±

[1] Anti-muramidase (lysozyme).
[2] − + + + + Semi-quantitayive score of number of positive cells.
[3] In the B-cell series the pattern of staining of the neoplastic cell varies e.g. myeloma cell-plasma cell; large amounts of cytoplasmic immunoglobulin present-chronic lymphocytic lymphocyte − small lymphocyte: little or no detectable cytoplasmic immunoglobulin, though surface immunoglobulin is present.

These final two tables illustrate some of the uses of immunohistochemical methods in an approach to lymph node diagnosis (Table 20) and give examples of staining patterns that might be expected in studies of immunoglobulin in lymphomas (Table 21).

BIBLIOGRAPHY

This annotated bibliography has been ordered in the style of the Vancouver declaration of 1978, but authors are cited in alphabetical order. The names of the first three authors only are listed here, so that the name of the real contributor may not always appear in the entry. We have omitted titles of articles and the number of the last page, but, believing it to be more useful, have indicated in a phrase the reason for the quotation.

Adami JG. Medical Contribution to the Study of Evolution. London: Macmillan, 1918:340
Concept of progressive hyperplasia; communicated to the Pathological Section of 17th International Medical Congress, London, August 1913

Ahlström CG. Acta Pathol Microbiol Scand 1933;10:241
Reticulosarcoma

Aisenberg AC. In: Zarafonetis CJD, ed. Proceedings of the International Conference on Leukemia-Lymphoma. Philadelphia: Lea and Febiger, 1968:377
Initial use of non-Hodgkin lymphoma

Aisenberg AC. N Engl J Med 1977;297:206
Comment on lymphoma classification

Aiuti F, Cerottini JC, Coombs RRA et al. Scand J Immunol 1974; 3:521
Identification of human B- and T- lymphocytes. Report of WHO/IARC workshop

Aiuti F, Papa G, Lacava V et al. Br J Haematol 1974; 27; 635
Lymphocyte markers in leukaemia

Akazaki J. Byorigaku Zasshi 1943;2:483
Reticulosarcoma

Akazaki K. In: Akazaki K, Rappaport H, Berard CW et al, eds. Malignant Diseases of the Hematopoietic System. Gann monograph on Cancer Research 15. Tokyo: University of Tokyo Press, 1973:71
Reticulosarcoma

Albrink WS, Brooks SM, Biron RE et al. Am J Pathol 1960; 36:457
Anthrax

Amano S, Hirata M, Fujii A. Trans Soc Pathol Jap 1944;34:28
Antibody production by plasma cells

Anagnostou D, Parker JW, Taylor CR et al. Cancer 1977;39:1032
Detailed structural study of lacunar cells

Anday GJ, Schmitz HC. Arch Intern Med 1952;89:621
Cleaved cells in follicular lymphoma

Anderson LG, Talal N. Clin Exp Immunol 1971;9:199
Lymphoproliferation in Sjögren's syndrome

André JA, Schwartz RS, Mitus WJ et al. Blood 1962;19:313,334
Morphology of homograft reaction

André-Schwartz J. Blood 1964;24:113
Response of lymphoid cells to homografts

Andrewes FW. Trans Pathol Soc (London) 1902;52:305
Histology of Hodgkin's disease

Archer RK. The Eosinophil. Oxford: Blackwells, 1968

Armitage JO, Dick FR, Corder MP. Cancer 1978;41:422
Richter's Syndrome

Aschoff L. Erg Inn Med Kinderheilkd 1924;26:1
Account of the reticulo-endothelial system

Baehr G. Trans Assoc Am Physicians 1932;47:330
Follicular lymphoma

Baehr G, Rosenthal N. Am J Pathol 1927;3:550
Follicular lymphoma

Baker GP, de Nevasquez S, MacLean KS. Guys Hosp Rep 1949; 98:95
Amyloidosis of lymph nodes

Banks PM, Long JC, Howard CA. Hum Pathol 1979;10:617
Techniques of lymph node biopsy

Barcos MD, Lukes RJ. In: Sinks LF, Godden JO, eds. Conflicts in Childhood Cancer. New York: Liss 1975; vol 4:147
Malignant convoluted cell lymphoma

Barr PD, Whang-Peng J, Perry S. Science 1975;190:284
Stem cells in peripheral blood

Barth RF, Vergam GG, Khuram SK et al. Lancet 1972;ii:503
Familial histiocytosis with eosinophilia

Basten A, Miller JFAP, Sprent J. J Exp Med 1972;135:610
Distribution of B- and T-lymphocytes in mice

Beard MEJ, Durrant J, Catovsky D et al. Br J Haematol 1976; 34:167
Blast crisis in chronic myeloid leukaemia

Bell RJM, Benfield AJE, Barnes ND et al. Arch Dis Child 1968;43:601
Familial haemophagocytic reticulosis

Bennett JH. Edin Med J 1845;64:413
Early account of leukaemia

Bennett MH. Br J Cancer 1975;31:Suppl. II:44
Nodular sclerotic lymphosarcoma

Bennett MH, Farrer-Brown G, Henry K et al. Lancet 1974; ii: 405
National Lymphoma Investigation classification

Bennett MH, Millett YL. Clin Radiol 1969;20:339
Nodular sclerotic lymphosarcoma

Berard CW, ed. Cancer Treat Rep 1977;61:1037
Round table discussion of histopathological classifications of lymphomas

Berard CW, Dorfman AF. Clin Haematol 1974;3i:39
Report of Chicago workshop on non-Hodgkin's lymphoma, June 1973

Berard CW, O'Connor GT, Thomas LB et al. Bull WHO 1969;40:601
Histopathology of Burkitt's tumour

Bergsma D, Good RA, eds. Immunologic Deficiency Diseases in Man. The National Foundation – March of Dimes 1968; 4 Birth Defects original articles Series IV

Bessis M. Living Blood Cells and their Ultrastructure. Berlin: Springer, 1973

Bessis M, ed. Blood Cells 1979;3:143
Pluripotent stem cells

Billingham RE, Defendi V, Silvers WK et al. J Natl Cancer Inst 1962;28:365
Morphology of the homograft reaction

Billroth CAT. Beiträge zur pathologischer Histologie. Berlin:Reimer, 1858
Giant cells

Billroth CAT. Wien Med Wochenschr 1871;21:1065
Introduction of 'malignant lymphoma' as a term

Biomedicine editorial. Biomedicine 1975;22:466
Report of workshop for the classification of non-Hodgkin's lymphoma. Warrenton, Virginia, September 1975

Black MM, Spear FO. Arch Pathol 1958;66:754
Metalophil cells

Blanden NV. Transplantation 1969;7:484
Morphology of activated macrophage

Bloch KJ, Lee L, Mills JA et al. Am J Med 1973;55:61
Gamma-heavy chain disease

Bodley Scott R. Br J Radiol 1951;24:475
Clinical features of the reticuloses

Bodley Scott R, Robb-Smith AHT. Lancet 1939;ii:154
First account of histiocytic medullary reticulosis

Bowling MC. Procedures of the Pathologic Branch of the NCI. Washington DC: US Govt Printing Office, 1967
Histological methods

Bowling MC. Lymph node specimens. Improved Service issue 20. Chicago: American Society of Clinical Pathologists, 1976
Histological methods

Brahim F, Osmond DG. Clin Exp Immunol 1976;24:515
Migration of lymphocytes in immune response

Braunstein H, Freiman DG, Gall EA. Cancer 1958;11:829

Braunstein H, Freiman DG, Thomas W Jr, et al. Cancer 1962;15:130
Enzyme histochemistry of lymph nodes

Braylan RC. Jaffe ES, Berard CW. In: Sommers SC, ed. Pathology Annual. New York: Appleton Century Crafts, 1975:213
Classification of malignant lymphomas

Braylan RC, Jaffe ES, Burbank JW et al. Blood 1975;46:1036
Surface characters of lymphocytes

Braylan RC, Rappaport H. Blood 1973;42:579
Immunoglobulin differentiation of reactive follicular hyperplasia and follicular lymphoma

Brill NE, Baehr G, Rosenthal N. JAMA 1925;84:668
Follicular lymphoma

Brittinger G. Recent Results Cancer Res 1978;65:197
Findings of Kiel Lymphoma Study Group

Broder S, Edelson RL, Lutzner MA, et al. J Clin Invest 1976;58:1297
Helper T-cells in Sézary's syndrome

Broome JD, Zucker-Franklin D, Wiener MS et al. Clin Immunol Immunopathol 1973;1:39
T-cells in Sézary's syndrome

Brouet J-C, Flandrin G, Sasporter M et al. Lancet 1975;ii:890
T-cell chronic lymphocytic leukaemia

Brouet J-C, Flandrin G, Seligmann M. N Engl J Med 1973;289:341
T-cells in Sézary's syndrome

Brouet J-C, Mason DY, Danon F et al. Lancet 1977;ii:280
α-Chain disease

Brouet J-C, Preud'homme JG, Flandrin G et al. J Natl Canc Inst 1976;56:631
Membrane markers in 'histiocytic' lymphomas

Brouet J-C, Valensi F, Daniel M-T et al. Br J Haematol 1976;33:319
Immunological classification of acute leukaemia

Brubacker DB, Whiteside TL. Am J Pathol 1977;88:323
Localization of T-cells in sections by rosetting technique

Butler JJ. In: Rebuck JW, Berard CW, Abel MR, eds. The Reticulo-endothelial System. Baltimore: Williams and Wilkins, 1975:184
Criteria for diagnosis of nodular sclerotic Hodgkin's disease

Butler JJ, Stryker JA, Schullenberger CC. Br J Cancer 1975;31 Suppl II:208
Trial of Lukes-Collins classification

Byrne GE Jr. Cancer Treat Rep 1977;6:935
Comparability study of non-Hodgkin's lymphoma classifications

Byrne GE Jr, Rappaport H. In: Akazaki K, Rappaport H, Berard CW et al, eds. Malignant Diseases of the Hematopoietic System. Gann monograph on Cancer Research 15. Tokyo: University of Tokyo Press, 1973:145
Malignant histiocytosis

Calderon C, Atias A, Saavedra P et al. Lancet 1973;ii:1264
Immunofluorescent identification of toxoplasma in lymph nodes

Callendar GR. Am J Pathol 1934;10:443
Lymph Node Registry classification

Carbone PP, Kaplan HS, Musshoff V et al. Cancer Res 1971;31:1860
Ann Arbor staging for Hodgkin's disease

Carswell R. An Album of Illustrations of Pathology. London: New Sydenham Society, 1898:fasc.12. [cf Dawson, 1968]
Drawings illustrating Thomas Hodgkin's original account

Carter RL. Lancet 1975;i:846
Morphogenesis of infectious mononucleosis

Catovsky D. Lancet 1975;ii:327
Acid phosphatase reaction of T-cell lymphoblasts

Catovsky D. Clin Haematol 1977;6:245
Nature of hairy cell leukaemia

Catovsky D, Cherchi M, Greaves MF, et al. Lancet 1978;i:749
Acid phosphatase reaction in acute lymphoblastic leukaemia

Catovsky D, Pettit JE, Galletto J et al. Br J Haematol 1974;26:29
Lymphocyte markers

Catovsky D, Pettit JE, Galton DAJ et al. Br J Haematol 1974;26:9
Hairy cell leukaemia

Chanana AO, Schaedeli J, Hess MW et al. J Immunol 1973;110:283
Distribution of B- and T- lymphocytes in newborn mice

Chandra P, Chaudhery SA, Rasner F et al. Arch Int Med 1975;135:985
'Transient' histiocytic medullary reticulosis

Chelloul N, Daniel MT, Flandrin G. Pathol Eur 1973;8:235
Hairy cell leukaemia

Chelloul N, Diebold J, Flandrin G et al. Ann Anat Pathol 1976; 21:301
Review of WHO classification of non-Hodgkin's lymphoma

Chessells JM, Hardesty RN, Rapson N et al. Lancet 1977;ii:1307
Classification of acute lymphoblastic leukaemia

Churg J, Strauss L. Am J Pathol 1951;27:277
Lymph nodes in polyarteritis nodosa

Clandy AL. Br J Dermatol 1974;91:597
Sézary cell

Cline MT, Golde DW. Nature 1979;277:177
Review of modern concept of pluripotent haemato-poietic cells

Coccia PF, Kersey JH, Kazamièra J et al. Am J Haematol 1976;1:405
Significance of marker studies in childhood leukaemias

Cohen S. Hum Pathol 1976;7:249
Lymphokines

Cohen S, Ward PA. J Exp Med 1971;133:133
Eosinophil chemotaxis

Cohnheim JF. Virchow's Archiv 1865;33:451
Pseudo-leukaemia

Congdon CC, Hannan MG Jr. In: Cottier H, Odartchenko N, Schindler R et al, eds. Germinal Centres in Immune Response. Berlin: Springer, 1967:1
Finding of germinal centres

Cooper MD, Peterson RDA, Gabrielson AE, et al. Cancer Res 1966;26:1165
Early suggestion of immunological relationship to lymphomas

Cooper MD, Gabrielson AE, Peterson RDA et al. In Cottier H, Odartchenko N, Schindler R et al, eds. Germinal Centres in Immune Response. Berlin: Springer, 1967:28
Ontogeny of immune system

Coppleson LW, Factor RM, Strum SW et al. J Nat Cancer Inst 1970;45:731
Observer error in lymph node diagnosis

Corbett EU. Am J Pathol 1945;21:905
Pseudo-appendicitis syndrome in measles

Cornil V. Arch Gen Med 1855;ii:206
Introduced 'lymphadenoma' as a term

Cottier H, Turk J, Sobin L. Bull WHO 1972;47:375
Lymph node analysis

Cottier H, Odartchenko N, Keiser G et al. Ann NY Acad Sci 1964;113:612
Germinal centres in immune response

Craddock GC, Vakali GS, Fukuta H et al. J Exp Med 1964;120:389
Thymidine study of change from small to large lymphocyte

Craddock CG, Longmire RL, McMillan R. In: Williams WJ, Beutler E, Eslev AJ et al. Hematology 2nd ed. New York: McGraw-Hill, 1977:902,920
Lymphocyte production and function

Cramer A. In: Taylor CR. Hodgkin's Disease and the Lymphomas, Vol. 3 Montreal: Eden Press, 1979; ch 10: 109
Review of lymphoid cytochemistry

Craver LF. Med Clin North Am 1934;18:703
Follicular lymphoma

Cross RM. J Clin Pathol 1968;21:303
Nodular sclerotic Hodgkin's disease

Cross RM. J Clin Pathol 1969;22:165
Histological classification of Hodgkin's disease

Cruikshank AH. J Clin Pathol 1965;18:891
Lympho-epithelial lesion of salivary gland

Crum ED, Ng ABP, Tsoa L-L et al. Am J Clin Pathol 1974;61:403
Survival in Hodgkin's disease in relation to histology

Custer RP. In: Rebuck JW, ed. The Lymphocyte and Lymphocytic tissue. New York: Hoeber, 1960: ch 15
Clinical pattern of lymph node malignancies

Custer RP, Bernhard WG. Am J Med Sci 1948;216:623
The relationship of Hodgkin's disease to other lymphoid disorders

D'Ablaing G, Rogers ER, Parker JH et al. Am J Clin Pathol 1970;54:667
Simple methyl-green pyronin stain

Dameshek W. Folia Haematol 1933;49:64
Review of reticulosis

Dameshek W. Blood 1963;21:243
Immunoblast concept

Dameshek W. In: Zarafonetis CJD, ed. Proceedings of the International Conference on Leukaemia-Lymphoma. Philadelphia: Lea and Febiger, 1968:212,501
Discussion on immunological aspect of lymphomas

Danon F, Clauvel JP, Seligmann M. Rev Fr Etud Clin Biol 1967;12:681
'Paraprotein' lymphomas

Davies AJS, Carter RL, Huchars E et al. Immunology 1969;17:111
Thymic origin of oxazalone stimulated cells

Davies JD, Stansfeld AG. J Clin Pathol 1972;25:689
Thrombosis of nodal vein inducing infarction

Davis JMA. Br J Exp Pathol 1967;48:377
Relationship of macrophages and fibroblasts

Dawson PJ. Arch Intern Med 1968;121:288
Carswell's drawings of Hodgkin's disease

Dawson PJ, Harrison CV. J Clin Pathol 1961;14:215
Benign Hodgkin's disease

Delbruck H. Klin Wochenschr 1978;56:539
Prognostic value of Kiel classification

Del Rio-Hortega P. Mem Soc Espan Hist Nat 1921;11:213
Silver techniques for histiocytes

De Vita VT, Canellos GP, Chabner B et al. Lancet 1975;i:248
Excellent chemotherapeutic response in 'diffuse histiocytic lymphoma'

Dewar G, Fabre J, Familiades J et al. Am J Clin Pathol 1978;69:646
Lympho-epithelioid (Peedell-Lennert) lymphoma

de Sousa MAB. See Sousa

Dhom G, ed. Verh Dtsch Ges Pathol 1980;64
Numerous papers on granulomas and granulomatosis

Diebold J. Ann Anat Pathol (Paris) 1975;20:35
Classification of lymphoma

Donohue WL, Thompson MW. Birth Defects 1972;8:105
Familial haemophagocytic reticulosis

Dorfman RF. In: Akazaki K, Rappaport H, Berard CW et al, eds. Malignant Diseases of the Hematopoietic System. Gann monograph on Cancer Research 15. Tokyo: University of Tokyo Press, 1973;177
Follicular lymphomas

Dorfman RF. Lancet 1974;i:1295;ii:961
Classification of lymphomas

Dorfman RF. In: Rebuck JW, Berard CW, Abell MR, eds. The Reticulo-endothelial System. Monographs in Pathology 16. Baltimore: Williams and Wilkins, 1975:262
Classification of lymphomas

Dorfman RF. Am J Surg Pathol 1977;1:167
Classification of lymphomas

Dorfman RF. Cancer Treat Rep 1977;61:945
Classification of lymphomas

Dorfman RF, Remington JS. N Eng J Med 1973; 289:878
Histological diagnosis of toxoplasmosis

Dorfman RF, Warnke R. Hum Pathol 1974;5:517
Lymph node diagnosis

Douglas SD. In: Richter GW, Epstein MA, eds. Int Rev Exp Path. New York, London: Academic Press, 1971;10:42
Lymphocytic transformation and immune proliferation

Downey H, Stasney T. Folia Haematol (Leipz) 1936;54:417
Histology of infectious mononucleosis

Ehrlich P. Arch Micro Anat Morph 1877;13:263
First account of mast cells

Enzinger FM, Helwig EB. Virchow's Arch 1963;336:238
Lymph node changes in Whipple's disease

Epstein E. Med Klin 1925;21:1501,1542
Lymphoproliferative disorders

Epstein EH, Levin DL, Croft JD et al. Medicine 1972;15:61
Mycosis fungoides

Ernström V. Acta Pathol Microbiol Scand Suppl 1965;178
Lymphoid development in germ-free animals

Evans ML, Butler JJ, Youness EL. Cancer 1978;41:1440
Intermediate lymphocytic lymphoma

Evans N. Arch Pathol 1914;37:175
Lymph node changes in secondary syphilis

Ewing J. J Med Res 1913;23:1
First use of 'reticulum cell sarcoma'

Ewing J. Neoplastic Diseases. 3rd ed. Philadelphia: W.B. Saunders, 1928:368
Discussion of 'reticulum cell sarcoma'

Fagraeus: A. Acta Med Scand Suppl 1948;130:Suppl 1:204
Antibody production by plasma cells

Farrer-Brown G. 1973
Lymphoma classification presented at workshop on non-Hodgkin's lymphoma, Chicago, June 1973, which was reported by Berard and Dorfman 1974: it is not identical with the NLI classification reported by Bennett et al 1974

Fayemi AO, Toker C. Arch Pathol 1975;99:170
Vascular transformation of the sinuses

Feremans WW, Neve D, Caudron M. J Clin Pathol 1978;31:250
IgM crystals in lymphocytic leukaemia

Feuermann ET, Sandbank M. Arch Dermatol 1972;105:233
Lymphomatosus papulosus

Fisher RI, Jaffe ES, Braylen RC et al. Am J Med 1976;61:553
Sarcomatous change in immunoblastic lymphadenopathy

Fite GL, Cambre PJ, Turner HH, Arch Pathol 1947;43:624
Staining technique for demonstrating lepra bacilli

Flandrin G. Recent Results Cancer Res 1978;64:246
Immunoblastic lymphadenopathy

Flemming W. Arch mikros Anat 1885;24:50
Germinal centres and tingible bodies

Fliedner TM, Kisse M, Cronkite EP et al. Ann NY Acad Sci 1964;113:578
Monocyte proliferation in immune response

Fox H. Ann Med Hist 1926;8:370
Re-examination of Hodgkin's material in the museum of Guy's Hospital

Frangione B, Franklin EC. Semin Hematol 1973;10:53
Review of IgG heavy chain disease

Franklin EC. Arch Intern Med 1973;135:71
IgM heavy chain disease

Freeman HJ, Weinstein WM, Shnilka TK et al. Am J Med 1977;63:585
Lymph nodes in sprue

Friedell GH, Soto EA, Kumaoka S et al. Lancet 1974;ii:1228
Sinus histiocytosis in breast cancer

Frizzera S, Moran EM, Rappaport H. Lancet 1974;i:1070; Am J Med 1975;59:803
Angio-immunoblastic lymphadenopathy

Fudenberg HH, Good RA, Goodman HC et al. Pediatrics 1971;47:929
WHO nomenclature of immune deficiency diseases

Galea JMP. University of Oxford: BSc thesis, 1952
Correlation of histological structure and natural history in Hodgkin's disease

Galian A, Lecestre M-J, Scotto J et al. Cancer 1977;39:2081
Evolution of α-chain disease

Gall EA. Minn Med 1955;38:674
Abandonment of 'reticulum cell sarcoma'

Gall EA. Ann NY Acad Sci 1958;73:120
Interrelationship of mesenchymal cells of lymphoid tissue

Gall EA. 1962. Personal communication to AHT Robb-Smith on classification

Gall EA. In: Pack GT, Ariel IM, eds. Lymphomas and Related Diseases. New York: Hoeber, 1964:28
Differential diagnosis of lymph nodes

Gall EA, Mallory TB. Am J Pathol 1942;18:381
Reticulum cell sarcoma includes clasmatocytic and stem cell types

Gall EA, Rappaport H. In: McDonald JR, ed. Proc 23rd Seminar on Diseases of Lymph Nodes and Spleen. Am Soc Clin Pathol 1958:107
Characterization of lymphadenopathies

Gall EA, Stout HA. Am J Pathol 1940;16:433
Lymph nodes in infectious mononucleosis

Galton PAG, Catovsky D, Wiltshaw E. Cancer 1978;42:901
Clinical spectrum of lymphoproliferative diseases

Gams RA, Neal JA, Conrad FG. Ann Intern Med 1968;69:557
Hydantoin lymphadenopathy

Garrett R, Ada AEW. Cancer 1957;10:173
Epithelial inclusions in lymph nodes

Gérard-Marchant R. Bull Cancer (Paris) 1974;61:1. Ann Anat
Pathol (Paris) 1974;19:149
Strong support for the Lennert-Lukes approach to the
lymphomas

Gérard-Marchant R, Hamlin I, Lennert K et al. Lancet
1974;ii:406
Kiel classification of non-Hodgkin's lymphoma

Glynn LE. Ann Rheum Dis 1968;27:105
Acute inflammatory response and granuloma formation

Goldner J. Am J Pathol 1938;14:237
Modification of Masson's trichrome stain

Goldzieher MA, Hornick OS. Arch Pathol 1931;12:773
Reticulosis

Good RA. Harvey Lectures. London: Academic Press, 1973;
vol 67:1
Lymphocytes and immunodeficiency

Good RA, Finstad J. In: Zarafonetis CJD, ed. Proceedings of
the International Conference on Leukaemia-Lymphoma.
Philadelphia: Lea and Febiger, 1968:175
First suggestion of B-and T-cells in relation to
lymphomas

Gordon H, Sweets HHJ. Am J Pathol 1936;12:545; also in:
Culling CFA. Handbook of Histopathological and Histochemical Techniques 3rd ed. London: Butterworth,
1974:427
Reticulin staining method

Gordon HA, Wostmann BS. Anat Rec 1960;137:65
Germfree rats and lymphoid follicles

Gordon MH, ed. Rose Research Studies on the Aetiology of
Lymphadenoma. Bristol: John Wright, 1932

Gow AE. Proc R Soc Med 1934;27:1039
Mononuclear reticulosis

Gowans JL, Knight ET. Proc R Soc Lond (B) 1964;159:257
Circulation of small lymphocytes

Gowans JL, McGregor DD, Cowen DM. Nature
1962;196:561
Transition from small to large lymphocyte

Gowing NFC. In: Sommers GC, ed. Pathology Annual. New
York: Appleton, 1975:1
Histopathology of infectious mononucleons

Graham RC, Karnovsky MT. J Histochem Cytochem
1966;14:291
Diaminobenzene reaction

Granger GA. Ser Haematol 1972;5.4:8
Lymphokines

Greaves MF, Brown G, Rapson NT et al. Clin Immunol
Immunopathol 1975;4:67
Specific anti-ALL serum

Greenfield WS. Trans Path Soc (London) 1878;29:292
Histology of lymphadenoma

Griffin FM Jr, Griffin JA, Silverstein SC. J Exp Med
1976;144:788
Phagocytosis

Haegert DG, Coombs RRA. Lancet 1979;ii:1051
Concept of 'B-major' and 'B-minor' lymphocytes

Haferkamp O, Rosenau W, Lennert K. Arch Pathol
1971;92:81
Vascular transformation of the sinuses

Hall J, Scollay R, Smith M. Eur J Immunol 1976;6:117
Homing of lymphocytes

Hall J, Hopkins J, Orlean E. Eur J Immunol 1977;7:30
Homing of lymphocytes

Hall JG, Morris B, Moreno G et al. J Exp Med 1967;125:91
Cells in lymph following antigen injection

Hanaoka M, Sasaki M, Matsumoto H et al. Acta Pathol Jap
1979;29:723
Adult T-cell leukaemia

Hanker JS, Yates PE, Metz CB et al. Histochem J 1977; 9:789
Non-carcogenic substitute for diaminobenzidine

Hansen JA, Good RA. Hum Pathol 1974;5:567
Review of immune deficiencies and malignant change

Hanson TAS. Cancer 1964;17:1595
Nodular sclerotic Hodgkin's disease

Harrison CV. J Path Bact 1952;64:513
Benign Hodgkin's disease

Harrison CV. Practitioner 1956;177:123
Classification of reticulosis

Harrison CV. In: Harrison CV, ed. Recent Advances in Pathology, Edition 8. London: Churchill, 1966:221
Lymphangiographic changes in lymph nodes

Harrison CV. J Clin Pathol 1972;25:12
Waldenström's disease

Harrison CV. In: Harrison CV, Weinbren K, eds. Recent Advances in Pathology. Edinburgh: Churchill, Livingstone,
1975:73
Lymph node diseases

Hartsock RT. Cancer 1968;21:632
Post-vaccinial lymphadenitis

Hartsock RT, Halling LW, King FM. Am J Clin Pathol
1970;53:314
Syphilitic lymphadenitis

Hay JB, Murphy MJ, Morris B et al. Am J Pathol 1972;66:1
Proliferation and differentiation of antibody producing
cells

Hay JB, Hobbs BB. J Exp Med 1977;143:31
Lymphocyte traffic in the immune response

Hayhoe FGJ. In: Zarafonetis CJD, ed. Proceedings of the
International Conference on Leukemia-Lymphoma.
Philadelphia: Lea and Febiger, 1968:354
Suggestion of an immunological classification of
lymphomas

Hellman TJ. Beitr Pathol Anat 1921;68:233
Lymphoid follicles

Hellman TJ. In:von Mollendorff W, ed. Handb Mikrosp Anat
des Menschen. Berlin: Springer, 1930
Lymphoid follicles

Henry K. Communication to 131st meeting of Pathological
Society of Great Britain and Ireland, 1975
Malignant hystiocytic lymphoma

Henry K, Bennett MH, Farrer-Brown G. Recent Results Cancer
Res 1978;64:38
Discussion on lymphomata

Henry K, Bennett MH, Farrer-Brown G. In: Anthony PP, Woolf N, eds. Recent Advances in Histopathology 10 Edinburgh: Churchill Livingstone, 1978:275
Descriptive review of lymphomas

Henry K, Farrer-Brown G. Histopathology 1977;1:53
Plasma cell tumours of the gastro-intestinal tract

Henry L. J Path Bact 1967;93:661;1968;96;337
Acute thymic involution

Hers HG, van Hoof F, eds. Lysosomes and Storage Diseases. New York: Academic Press, 1973
General review

Hertel BF, Rosai J, Dehner LP et al. Lab Invest 1977;36:12
Lymphoproliferative lesions in transplant recipients

Heudorfer K. Z Anat Entwicklungsgesch 1921;61:365
Lymph node morphology

Higgy KE, Burns GE, Hayhoe FGJ. Scand J Haematol 1977;18:437
Differentiation of lymphocytes by esterase cytochemistry

Hinrichson K. In: Cottier H, Odartchenko N, Schindler R et al, eds. Germinal Centres in Immune Responses. Berlin: Springer, 1967:152
Study of developing germinal centres

His W. Z Wiss Zool 1862;11:65
Recognition of medulla and cortex in lymph nodes

Hodgkin T. Med Chir Trans 1832;17:68
Original account of Hodgkin's Disease

Holt JM, Robb-Smith AHT. J Clin Pathol 1973;26:649
Sarcomatous change in myeloma

Hurez P, Flandrin G, Preud'homme JL et al. Clin Exp Immunol 1972;10:223
IgM crystals in chronic lymphocytic leukaemia

Isaacs R. Proc Central Soc Clin Res 1939;72:37
First mention of notched leukaemic cells

Isaacson P, Jones DB, Millward-Sadler GH et al. Proc Path Soc Great Britain and Ireland 140th meeting 1980; item 96:63
α'-antitrypsin in histiocytes

Isaacson P, Wright DH. Hum Pathol 1978;9:661
'Malignant histiocytosis' of the intestine

Isaacson P, Wright DH, Judd MA et al. Cancer 1979;43:1805
Primary gastro-intestinal lymphoma

Isaacson P, Toms DB, Judd MA. Cancer 1979;ii:964
α'-antitrypsin in normal and malignant histiocytes

Isaacson P, Wright DH. Lancet 1978;i:67;i:485
Histiocytic tumours

Isobe T, Osserman EF. N Engl J Med 1974;290:423
Amyloid and plasma cell tumours

Jackson H. Surg Gynecol Obstet 1937;64:465
Subdivisions of Hodgkin's Disease

Jackson H, Parker F. Hodgkin's Disease and Allied Disorders. New York: OUP 1947
Classification and characterization of lymphadenopathies

Jaffe ES, Berard CW. Ann Intern Med 1978;89:417
Revival of lymphoblastic lymphoma

Jaffe ES, Shevach EM, Frank MM et al. N Eng J Med 1974;290:813
B-lymphocytic origin of nodular lymphoma

Janossy G, Greaves MF, Revesz T et al. Brit J Haematol 1976;
Blast crisis in chronic myeloid lymphoma

Jellife AM: Thomson AD. Br J Cancer 1955;9:21
Benign Hodgkin's disease

Job TT. Am J Anat 1922;31:123
Lymph node studies

Jones DB, Castleden M, Smith JL et al. Br J Cancer 1978;37:1053
Angio-immunoblastic lymphadenopathy

Jones SE, Godden T, eds. Cancer Treat Rep 1977;61:1937
Conference on Non-Hodgkin's Lymphoma, California Sep 30/Oct 2 1976
Informative round table conference in which Henry Rappaport and Robert Lukes, amongst others, discuss their views with freedom

Kadin ME, Glatstein E, Dorfman RF. Cancer 1971;27:1277
Cellular phase of nodular sclerotic Hodgkin's disease

Katayama I, Finkel HE. Am J Med 1974;57:115
Hairy cell leukaemia

Katayama I, Yang JPS. Am J Clin Pathol 1977;68:268
Histochemistry of hairy cells

Kay HSM. Lancet 1974;ii:586
Classification of non-Hodgkin's lymphomas

Keller AR, Hochholzer L, Castleman B. Cancer 1972;29:678
Plasma cell form of giant lymph node hyperplasia

Keller AR, Kaplan HS, Lukes RJ et al. Cancer Res 1968;16:422
Correlation of histopathology of Hodgkin's disease

Kelsall SRH, Blackwell JB. Pathology 1969;1:211
Lipogranulomatosis of lymph nodes

Keuning FJ. Oncologica 1965;19:180
Homograft response of lymphoreticular system

Kim H, Dorfman RF, Rappaport H. Am J Surg Pathol 1978;2:119
Signet-ring cells in follicular lymphoma

Kim H, Jacobs C, Warnke RA et al. Cancer 1978;41:620
Lympho-epithelioid (Peedell-Lennert) lymphoma

King LJ. J Exp Med 1939;70:303
Gordon's test for Hodgkin's disease

Klein MA, Jaffe R, Neiman RS. Am J Clin Pathol 1977;68:601
Lympho-epithelioid (Peedell-Lennert) lymphoma

Kojima M. Trans Soc Path Jap 1969;58:3
Follicular lymphoma

Kojima M, Imai Y, Mori N. In: Akazaki K, Rappaport H, Berard CW et al, eds. Malignant Diseases of the Hemato-poietic System. Gann monograph on Cancer Research 15. Tokyo: University of Tokyo Press, 1973:195
Follicular lymphoma

Kramer H, Windrum GM. J Histochem Cytochem 1955;3:227
Metachromatic Technique

Krasnazi G, Szegedi G. Acta Morph Acad Sci Hung 1969;17:175
Drug induced lymphadenopathy

Krueger GRF. Z Krebsforsch 1977;89:253
Comparative pathology of malignant lymphomas

Kundrat H. Wien Klin Wschr. 1893;6:211
Change in meaning of lymphosarcoma

Lainport F, Lennert K. Cancer 1976;37:783
Sinus histiocytosis and massive lymphadenopathy

Lame E. Radiology 1953;61:764
Fluidity of lymphomas

Lampert LA, Catovsky D, Bergier N. Br J Haematol 1978;40:65
Histiocytic medullary reticulosis

Lancet editorial. Lancet 1979;i:306
Premalignant to malignant lymphomas

Lange P. Acta Obstet Gynecol Scand 1955;34:111
Endometrium in inguinal lymph nodes

Lawrence EC, Broder E, Jaffe ES et al. Blood 1978;52:48
Helper T-cells in Sézary's syndrome

Lawrinson W, Gross S. Lab Invest 1964;13:1612
Aryl sulphatase reaction in lymphocytes

Leclerc JL, Hould F, Lelièvre M et al. Laval Médical 1971;42:461
Wolman's disease

Leder L-D. Verh Dtsch Ges Path 1964;48:317
Naphthol-AS-D-Chloracetate esterase technique

Leder L-D. Klin Wschr 1965;43:795
Focal acid phosphatase reaction in primitive cells

Lennert K. Frank Z Path 1953;64:343
Early reference to lympho-epithelioid (Peedell-Lennert) lymphoma

Lennert K. Verh Dtsch Ges Pathol 1953;37:176
Hodgkin's disease

Lennert K. In: Lubarsch O, Henke F, Rössle R et al, eds. Lymphknoten Diagnostik in Schnitt und Austrich. Bandteil A: Lymphadenitis. Handb Spez Path Anat Hist Bd 1 Teil 3. Berlin: Springer, 1961
Excellent account of lymphadenopathies; details of Giemsa Technique

Lennert K. Strahlentherapie 1964;57:48.
Pathological Anatomy of the Reticuloses. (Mainz: Cancer Committee, Sep 1963

Lennert K. In: Rüttiman A, ed. Progress in Lymphology. Stuttgart: G. Thieme, 1967:103
European concept of classification of lymphomas

Lennert K. In: Proc European Div Int Soc Haematol, Milan. Milan: Fratelli Ferrari, 1971;109
Follicular lymphomas

Lennert K. In: Akazaki K, Rappaport H, Berard CW et al, eds. Malignant Diseases of the Hematopoietic System. Gann monograph on Cancer Research 15. Tokyo: University of Tokyo Press, 1973:217
Follicular lymphomas

Lennert K. In: Stacher A, ed. Leukämien und maligne Lymphone. Munich: Urban and Schwarzenberg, 1973:181
Classification of malignant lymphomas; discusses lymphogranulomatosis (angio-immunoblastic lymphadenopathy) and lympho-epithelioid (Peedell-Lennert) lymphomas

Lennert K. Patologia 1974;7:35
Reticuloses and reticulosarcoma

Lennert K. Lancet 1974;ii:586
Immunoblast

Lennert K. In: Jellinger K, Seitelberger F, eds. Malignant Lymphomas of the Nervous System. Berlin: Acta Neuropath, 1975;suppl 6:2
Discussion of Kiel Classification and lympho-epithelioid (Peedell-Lennert) lymphoma. (Congress in Vienna, Aug 29/31, 1974)

Lennert K. In: Löffler H, ed. Maligne Lymphome und Monoklonale Gammopathie. Blut 18. Sonderband. Munich: Lehmann, 1975:145
Discussion of Kiel Classification and Waldenström's disease. First account of T-zone lymphoma

Lennert K. Recent Results Cancer Res 1978;64:31
Frequency distribution of lymphadenopathies by the Kiel Classification

Lennert K, Kaiserling E, Müller-Hermelink HK. In: Clarkson B, Marks PA, Till JE, eds. Differentiation of Normal and Neoplastic Hematopoietic Cells (Conference on Cell Biology V). New York: Cold Spring Harbour Laboratory, 1978;Book B:897
Discusses relationship of dendritic and interdigitating reticulum cells to morphology of lymphomata

Lennert K, Knecht H, Burkert M. Verh Dtsch Ges Pathol 1979;63:170
Pre-neoplastic phases of lymphoma

Lennert K, Mestdagh J. Virchow's Arch 1968;344:1
Lympho-epithelioid (Peedell-Lennert) lymphoma

Lennert K, Mohri N, Stein H et al. Br J Haematol 1975; 31 (Suppl):163
Histopathology of lymphomas

Lennert K, in collaboration with Mohri K, Stein H et al. In: Lubarsch O, Henke F, Rössle R et al. Handb Spez Path Anat Hist. Bd 1 Teil 3 Bandteil B. Berlin: Springer, 1978, Malignant Lymphomas other than Hodgkin's Disease
A masterly account embracing all aspects

Lennert K, Niedorf HR. Virchow's Arch 1969;134:148
Follicular lymphoma

Lennert K, Parwaresch MR. Histopathology 1979;3:349
Review of mast cell disease

Lennert K, Stein H, Kaiserling E. In: Libansky J, Donner L, eds. Present Problems in Haematology. Amsterdam: Excerpta Medica, 1974:113
This incorporated a report by Lennert at the workshop on the classification of non-Hodgkin's lymphoma held at Chicago on June 25/29 1973, and at the second meeting of the European and African division of the International Society of Haematology at Prague August 27/29, 1973. Discusses use of immunoglobulin methods in the classification of lymphomas

Lennert K, Stein H, Kaiserling E. Br J Cancer 1975;31 Suppl II:29
Cytological and functional criteria for classification of lymphoma

Letterer E. Frank Z Pathol 1924;30:377
First use of 'reticulosis' in a case of acute reticulosis of infancy (Letterer-Siwe syndrome)

Letterer E. Veröff Gewerb Konstitut Path 1934;8:4
States that in 1924 reticulosis was used in a specific not generic sense

Levine GD, Dorman RF. Cancer 1975;35:148
Accepts germinal centre origin of follicular lymphoma

Lewis MR. Am J Pathol 1925;1:91
Transition of macrophage to epithelioid and giant cells

Li C-Y, Harrison EG. Am J Clin Pathol 1978;70:721
Analysis of large cell lymphomas

Li C-Y, Lam KW, Yam LT. J Histochem Cytochem 1973;21:1
Esterases in leucocytes

Li C-Y, Yam LT, Crosby WH. J Histochem Cytochem 1972;20:1049
Histochemistry of spleen

Li C-Y, Yam LT, Lam KW. J Histochem Cytochem 1970;18:473
Acid phosphatase in leucocytes

Lie JT, Holley KE, Kampa WN et al. Mayo Clin Proc 1971;46:319
Modified haematoxylin technique

Liebow AA, Carrington CRB, Friedman PJ. Hum Pathol 1972;3:457
Lymphomatoid granulomatosis

Lillie RD. Histopathologic Technic and Practical Histochemistry, 4th ed. New York: McGraw-Hill, 1976:451
Inter alia provides details of the Graham α-naphthol pyronine reaction

Long JC. N Engl J Med 1977;297:206
Quotes Noel, Helbron and Lennert (1979) on lympho-epithelioid (Peedell-Lennert) lymphoma

Longcope WT. Bull Ayer Clin Lab Pennsylvania Hosp 1903;1:4
Characterization of Hodgkin's disease

Longo S. Hum Pathol 1976;7:349
Benign epithelial lymph node inclusions

Lubin J, Rywlin AM. Arch Pathol 1971;92:338
Kaposi's sarcoma in lymph nodes

Lukes RJ. Am J Roentgenol 1963;90:944
First account of nodular sclerotic Hodgkin's disease

Lukes RJ. In: Rüttiman A, ed. Progress in Lymphology. Stuttgart: G. Thieme, 1967:109
American concept of the classification of lymphoma

Lukes RJ. In: Zarafonetis CJD, ed. Proceedings of the International Conference on Leukemia-Lymphoma. Philadelphia: Lea and Febiger, 1968:331,354
Classification of lymphoma

Lukes RJ. Cancer Res 1971;31:1755
Histological characters of Hodgkin's disease; criteria for cellular nodular sclerosis

Lukes RJ, Butler JJ. Cancer Res 1966;26:1063
Histological classification of Hodgkin's disease

Lukes RJ, Butler JJ, Hicks GB. Cancer 1966;19:317
Classification of Hodgkin's disease

Lukes RJ, Collins RD. In: Akazaki K, Rappaport H, Berard CW et al, eds. Malignant Diseases of the Hematopoietic System. Gann monograph on Cancer Research 15. Tokyo: University of Tokyo Press, 1973:209
Follicular lymphoma; recognition of cleaved and non-cleaved follicular cells

Lukes RJ, Collins RD. Recent Results Cancer Res 1974;46:18
Functional classifications of lymphomas; recognition of immunoblast

Lukes RJ, Collins RD. Br J Cancer 1975;31:Suppl II,1 Classification of lymphoma based on paper given in London in Sept 1973

Lukes RJ, Collins RD. Cancer 1975;34:1488
Classification of non-Hodgkin's lymphoma, based on paper given in New York, November 1973

Lukes RJ, Collins RD. In: Rebuck JW, Berard CW, Abell MR, eds. The Reticulo-endothelial system. Monographs in Pathology 16. Baltimore: Williams and Wilkins, 1975:213
Function classification of lymphoma

Lukes RJ, Collins RD. Cancer Treat Rep 1977;61:97
Review of Southern Californian and Vanderbilt series of lymphoma cases

Lukes RJ, Craver LF, Hall TC et al. Cancer Res 1966;26:1311
Rye classification of Hodgkin's disease

Lukes RJ, Gompel C, Nezelof C. Nouv Rev Franc Hematol 1966;6:11
Reproducability of Rye classification of Hodgkin's disease

Lukes RJ, Parker JW. In: Twomey JJ, Good RA, eds. Immunopathology of Lymphoma. New York: Plenum Press, 1978:239
General review of the pathology of lymphoreticular neoplasms

Lukes RJ, Parker JW, Taylor CR et al. Semin Hematol 1978;15:322
Review of multiparameter studies in a series of cases of lymphoma

Lukes RJ, Taylor CR, Parker JW. Am J Pathol 1978;90:461
An earlier analysis of a smaller series

Lukes RJ, Tindle BH. Proc 8th World Congress of Anatomic and Clinical Pathology. International Congress Series 262:86. Amsterdam: Excerpta Medica, 1972
Technique for examination of bone marrow

Lukes RJ, Tindle BH. (a) Communication at Pathology Panel for Clinical Trials. National Cancer Institute, Jan 1973. (b) Communication at workshop on classification of non-Hodgkin's lymphoma at University of Chicago, June 1973.
Neither of these communications on angio-immunoblastic lymphadenopathy was published

Lukes RJ, Tindle BH. N Engl J Med 1975;292:1
Angio-immunoblastic lymphadenopathy and sarcoma

Lumb G. Tumours of Lymphoid Tissue. Edinburgh: Livingstone, 1954
Benign Hodgkin's disease

Lutzner M, Edelson R, Schein P et al. Ann Intern Med 1975;83:534
Cutaneous T-lymphomas

Lutzner MA, Jordan HW. Blood 1968;31:719
Sézary cell

Mackaness GB. J Exp Med 1964;120:105
Macrophage response

Mackaness GB. Am Rev Respir Dis 1968;97:337
Macrophage response

Mackaness GB. In:van Furth R, ed. Mononuclear Macrophages. Oxford: Blackwell, 1970:461
Macrophages in delayed sensitivity

Mackenzie DH. Br Med J 1963;ii:1449
Amyloidosis of lymph nodes

MacLennan ICM, Harding B. Br J Cancer 1973;28:Suppl I,7.
Two types of cytotoxic lymphocyte

McDonald S. North Engl Clin J 1911;1:38
Greenfield's teaching on Hodgkin's disease

McWhirter R. Br J Radiol 1951;24:503
Chemotherapy for the reticuloses

Maldonado JE, Bayard ED, Brown AL Jr. Am J Clin Pathol 1965;44:605
Plasma cell variants

Maldonado JE, Kyle RA, Brown AL Jr et al. Blood 1966;22:212
Intermediate cell types in myeloma

Maldonado JE, Brown AL Jrs, Bayard ED.
Cancer 1966;19:1613
Electron microscopic studies of myeloma

Mallory FB. The Principles of Pathological Histology.
Philadelphia: Saunders, 1914
Discussion of lymphoblastoma

Mann RB, Jaffe ES, Berard CW. Am J Pathol 1979;94:105
Excellent review of lymphomas

Mann RB, Jaffe ES, Braylan RC et al. N Engl J Med
1976;295:685
Burkitt's lymphoma

Marchand FJ. Verh Dtsch Ges Pathol 1913;16:5
Nature of lymphoid follicles

Marchesi VT, Gowans JL. Proc R Soc Lond (Biol)
1964;159:283
Electron microscopic study of lymphocytes and post-
capillary venules

Mark I, Fehér J. Zbl Allg Path Pathol Anat 1959;99:369
Lymph nodes in allergic granulomatosis

Marks SM, Yanovich S, Rosenthal DS et al.
Blood 1978;51:435
Chronic T-cell lymphatic leukaemia

Marschalko T von. Arch Dermatol Forsch 1895;30:241
Morphology of plasma cells

Marshall AHE. J Pathol Bact 1948;60:515
Argyrophil (metalophil) cells

Marshall AHE. Outline of the Cytology and Pathology of the
Reticular Tissue. Edinburgh and London: Oliver and
Boyd, 1956
A useful review

Mason DY, Farrell C, Taylor CR. Br J Haematol 1975;31:361
Detection of antigens in lymphocytes

Mason DY, Taylor CR. J Clin Pathol 1975;28:124
Distribution of muramidase containing cells

Matas AJ, Hertel BF, Rosai J et al. Am J Med 1976;61:716
Post-transplant malignant lymphoma

Mathé G. Biomedicine 1977;26:377
Excellent review of WHO lymphoma classification

Mathé G, Belpomme D, Dantchev D et al. Biomedicine
1975;22:177
Classification of leukaemias and reticulosarcoma

Mathé G, Pouillart P, Schwarzenberg L, eds. Nomenclature,
Methodology and Results in Acute Leukaemias. Recent
Results Cancer Res 1973;43
Useful review

Mathé G, Rappaport H, O'Connor GT et al. Histological and
Cytological Typing of Neoplastic Diseases of Haematopoietic and Lymphoid tissues. International Classification
of Tumours No. 14. Geneva: WHO, 1976
The WHO classification of lymphoma

Mathé G, Seligmann M, Tubiana M, eds. Recent results Cancer Res 1978;64:65
Report of EORTC/CNRS International Colloquium of
lymphoid neoplastic diseases held in Paris, July 1977

Maximow AA. In: von Mollendorf W, ed. Handbuch der Mikrosp Anat des Menschen. Berlin: Springer, 1927:II,1,359
General account of the Maximow concept

Maximow AA. In: Cowdry EV, ed. Special Cytology 2nd ed.
New York: Hoeber, 1932:602
Lymphocyte types

Mellors RC, Korngold L. J Exp Med 1963;118:387
Fluorescent labelling with IgG

Mendelsohn G, Eggleston J, Mann RB. Cancer 1980:45:273
Lysozyme activity in relation to histiocytic proliferation

Meugé C, Hoerni B, de Mascurd A et al. Eur J Cancer
1978;14:587
Review of a series of cases classified according to 'Kiel'

Möbius W, Hennekenser HH, Westerhausen M et al. Acta
Haematol 1975;53:1
Hairy cell leukaemia

Moeschlin S. Proc Int Soc Haematol 1951;3:266
Mononuclear cells in Hodgkin's disease

Möller G, ed. T- and B- Lymphocytes in Humans. Transplant
Review 1973;16:3

Moore DF, Migliore PJ, Shullenberger CC et al. Ann Intern
Med 1970;72:43
Macroglobulin production of malignant lymphomas

Moore PD, Weisberger AS, Bowerfind ES. Arch Pathol
1956;62:472
Lymph nodes in disseminate lupus erythematosus

Moran EM, Ultmann JE, Ferguson DJ et al. Br J Cancer
1975;31:Suppl II,228
Modification of Ann Arbor staging for non-Hodgkin's
lymphomas

More RH, McMillan GC, Duff GL. Am J Pathol 1942;22:703
Pathology of sulphonamide allergy

Morris B. Blood Cells 1980;6:3
Lymphocyte homing

Motoi M, Schwanze E-W, Stein H et al. Verh Dtsch Ges Pathol
1978;62:514
Enzymic identification of histiocytic reticulosarcoma

Mott FW. Proc R Soc Lond B 1905;76:235
'Mott' plasma cells

Mueller J, Brun del Re G, Buerki H et al. Eur J Immunol
1975;5:270
Histochemical differentiation of T- and B-lymphocytes

Murphy MJ, May JB, Morris B et al. Am J Pathol 1972;66:25
Ultrastructural analysis of antibody synthesis in lymphoid cells

Müller-Hermelink HK, Heusermann V, Stutte HJ. Cell Tissue
Res 1974;154:167
Enzyme histochemistry in lymphoid tissue

Naji AF, Carbonell F, Barker HJ. Am J Clin Pathol
1962;38:513
Cat-scratch disease

Nakane PK. Ann NY Acad Sci 1975;254:203
Advances in the peroxidase-labelled antibody technique

Nathwani BN. Cancer 1979;44:347
Critical review of the various classifications of non-
Hodgkin's lymphomas

Nathwani BN, Kim H, Rappaport H. Cancer 1976;38:964
Lymphoblastic lymphoma

Nathwani BN, Rappaport H, Moran AM et al. Cancer
1978;41:578
'Malignant change' in angio-immunoblastic
lymphadenopathy

Neimann RS, Dervan D, Haudenschild C et al. Cancer
1978;41:507
Detailed cytological study of angio-immunoblastic
lymphadenopathy

Nemerov H. Encyclopaedia Britannica 1975;14:595
  The quality of definition

Niemi M, Korhonen LK. Bull Int Acad Pathol 1972;13/2:11
  Histochemical methods for diagnostic pathology

Nixon RK. Ann Intern Med 1966;64:856
  Mast cells

Noel H, Helbron D, Lennert K. In:Stacher A, Höcker P, eds.
  Lymphknoten Tumoren. Munich: Urban and Schwarzenberg, 1979;40
  Analysis of a series of cases of lympho-epithelioid (Peedell-Lennert) lymphoma

Nossal GTV, Ada GL. Antigens, Lymphoid Cells and the Immune Response. New York and London: Academic Press, 1971
  Review of lymphocyte function

Ober WB. NY State J Med 1977;77:126
  History of Hodgkin's disease

Oberling C. Bull Cancer 1928;17:259
  Reticulosarcomas

Occam G. Quodlibet septem. Strasburg: G. Husner 1491 m2^{V}
  Razor quotation

O'Connell KM. J Clin Pathol 1977;30:696
  Lymph node lesions in Kaposi's sarcoma

O'Connor GT, Sobin LH in Mathé G, et al, eds:
  Recent Results Cancer Res 1978

Omenn GS. N Engl J Med 1965;273:427
  Familial histiocytosis with eosinophilia

Palutke M, Varadacheri C, Weise RW. Am J Clin Pathol 1978;69:643
  Evidence that lympho-epithelioid (Peedell-Lennert) lymphoma may be a T-cell condition

Pangalis GA, Nathwani BN, Rappaport H. Cancer 1977;39:999
  Well-differentiated lymphocytic lymphomas

Pangalis GA, Rappaport H. Lancet 1977;ii:880
  α-chain disease

Papadimitriou JM, Wee SA. J Pathol 1976;120:153
  Epithelioid giant cell histiocytic response

Parrott DMV, de Sousa MAB. Clin Exp Immunol 1971;8:663
  Thymus dependent and independent lymphocyte populations

Parrott DMV, de Sousa MAB, East J. J Exp Med 1966;123:191
  T-cell areas in lymphoid tissue of thymectomized mice

Patchefsky AS, Bradovsky H, Southard M et al. Cancer 1973;32:150
  Cellular nodular sclerotic Hodgkin's disease

Pattengale PK, Taylor CR, Panke T et al. Acta Neuropathol (Berlin) 1979;48:165
  X-linked lympho-proliferative syndrome with central nervous system malignant lymphoma

Pernis B. In: Cottier H, Odartchenko N, Schindler R et al, eds. Germinal Centres in Immune Responses. Berlin, New York: Springer 1967:112
  Immunoglobulin in germinal centres

Peters MV. Am J Roentgenol Radium Ther Nucl Med 1950;26:1232
  Treatment of Hodgkin's disease

Pierce CW, Pevy DL, Tadakuma T. Ann NY Acad Sci 1975;256:365
  Suppressor T-cells

Pinkus GS, Said JW. Am J Pathol 1979;94:349
  Value of marker studies in lymphomas

Plato. Dialogues of Plato translated by B. Jowett. Charmides 2nd ed. Oxford: OUP, 1875;I:21 (Stephens ii 163D)
  Definitions

Pollard M. In: Cottier H, Odartchenko N, Schindler R et al, eds. Germinal Centres in Immune Responses. Berlin, New York: Springer, 1967:343
  Germinal centres in germ free animals

Polliack A, De Herven E. Clin Immunol Immunopathol 1975;3:412
  Lymphocyte surface features

Polliack A, Hammerling U, Lampen N et al. Eur J Immunol 1975;5:32
  Surface morphology of lymphocytes

Polliack A, Lampen N, Clarkson BD et al. J Exp Med 1973;138:607
  Electron microscopy of lymphocytes

Poppema S, Kaiserling E, Lennert K. Histopathology 1979;3:412
  Nodular lymphocyte preponderant Hodgkin's disease, a distinct entity

Porter KA. Br Med Bull 1956;21:171
  Morphology of graft reaction

Preud'homme JL, Labaume S. Ann NY Acad Sci 1975;254:254
  Detection of surface immunoglobulins of lymphocytes

Pullinger BD. In: Gordon MH, ed. Rose Research on Lymphadenoma. Bristol: John Wright and Sons, 1932:117
  Histology of Hodgkin's disease

Purtilo DT, Bhawan J, Hutt LM et al. Lancet 1978;i:798
  X-linked lympho-proliferative syndrome

Purtilo DT, Hutt LM, Bhawan J et al. Clin Immunol Immunopathol 1978;9:147
  X-linked lympho-proliferative syndrome

Purtilo DT, Yang JDS, Cassel CK et al. Lancet 1975;i:935
  Duncan's disease. X-linked lympho-proliferative syndrome

Quattrin N, de Rosa L, Quattrin S. Klin Wschr 1978;56:17
  Sea blue histiocytes

Radaszkiewicz T, Lennert K. Dtsch Med Wschr 1975;100:1157
  Angio-immunoblastic lymphadenopathy

Raff MC. Immunology 1970;19:637
  Distinct populations of peripheral lymphocytes identified by immuno-fluorescence

Raff MC. Am J Pathol 1971;65:467
  Study of T- and B-mouse lymphocytes

Raff MC, Nase S, Mitchison N. Nature 1971;230:50
  Lymphocyte antigens in mice

Raff MC, Sternberg M, Taylor RB. Nature 1970;225:553
  Immuno-fluorescent display of lymphocyte surface antigens

Randerath E, Ullbricht H. Frankf Zeit Pathol 1952;63:60
  Dermatopathic lymphadenopathy

Rappaport H. In: Roulet FC, ed. Symposium on Lympho-reticular Tumours in Africa, Paris 1963. Basel: Karger, 1964:174
Histology of malignant lymphoreticular neoplasms

Rappaport H. Tumors of the Hematopoietic System. Atlas of Tumor Pathology. Washington DC: Armed Forces Institute of Pathology, 1966;Section III Fasc 8
The text of the Rappaport classification

Rappaport H. Cancer Treat Rep 1977;61:1037. cf Jones and Godden (1977)
Round table discussion of histopathological classification of lymphomas

Rappaport H, Moran EM. N Engl J Med 1975;292:42
Angio-immunoblastic lymphadenopathy

Rappaport H, Thomas LB. Cancer 1974;34:1198
Extradermic manifestations of mycosis fungoides

Rappaport H, Winter WT, Hicks EB. Cancer 1956;9:79.2
Follicular lymphoma

Rather LJ. Bull NY Acad Med 1972;48:943
History of the Hodgkin giant cell

Rausch E, Kaiserling E, Goos M. Virchow's Arch B 1977;25:327
Relationship of Langerhans and interdigitating reticulum cells

Ravel R. Am J Clin Pathol 1966;46:355
Lymph node changes in lymphangiography

Rebuck, Berard and Abell see Dorfman RF, 1975

Recklinghausen F von. Die Lymphgefässe und ihre Beziehung zum Bindegewebe. Berlin: Muschwald, 1862
Variability of lymph node structure

Reed DM. Johns Hopkins Hosp Rep 1902;10:133
Dorothy Reed Hodgkin cell

Reid H, Fox H, Whittaker JS. Histopathology 1977;1:31
Eosinophil granuloma of lymph node

Rhoads CP. N Engl J Med 1928;198:76
Reticular cell is a phagocytic cell

Rhoads CP. J Mt Sinai Hosp 1946;13:6
The nitrogen mustard incident in Bari harbour

Richter MN. Am J Pathol 1928;4:283
Richter's syndrome

Rilke F, Carbone A, Musumeci R et al. Tumori 1978;64:211
Histiocytic medullary reticulosis

Rilke F, Pilotti S, Carbone A et al. J Clin Pathol 1978;31:1009
Excellently illustrated cytological account of the various lymphomas

Ringertz N, Adamson CA. Acta Pathol Microbiol Scand (Suppl) 1950;86:
Nodal response to antigen

Risdall RJ, McKenna RW, Nesbet ME et al. Cancer 1979;44:993
Reactive haemophagocytic syndrome

Roath S, Newell DG. Lancet 1975;i:284
Scanning electron microscopy of hairy cells

Robb-Smith AHT. J Path Bact 1937;43:312
Reticulin impregnation

Robb-Smith AHT. J Path Bact 1938;47:437
Classification of reticulosis and reticulosarcoma

Robb-Smith AHT. Br J Dermatol 1944;56:151
Dermic manifestations of lymphoid disorders

Robb-Smith AHT. In: Dyke SC, ed. Recent Advances in Clinical Pathology. London: Churchill, 1947:350
Lymph node diagnosis and natural history

Robb-Smith AHT. La Réticulose Lymphoide Folliculaire. Réunion internationale d'hématologie, Paris, May 1948

Robb-Smith AHT. Lancet 1953;ii:619
Discussion of the reticuloses

Robb-Smith AHT. In Pack GT, Ariel IM. Treatment of Cancer and Allied Diseases Vol. 9, Lymphomas and Related Diseases. New York: Hoeber, 1964:1
Review of lymph node disorders

Robb-Smith AHT. A Cool Look at the Reticuloses. Honyman-Gillespie Lecture. Edinburgh: University of Edinburgh, 1970

Robb-Smith AHT. Lancet 1974;i:513
Immuno-topography of lymphoreticular disorders

Robb-Smith AHT. Lancet 1976;ii:970
Lympho-epithelioid (Peedell-Lennert) lymphoma

Robb-Smith AHT. In: Finckh ES, Clayton-Jones E, eds. Proc 9th World Congress of Anatomic and Clinical Pathology, Sydney, Oct 1975. International Congress Series 384: 165 Amsterdam-Oxford: Excerpta Medica, 1976
Lymphoreticular hyperplasia and neoplasia

Rosai J, Dorfman RF. Cancer 1972;30:1174
Sinus histiocytosis and massive lymphodenopathy

Rosen PJ, Feinstein DL, Pattengale PK et al. Ann Intern Med 1978;89:319
Convoluted lymphoma in adults

Rosenberg SA. Cancer Res 1966;26:1310
Rye clinical staging

Rosenberg SA. Cancer Treat Rep 1977;61:1023
Defects of Ann Arbor staging in non-Hodgkin's lymphoma

Rosenberg SA, Diamond HD, Jaslowitz B et al. Medicine 1961;40:31
Review of lymphosarcoma

Rosenthal SR. Arch Pathol 1936;21:628
Influence of lymphoid content on prognosis in Hodgkin's disease

Ross R. Biol Rev 1968;43:51
Fibroblasts

Roth LM. Cancer 1965;18:1
Thyroid tissue inclusions in lymph nodes

Roth S, Riecken EO. In: Frick P, van Harnack GA, Martini GA et al, eds. Advances in Internal Medicine and Paediatrics. Berlin: Springer, 1977:79
α-chain disease

Roulet F. Virchow's Arch 1930;277:15. 1932;286:701
Retothel sarcoma

Russell W. Br Med J 1890;ii:1356
Russell body of plasma cells

Sainte-Marie G. J Histochem Cytochem 1962;10:250
Dendritic reticular cells

Sainte-Marie G, Sin YM, Chan C. Rev Can Biol 1967;26:141
Function of post-capillary venules

Saltzstein SL. Surgery 1965;58:659
Outcome of non-diagnostic biopsies

Saltzstein SL, Ackerman LV. Cancer 1959;12:164
Drug induced lymphadenopathy

Saxe N, Kahn LB, King H. J Cutan Pathol 1977;4:111
Mycosis fungoides

Schittenhelm A. Die Klinik des Reticulo-endothelial Systems.
Berlin: Springer, 1925
Reticulo-endothelioses

Schnaidt U, Krmpotic E, Stünkel K et al. Verh Dtsch Ges
Pathol 1979;63:379
Cytological characters indicative of invasive and sarcomatous change in angio-immunoblastic
lymphadenopathy

Seligmann M. Arch Intern Med 1975;135:78
α-chain disease

Seligmann M, Brouet J-C, Preud'homme JL. Cancer Treat Rep
1977;61:1179
Immunological diagnosis of lymphomas

Selye H. The Mast Cells. Washington: Butterworth, 1965

Shimoyama M, Watanabe S, eds. Symposium on T-cell malig-
nancies. Jap J Clin Oncol 1979;9 Suppl 1:315
This is an excellent, well-illustrated symposium held in
Tokyo Dec 1979

Shirakura T, Kobayashi Y, Murai Y. Scand J Haematol
1976;10:387
Gamma-heavy chain disease

Slaughter DP, Economou SG, Southwick HW. Ann Surg
1958;148:705
Block dissection in Hodgkin's disease

Sluiter JTF. De histologie van der Ziekte van Brill in haar
verschittende phasen. Amsterdam: Diss. Med, 1956
Follicular lymphoma

Smetana HF. Am J Pathol 1969;98:231
Follow up of Hodgkin's disease in U.S. Forces

Smetana HF, Cohen BM. Blood 1956;11:211
Hodgkin's disease in U.S. Forces

Smith JL, Klein CP, Barker CR et al. Lancet 1973;i:74
First report of convoluted cell sarcoma

Söderström N. Scand J Haematol 1967;4:411
Post-capillary venules

Sordat B. J Exp Med 1970;131:77
Antibody production in germinal centres

Sorkin E, Boyden SV. J Immunol 1954;82:332
Immune complexes and macrophage

Sousa MAB de. Clin Exp Immunol 1971;9:371
Ecotaxis or homing of lymphocytes

Sousa MAB de. In: Twomey JT, Good RA, eds.
Immunopathology of Lymphoreticular Neoplasms.
New York: Plenum Medical Books, 1971:325
Ecotaxis of lymphocytes

Spain DM. Arch Pathol 1957;64:59
Lipogranulomatosis; pseudo-sarcoid

Spector WG. Int Rev Exp Pathol 1969;8:1
Macrophage potentialities

Spector WG, Heesom N. J Path Bact 1969;98:31
Immune complexes and granuloma formation

Spector WG, Lykke AWJ. J Path Bact 1966;92:163
Relationship of histocytes to small round cells

Spector WG, Ryan BG. In: van Furth R, ed. Mononuclear
Phagocytes. Oxford: Blackwell, 1970:219
Macrophages in granulomas are marrow derived

Spector WG, Willoughby DA. J Pathol 1968;96:389
Inflammatory macrophages are marrow derived

Spiers RS. Ann NY Acad Sci 1958;73:283
The eosinophil

Spiro S, Galton DAG, Wiltshaw E. Br J Cancer
1975;31:Suppl II 60
Follicular lymphoma natural history

Staiger J, Westerhausen M. Med Welt 1975;26:223
Waldenström's disease

Stathopoulos G, Davies AJS, Papamichail M et al.
Lancet 1974;i:927
Sternberg's sarcoma may be of T- or B-cell origin

Stansfeld AG. J Clin Pathol 1961;14:565
Diagnosis of toxoplasmosis

Stein H, Kaiserling E, Lennert K. Virchow's Arch 1974;364:51
B- cell origin of reticulum cell sarcoma

Stein H, Lennert K, Parwaresch MR. Lancet
1972;ii:855
B- cell lymphomas

Stein H, Petersen N, Gaedicke G et al. Int J Cancer
1976;17:292
T- cell origin of convoluted acid phosphatase lymphoma

Sternberg C. Z Heilk 1898;19:21
Relationship of Hodgkin's disease and tuberculosis

Sternberg C. Erg Allg Pathol Pathol Anat 1903;9:502
Hodgkin's giant cells

Sternberg C. Beitr Pathol 1916;61:75
Mediastinal leucosarcoma

Sternberg C. In: Lubarsch O, Henke F, ed Handb Spez Path
Anat Hist. Berlin: Springer, 1926; Bd. 1, Teil 2:8
There are seven pages devoted to lymphoma in this
edition compared to nearly a thousand pages in Lennert's volume (1978)

Sternberg TH, Ashley FL, Winner LH et al. Hautarzt
1964;15:281
Silicone granuloma

Sternberger LA. Immunocytochemistry. New Jersey: Prentice-
Hall, 1979
Technical details

Strauchen JA, Young RC, De Vita VT et al. New Engl J Med
1978;299:1382
Morphological analysis of 'diffuse histiocytic
lymphoma'

Straus W. J Histochem Cytochem 1968;16:237
Use of horseradish peroxidase

Strum SB, Park JK, Rappaport H. Cancer 1970;26:176
Reed-Sternberg-like cells in various conditions

Strum SB, Rappaport H. Arch Pathol 1971;91:127
Cellular nodular sclerotic Hodgkin's disease

Suchi T, Tajima K, Nanba K et al. Acta Pathol Jap
1979;29:755
Japanese classification of lymphoma including adult T-
cell leukaemia

Symmers WStC. Br J Radiol 1951;24:450
Review of reticulosis concepts

Symmers WStC. In: Welsch M, Dustin P, Dagnelie J. Eight
Colloquia on Clinical Pathology. Brussels, 1958:749
Lymph nodes in disseminate lupus erythematosus

Symmers WStC. In: Raven RW, ed. Cancer. London: Butterworth, 1958;2:478
Benign Hodgkin's disease

Symmers WStC. J Clin Pathol 1968;21:650
Review of 600 reputed cases of Hodgkin's disease

Symmers WStC. Br Med J 1968;ii:19
Silicone lymphadenitis

Symmers WStC. Br Med J 1970;ii:763
Leprous lymphadenitis

Symmers WStC. In: Symmers WStC, ed. Systemic Pathology. Edinburgh: Churchill Livingstone, 1978 2nd ed;2:693
Lymph nodes in polyarteritis nodosa. The whole chapter is an excellent review of lymph node disorders, in particular the inflammatory lymphadenopathies

Takahashi M, Yagi Y, Moore GE. J Immunol 1969;103:834
Immunoglobulin synthesis in the lymphocyte cycle

Tanaka N. In: Akazaki A, Rappaport H, Berard CW, eds. Malignant Diseases of the Hematopoietic system. Gann monograph on Cancer Research 15. Tokyo: University of Tokyo Press, 1973:123
Example of reticulosis

Tanaka N. Arch Pathol 1976;100:81
Mucocutaneous lymph node syndrome

Taylor CR. J Pathol 1973;110:221
Identification of cells reacting by anti-lymphocytic sera

Taylor CR. Lancet 1974;ii:802
Identifying 'reticulum cells' with immunoperoxidase methods in paraffin sections

Taylor CR. An immuno-histological study of human and murine lymphomata. University of Oxford, 1974; D Phil thesis

Taylor CR. Eur J Cancer 1976;12:61
Immuno-histological study of lymphomata

Taylor CR. J Pathol 1976;118:201
Characters of reticulum cell sarcoma in the mouse

Taylor CR. In: Horrobin DF, series ed. Annual Research Reviews. Hodgkin's Disease and the Lymphomas, Vols 1,1976;2,1977;3,1978. Montreal: Eden Press, 1977, 1978, 1979
The first of these volumes is undated and has no volume number but has ISBN O 904406 482. In the Introduction p4 it is stated that it is based on the twelve volumes of the Index Medicus for 1975 and includes a small number of 1977 references; the advertising brochure states that it was published in October 1976, and 1976 is given as the reference date in the bibliography to Vol 2, 1978, but in fact it did not appear until April 1977. In this first volume the English publisher is given as 'Lunesdale House, Hornby, Lancaster'. Subsequent volumes are dated clearly and the publisher outside North America is given as: Edinburgh, Churchill Livingstone. Volume 3 includes chapters by other authors. Invaluable reviews

Taylor CR. Arch Pathol 1978;102:113
Immunoperoxidase techniques. General review

Taylor CR. J Histochem Cytochem 1978;26:496
Immunocytochemical methods in the study of lymphomata

Taylor CR. Oncology 1978;35:189
Immunohistology in tumour diagnosis

Taylor CR. Arch Pathol Lab Med 1978;102:549
Classification of lymphomas

Taylor CR. Am J Clin Pathol 1979;72:Suppl 687
Analysis of B- lymphomas by surface markers and immuno-histological methods

Taylor CR, Burns J. J Clin Pathol 1974;27:14
Application of immunoperoxidase technique to paraffin-embedded material

Taylor CR. Mason DY. Clin Exp Immunol 1974;18:417
Value of immunoperoxidase methods in studies of myeloma etc.

Taylor CR, Parker JW, Pattengale PK et al. Proc XII Internat Cancer Congress, Buenos Aires, Oct 1978. New York: Plenum Press, 1979
Immunopathological study of lymphomas

Taylor CR, Russell R, Lukes RJ et al. Cancer 1978;41:2197
Immunoglobulin content of central nervous system lymphomas

Taylor RB. Br J Exp Pathol 1965;46:376
Pluripotent stem cells in embryonic liver

Templeton AC. Cancer 1972;30:854
Kaposi's sarcoma in lymph nodes

Terashima K, Takahashi K, Kojima M et al. Acta Pathol Jap 1978;28:111
Kappa light chain crystals in histiocytes with minimal plasma cell proliferation

Thorbecke GT. Ann NY Acad Sci 1959;78:237
Lymphoid reactions in germ free animals

Tindle BH, Parker JW, Lukes RJ. Am J Clin Pathol 1972;58:607
Reed-Sternberg-like cells in infectious mononucleosis

Toben HR, Smith RG. Clin Exp Immunol 1977;27:292
Chronic T-cell lymphatic leukaemia

Transplantation Reviews (Kobenhavn). Transplant Rev 1973:16
T- and B-lymphocytes in man

Tschistowitch T, Bykowa O. Virchow's Arch 1928;269:91
Early use of the term 'reticulosis'

Turk JL. Br Med Bull 1967;23:3
Cytology of early hypersensitivity reaction

Turk JL, Stone SH. In: Amos B, Koprowski H, eds. Cell Bound Antibodies. New York: Wistar Institute Press, 1963
Histology of hypersensitivity reaction

Turk JL, Waters MFR. Clin Exp Immunol 1971;8:363
Leprous lymphadenitis

Turner DR, Wright DJM. J Pathol 1973;110:305
Syphilitic lymphadenopathy

Uehlinger E. Beitr Pathol 1930;83:719
Early classification of reticuloses

Unanue ER, Dixon FJ. Adv Immunol 1967;6:1
Immune complexes and granuloma formation

Undritz E. Sandoz Atlas of Haematology. Basel, 1952:91
Variants of the plasma cell

Van Bekkum DW, van Noord MJ, Maat B et al. Blood 1971;38:547
Identification of haematopoietic stem cells in the mouse

Van den Berg FWT, Kaiserling E, Lennert K. Virchow's Arch 1976; 371:27
Glomangioma in lymph nodes

Van den Tweel JG, Lukes RJ, Taylor CR. Am J Clin Pathol 1979;71:509
Nature of so-called composite lymphoma

Van den Tweel JG, Taylor CR, Parker JW et al. Am J Clin Pathol 1978;69:306
Dutcher bodies in Waldenström's syndrome

Van Neil CB. Cold Spring Harbour Symposia 1946;11:285
Classification of bacteria

Videbaek A. Acta Hamatol 1949;2:201
The problem of fluidity in the lymphadenopathies

Virchow R. Die Krankhaften Geschwülste. Berlin: Hirsch-wald, 1864/5.
Bd 2 erstes Hefte:212, lymphosarcoma; Bd 2 zweites Hefte: 618, giant cells

Virchow R. Klin Wochenschr 1892;i:289
'Mishmash' of pseudoleukaemia

Volkman A. J Exp Med 1966;124:241
Origin and turnover of peritoneal mononuclear cells

Volkman A, Gowans JL. Br J Exp Pathol 1965;46:50
Formation of macrophages

von Marschalko T, see Marschalko

von Recklinghausen F. see Recklinghausen

Waksman BH, Namba Y. Cell Immunol 1976;21:161
Lymphokines

Waldmann TA, Broder S, Durma M et al. In Oppenheim JJ, Rosenstreich DL, eds. Mitogens in Microbiology. New York: Academic Press, 1976:59
Suppressor T-cells

Waldron TA, Leech JA, Glick AD et al. Cancer 1977;40:1604
T- zone lymphoma

Warner NL. Adv Immunol 1974;19:67
Membrane immunoglobulins on lymphocytes

Warnke RH, Kim H, Dorman RF. Cancer 1976;3:215
Malignant histiocytosis

Warthin AS. Ann Surg 1931;93:153
'Fluid' school of lymphomas

Waugh TR. Am J Med Sci 1937;193:337
Interrelationship of haematopoietic disorders

Wegmann W, Siebermann R, Amman R. Verh Dtsch Ges Pathol 1976;60:263
Relation of adult Niemann-Pick disease and sea blue histiocyte

Whitehead R. Gut 1968;9:569
Steatorrhoea lymphadenopathy

Wilks S. Guys Hosp Rep 1856;Series 3,2:103
Hodgkin's disease and the eponym. Emphasized Hodgkin's achievements, but 'Hodgkin's Disease' first appears as a subtitle in a later paper (ibid. 1865; Series 3,11:56)

Williams AH, Taylor CR, Higgins SR et al. Cancer 1978;42:121
Childhood leukaemia and lymphoma

Willis RA. Pathology of Tumours, 3rd ed. London: Butterworth, 1960

Wiltshaw E. Medicine 1976;59:217
Extra-medullary plasmacytoma

Winkelmann RK, ed. Mayo Clin Proc 1974;49:513
Symposium on the Sézary cell and syndrome

Wright CJE. Am J Pathol 1956;32:201
Germinal centre origin of follicular lymphoma

Wright DH, Jones DB, Smith JL et al. Proc Path Soc. Newcastle-on-Tyne, July 1976; item 51
Angio-immunoblastic lymphadenopathy

Wunderlich CRA. Arch Physiol Heilk 1856;12:123
Suggested 'lymphadenoma' after Cornil's proposal

Yam LT, Li C-Y, Crosby WH. Am J Clin Pathol 1971;55:283
Cytochemical identification of granulocytes and monocytes

Yam LT, Mitus WJ. Blood 1968;31:480
B-glucoronidase activity in lympho-proliferative disorders

Yoffey JM. In: Yoffey JM, ed. The Lymphocyte in Immunology and Haemopoiesis. London:Arnold, 1966
Lymphocyte circulation

Yoffey JM, Courtice FC. Lymphocytes, Lymph and the Lympho-myeloid Complex. New York: Academic Press, 1970

Yoffey JM, Reinhardt WO, Everett NB. J Anat 1971;95:293
T³ flash labelling of lymph nodes

Ziegler K. Die Hodgkinsche Krankheit, Jena, 1911

Zucker-Franklin D, Franklin EC. Blood 1971;37:257
Morphology of IgM heavy chain disease

Zulman J, Jaffe R, Talal N. N Engl J Med 1978;299:1215
B-cell neoplasm in Sjögren's syndrome

Terminology of Lymph Node Disorders

The nomenclature used in this book is eclectic, the endeavour being to adopt terms that are brief and meaningful. If a well-established term fulfilled these criteria, it was accepted preferentially; in other instances a newer descriptive term was simplified. No neologisms have been introduced, but as was mentioned in the Preface, malignant lymphoma or sarcoma was reserved for overtly sarcomatous conditions manifesting invasive characters with stromal destruction and potentialities for lymphatic and haematogenous metastatic spread (Pathological dissemination of Galton et al, 1978).

Hodgkin's Disease

Diffuse epithelioid form (92, 212; *V.39*)
Lymphocytic depleted form (217; *V.20, 42*)
Lymphocytic and histiocytic predominant form [nodular or diffuse] (113, 212; *III.14, V.39*)
Lymphocytic predominant form [nodular or diffuse] (112, 150; *III.13*)
Mixed cellular form (205; *V.38*)
Nodular sclerotic form (116; *III.15*)

Lympho-reticular Proliferative Conditions

Acute reticulosis of infancy [Letterer-Siwe syndrome] (188; *V.26*)
Alpha [α] chain disease[1] (192; *V.33*)
Angio-follicular lymphadenopathy (100; *III.4*)
Angio-immunoblastic lymphadenopathy[2] (200; *V.37*)
Chronic lymphocytic leukaemia[2] [small lymphocytic lymphoma] (148; *V.1*)
Chronic myeloid leukaemia[3] (184; *V.24*)
Dermatopathic lymphadenopathy (72; *II.10*)
Eosinophilic granuloma (77, 94; *II.15*)
Familial haemophagocytic reticulosis (140; *IV.9d*)
Follicular lymphoma[4] (56, 101; *II.3, III.6*)
Gamma [γ] heavy chain disease (198; *V.33*)
Hairy cell leukaemia (156; *V.6*)
Histiocytic medullary reticulosis[5] (137; *IV.9*)
Histiocytosis X (77, 94, 188; *II.15, V.26*)
Letterer-Siwe syndrome (188; *V.26*)
Lympho-epithelioid [Peedell-Lennert] lymphoma[2] (92, 212; *V.39*)
Lymphomatoid granulomatosis (222)
Lymphoplasmacytoid lymphoma[2] (196; *V.34*)
Mast cell disease[3] (184; *V.25*)
Monocytic leukaemia (188)
Mu [μ] heavy chain disease (198)

Mycosis fungoides[6] (213)
Myeloid metaplasia (184; *V.24*)
Myelosclerosis (213; *V.14*)
Plasmacytoma[1] (189; *V.28, 30*)
Reticulum celled medullary reticulosis (188; *V.26*)
Sézary's syndrome[6] (152; *V.3, 5*)
Sinus histiocytosis with massive lymphadenopathy (132; *IV.4*)
Sjögren's lymphadenopathy (216; *V.41*)
Small lymphocytic lymphoma (148; *V.2*)
Steatorrhoea lymphadenopathy[5] (73, 130; *II.11, IV.2a*)
T-cell chronic lymphocytic leukaemia[6] (149)
T-zone lymphoma[6] (72)

Sarcomatous Conditions

Acute lymphoblastic leukaemia (166; *V.8*)
Acute myeloid/myelomonocytic leukaemia (109; *V.10*)
Burkitt's lymphoma (164; *V.12*)
Centroblastic sarcoma [diffuse] (180; *V.15*)
Convoluted cell malignant lymphoma (162; *V.11*)
Follicular centroblastic sarcoma (108; *III.7*)
Granulocytic sarcoma (184)
Histiocytic sarcoma (177; *V.21, 22*)
Immunoblastic sarcoma (168; *V.14, 32*)
Kaposi's angio-sarcoma (141)
Large cleaved cell malignant lymphoma (180; *V.23*)
Large non-cleaved cell malignant lymphoma (169, 181; *V.15*)
'Lymphoblastic' malignant lymphoma (157; *V.9*)
Nodular sclerotic lymphosarcoma (109, 218; *III.8, V.33, 34*)
Small cleaved cell malignant lymphoma (152; *V.7*)
Small non-cleaved cell malignant lymphoma (161; *V.10*)
Plasma cell sarcoma (172; *V.17, 44*)
Plasmacytoid immunoblastic sarcoma (172; *V.16, 31*)
Pleomorphic immunoblastic sarcoma (173; *V.18, 46*)
Richter's syndrome (151; *V.14c*)
T-cell immunoblastic sarcoma (172)

---

[1]Liable to undergo plasma cell sarcomatous change
[2]Liable to undergo immunoblastic sarcomatous change
[3]Liable to undergo 'blastic' sarcomatous change

[4]Liable to undergo centroblastic sarcomatous change
[5]Liable to undergo histiocytic sarcomatous change
[6]Liable to undergo T-cell malignant lymphomatous change

The photomicrographs are either low power views (usually ×40)
or high power details (of the order of ×750)

The Roman and Arabic numbers in italics *in this Index refer to the illustrations and the abbreviation m.l. stands for 'malignant lymphoma'.*

The terms in italics *are those used in the six classifications discussed on pp. 238–259, and set out as footnotes on pp. 101, 148, 152, 157, 162, 164, 169, 177, 180, 196, where they are related to the preferred terms used in this book. These preferred terms are shown in* Roman *type here.*

This Index does not include authors, as it seemed that the Bibliography displayed adequately the names of the referred authorities. However, there are a few references, mainly to the Appendices, to those who made particular contributions or who have been involved in the various classifications.

The terms in italics are those used in the six classifications discussed on pp. 238–259, and set out as footnotes on pp. 101, 148, 152, 157, 164, 169, 177, 180, 196, where they are related to the preferred terms used in this book. These preferred terms (see p. 297) are shown in Roman type here.